The Land Homeopathi METHOD

Exploring the breadth, context and application of different clinical approaches in the practice of homeopathy

Volume 2

Alastair C. Gray

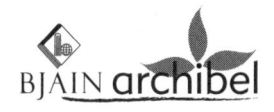

BJAIN archibel

B. Jain Archibel s.p.r.l.
Rue Fontaine St. Pierre 1E, Zoning Industriel de la Fagne,
5330 Assesse, Belgium, Europe

THE LANDSCAPE OF HOMEOPATHIC MEDICINE - METHOD

First Edition: 2011
1st Impression: 2011

All rights reserved. No part of this book may be reproduced, stored in a retrieval system or transmitted, in any form or by any means, mechanical, photocopying, recording or otherwise, without any prior written permission of the publisher.

© with the author

Published by
B. Jain Archibel s.p.r.l.
Rue Fontaine St. Pierre 1E, Zoning Industriel de la Fagne,
5330 Assesse, Belgium, Europe
Ph.: +32 82 66 05 00; *Fax:* +32 83 65 62 82
Email: info@bjain.com; *Website:* www.archibel.com

ISBN: 978-2-87491-021-0

Printed in India

Foreword

When I first met Alastair Gray, not even a year ago, I was simultaneously impressed with his fine understanding of homeopathy and with his humble demeanor. Having read the first book of this series (*Case Taking 2010*), I had invited him to speak at the Joint American Homeopathic Conference in Alexandria, Virginia. With self-effacing candor, Alastair had the audience laughing about his practice and his encounters with patients in a well-used neighborhood of Sydney, where he treated predominantly addicts and other non-traditional homeopathic clients. It was quickly apparent to me that Alastair combined clarity of thought and depth of knowledge with the objectivity required to aim a critical lens at himself and his modality. Time has only strengthened my impression of a mind deeply rooted in the principles of the *Organon*, yet spread wide to new ideas in homeopathy.

It gives me great pleasure to introduce the second book in a series that, simply for its breadth and objectivity, is certain to become a classic. *Method* surveys with a scientific eye the prescribing techniques of the best-known teachers and practitioners of homeopathy. From Hahnemann to Sankaran, sixteen different methods of settling on a remedy based on different understandings of the phrase, "totality of symptoms." Included in this volume are critical looks at Hahnemannian and Kentian prescribing (not the same thing!), so-called "constitutional" prescribing, as well as isopathic and tautopathic prescribing, miasmatic and other types of intercurrent prescribing, group and family analyses and vital sensation prescribing, among others.

Alastair begins with the theory behind each method and compares the different approaches. The *Organon of Medicine*, for example, dictates that we should prescribe for the totality of the disease picture since the patient was last well. This differs substantially from Kent's idea that we should prescribe for the totality of the person. It differs even more from a constitutional prescription that incorporates the totality of a patient's strengths and weaknesses, their typology and their temperament, as well as from a prescription in which the totality is encompassed by a vital sensation. What are the implications of these various approaches? How would we expect the practitioners of these methods to prescribe? Did their actual prescribing line up with their writings?

Alastair examines these questions as they apply to a dozen different methods of homeopathic prescribing. And he examines the casebooks of these homeopaths to see how their prescribing matched their own writings or differed from their fellows. Where his own understanding of particular methods is not well developed, Alastair brings in three experts in their methods to lead the discussion. Shilpa Bouraskar, a Sydney homeopath and the developer of the HomeoQuest software, writes on the vital sensation method, when it is best applied, and includes one of her own cases. Jennifer Osborne, who practices and teaches in Brisbane, gives an overview of miasmatic prescribing. And Greg Cope, a Brisbane homeopath and lecturer at Endeavor College of Natural Health, explains the group analysis approach of Jan Scholten.

The upshot, of course, is that we now have a broad

prescribing tradition on which to draw, one that allows the homeopath to individualize method in the same way we individualize the remedy. Any homeopath who has been in practice knows that not everyone with a rash is willing to sit for a two-hour probe into the subconscious. Some patients will need a remedy for the lesion. Later, perhaps they will accept an organopathic remedy, and maybe after months or years will consider a more in-depth prescription.

On the other end of the spectrum, what are your options when, having taken the case, you have no physical or even functional pathology on which to prescribe? One might approach the case from several different angles, so what are the strengths and weaknesses of, say, Kentian, constitutional and vital sensation approaches? Each might be a good choice, but each grows from a different understanding of the totality of symptoms. Therefore, each method will incorporate different information in its analysis and require a different use of the research tools at hand, whether those be repertory, materia medica or online tools. If we are to use these different methods, we must know what each requires.

This is valuable information for the modern clinician wishing to hone her prescribing skills. For the student venturing into clinical work for the first time, *Method* will help to reconcile what has been taught with what he sees in the exam room. The great theorists have much to teach us about how homeopathy works ideally, but it often looks different in practice. A good practitioner will be able to navigate the different methods of prescribing, to know which is best for the individual patient and to apply these effectively.

Alastair Gray makes a rare figure in homeopathy today, a practitioner and teacher with the objectivity to analyze the disparate methods of homeopathy without favoring one approach. Alastair has mapped here the entire terrain of homeopathic prescribing, from Kentian to polypharmacy. He surveys this landscape with an honest and critical eye, giving both the new and the seasoned practitioner an opportunity to reflect on what it is we do. I expect this book and its mates will become required reading for all students of homeopathy.

Kim Elia
Toronto, November 2011

Acknowledgements

In the completion of this second part of the *Landscape Project*, some significant thanks are warranted. To offset my lack of an eye for detail, a massive thanks to Helen Vuletin for her extraordinary editorial support. She had the firmness, the clarity and the style guide to keep the author on message when he was often well off. She also has perseverance and patience in abundance. Much gratitude.

It's a little difficult to remember every conversation, because there have been many over the years in relation to method in homeopathic medicine, but nevertheless there are some specific ones related to the contents of this book that stick in the mind. To Val Probert, Julie Andrews, Rachel Roberts, Judy Coldicott, Barbara Seideneck, Kate Chatfield, Frederik Schroyens, Richard Pitt, Simon Taffler, Greg Cope, David Levy, Carmen Nicotra, Misha Norland, Peter Tumminello, Ben Gadd, and Jen Osborne, many thanks for your insights, openness and robustness in expressing your opinions.

With averaging over three hundred lectures a year for the last decade or more I have been fortunate to have had a lot of opportunity to formulate and test my ideas. Thank you to the multitude of students who have listened to, and engaged in my lectures and conversations, and were ultimately responsible for the formation of many of the ideas expressed here. Thanks also for the challenges.

To the B. Jain team, especially Nishant and Geeta, and the Archibel team, Dale Emerson in particular, many thanks.

Contributors

Ben Gadd runs a homeopathic practice in inner southeast Melbourne Australia. Prior to becoming a homeopath he worked as a Registered Nurse in a variety of mental health settings. He lectures at the Melbourne campus of Endeavour College of Natural Health, and has a strong interest in the application of research to clinical practice.

Greg Cope graduated from the Australian College of Natural Medicine in 2004 with a Bachelor Degree in Health Science (Homeopathy) and Advanced Diploma of Health Science (Acupuncture). At graduation he was awarded the prize for excellence in clinical practice. Since then Greg has been in private practice, and was fortunate to spend 5 years working from a devoted homeopathic clinic with some of the leading homeopathic practitioners in Queensland Australia. Greg's clinical interest has a special focus on acute prescribing, childhood asthma and anxiety disorders. After graduating, Greg started working with Archibel the producers of RADAR software, and with Frederik Schroyens, the editor of Synthesis Repertory on the development of homeopathic information and technologies. This has given him opportunity to interact with many of Australia's, New Zealand's and the world's leading homeopathic teachers, as well as to interact with local practitioners on new developments in homeopathic practice and the application of new information and technologies. Greg has been a homeopathic teacher since 2008 and is Senior Lecturer on the Brisbane campus at Endeavour College. Greg is currently the President of the Australian Homeopathic Association, and has been a member of the AHA's committee since 2004 when he started in the role of Secretary. His special interest in homeopathic education and his role with the AHA is to increase practitioner confidence on entering clinical practice.

Jennifer Osborne has been a homeopathic practitioner since 2000. Trained under the guidance of Dr Isaac Golden at the original Melbourne College of Natural Medicine, Jennifer is currently pursuing post-graduate studies in the area of chronic disease progression and miasmatic history. Prior to this, her former career was within the medical field of general nursing and she lectured within the Bioscience department in her earlier associations with the college. She has been lecturing at Endeavour College of Natural Health since 2003 and is a current Senior lecturer within the Homeopathic Department for Brisbane campus. Jennifer's clinical expertise is within the area of chronic disease and genetic predispositions. Her private practice has been relocated from Melbourne to Brisbane within the last 18 months and continues to thrive. She has been published in *Similia*, The Journal of the Australian Homeopathic Association on infertility and *H.pathy* discussing a case of chronic polyneuropathy disease. She continues to enjoy and is passionate about delivering high quality education for future aspiring homeopaths for Endeavour.

Shilpa Bhouraskar graduated as a Bachelor of Homeopathic Medicine and Surgery from India in 1997. Further, she trained under some of the most experienced homeopaths in Homeopathic hospitals and Clinics and practiced as a homeopathic GP in India before she moved to Sydney, Australia in 2004 where she is currently in practice. She is a passionate teacher and a clinical supervisor. Her lectures and seminars have been popular for simplifying and deepening the understanding of complex homeopathic strategies gathered from her wealth of experience and real cases. She also runs

Contributors

The Argentum Mentoring, the first comprehensive homeopathic mentoring program which offers personalised one on one case mentoring by homeopathic experts to guide homeopaths past the many obstacles in homeopathic case management. Visit; http://www.homeopathy-mentoring.com/. She is the author of the ebook series *The Quest for Simillimum* which elaborates the simple yet effective Stages concept which is a distillation of the success strategies of the world's most successful homeopaths. The Stages concept demystifies the entire homeopathic case management which leaves the reader saying 'I wish I'd heard all of this sooner'. She has also created the user friendly homeopathic software 'HomeoQuest'. For details visit www.homeoquest.com.

Richard Pitt has been a pivotal figure in USA homeopathy for more than a decade,. Running a college in the Bay area, practicing and being involved in education and professionalisation, he's made a considerable mark. What struck me when I first met Richard was not just his scholarship but his openness. What is striking about Richard is that he maintains his critical thinking capacity while remaining open to the new. His work with individual remedies such as tobacco, and his perspective on broad issues impacting heavily on homeopathy are incredibly valuable at a time where (not only in homeopathy) anyone can have an opinion or a blog about anything and express it. I'm deeply grateful for Richard's permission to publish his article on method and the way forward in homeopathic education, which to me go hand in hand.

Researchers

Dr. Parag Singh completed his BHMS in 2003 from Delhi and did his MD in Organon of Homoeopathic Medicine from

National Institute Of Homoeopathy, Calcutta, in December 2006. He has been practicing homeopathy since 2007 at his private clinic. He is a classical homeopathic practitioner and is a follower of Dr. L.M. Khan from NIH, Calcutta. He has contributed significantly in researching this work.

Dr. Surender Agnihotri is a homeopathic practitioner from Uttar Pradesh, India and has clinical experience of more than 5 years. He also researched finding sources and material for this project.

Publisher's Note

After the successful launch of the series of *The Landscape of Homeopathic Medicine* with his first book, *Case Taking*, by Alastair Gray, we are happy to launch the second volume of this series. The idea of this series of books is to gather all the research available on homeopathic practice, from Hahnemann to the present, deconstruct it, explore, re-develop, and discuss it in a way it can be understood and used by homeopaths the world over in order to develop a deeper understanding of the broad landscape of homeopathy.

This volume *"Method"* focuses on the methodology of homeopathic practice which differs world-wide. Some homeopaths argue that this difference reflects individuality, but in actuality it can also highlight a negative aspect of homeopathy. Any new person coming to homeopathy, be it as a patient or as a student can get confused, lost and disorientated.

Yet the different ways that homeopathy can be practiced can also have advantages. What Alastair Gray does in this volume is to analyze the vast literature accumulated over 200 years on the subject. The works of the old masters, stalwarts and the new teachers, all have been brought to life in this one platform, in a beautiful way, and with all aspects of these various methods covered with intricate detail.

To complete this task, Alastair calls on homeopaths from many different backgrounds who practice these different methods and identify the issues for discussion and analysis. The unique feature of this work is that the homeopaths most familiar with these differing styles of prescribing, who use them on a daily basis, are called on to pass on the purest message possible and articulate clearly to the reader their thoughts and ways of practice.

We sincerely hope that with this book we are able to, as a united profession, move forwards towards a better understanding of the methodologies advocated by different homeopaths, put them to better use, and in doing so, develop a standardisation of homeopathy that can be explained to a wider audience and thus increase its global acceptability and appeal.

B. Jain Archibel

Contents

Foreword   *iii*
Acknowledgements   *vii*
Contributors   *ix*
Publisher's Note   *xiii*

Chapters

1. **Introduction**   **3**
   - Why This Book   6
   - Literature Review   9
   - Watson's Methodologies   10
   - Nomenclature, Method and Methodology   15
   - The Different Methods and Their Classification   16
   - Method at the Coalface of Homeopathy - A Personal Story   17
   - Flexibility with Principle   21
   - Culture, Football and Buddhism   22
   - What Authors Say, What They Do, and Change over Time   24

2. **Hahnemann, Bönninghausen and the Totality of Characteristic Symptoms of the Disease**   **29**
   - Totality of the Characteristic Symptoms of the Disease   31
   - Samuel Hahnemann 1755-1843   33

- Hahnemann in Paris ... 42
- His Cases / How He Practiced ... 44
- Cases Illustrative of Homeopathic Practice ... 45
- Some other cases ... 53
- Underpinnings of Hahnemannian Homeopathy ... 57
- Peculiarity ... 57
- Totality ... 58
- Causation ... 59
- Health ... 59
- Disease ... 61
- Cure ... 61
- von Bönninghausen 1785-1864 ... 62
- Complete Symptom ... 63
- The Therapeutic Pocketbook ... 65
- Cases ... 66
- Disadvantages of the Method ... 69
- Advantages of the Method ... 71
- Method in Epidemic Diseases ... 73
- Further Reading ... 76

3. **Kent and the Totality of the Characteristics of the Person** ... 77
   - The Person not the Disease ... 79
   - Totality of the Characteristics of the Person ... 80
   - James Tyler Kent, 1849-1916 ... 82
   - Kent's Legacy ... 84
   - Swedenborg ... 86
   - What Is Disease? ... 90
   - Kentianism ... 92
   - Kent's Other Influences on Homeopathy ... 95
   - Repertory ... 95
   - Types ... 96
   - Books ... 96

- Potency and Remedies — 96
- Waiting and Waiting — 97
- Kent's Hierarchy — 97
- The Mind — 98
- Kent's Case Work — 100
- Subtle Changes — 106
- Case Examples — 107
- Strategy — 109
- Further Reading — 110

4. Constitution and Constitutional Prescribing — 111

- Introduction — 113
- The Confusion — 114
- The Prescribing Style in a Nutshell — 116
- The Disadvantages of Constitutional Prescribing — 118
- Kent, Watson and Constitution — 119
- Massive Totality — 121
- Limitations — 121
- Definitions of Constitution — 125
- Etymology of the Word 'Constitution' in the Context of Homeopathy — 127
- Advocates of Constitutional Prescribing — 129
- Hydrogenoid Constitution — 135
- From von Grauvogl's practice — 135
- Oxygenoid — 144
- Carbo-nitrogenoid Constitution — 145
- From von Grauvogl's Practice — 146
- Lesser and Nebel — 149
- Carbonic — 151
- Phosphoric — 152
- Flouric — 152
- Vannier's Constitution and Types — 152
- Constitutional Prescribing in Light of a True Understanding of Constitution — 155

- Ingredients Needed for a Constitutional Prescription ... 160
- Mappa Mundi and Temperaments ... 163
- Little on the Phlegmatic Temperament ... 167
- The Temperament of the Phlegmatic ... 168
- Phlegmatic Bodily Constitution (Generals) ... 170
- Phlegmatic Predispositions (Diathesis and Miasms) ... 172
- Phlegmatic Remedies ... 174
- Conclusions ... 175
- Of Practical Use ... 177
- Further Reading ... 179

5. Vital Sensation Shilpa Bhouraskar ... 181

- Introduction ... 185
- The Evolution of Homeopathy in Stages ... 188
- Comparison of Stages, Disease and Medicine Understanding ... 193
- Application of the Stages in Practice ... 193
  - Confirm Your Prescription Through All the Four Stages ... 193
- A Case Example Incorporating All Stages ... 194
- Which Approach to Use and When ... 212
- The Sensation Method Compared With the Earlier Methods ... 215
- Conclusion ... 218
- Further Reading ... 218

6. Miasmatic Prescribing Jennifer Osborne ... 219

- The Use of Nosodes ... 219
- The use of anti-miasmatic remedies ... 220
- Faithfulness in Tracing the Picture of the Disease ... 225
- What Is Miasmatic Prescribing? ... 230
- Nosodes as the Simillimum and Intercurrents ... 230

- Other Application of Intercurrents ... 234
- Other Benefits of a Knowledge and Understanding of Miasms ... 236
- References ... 240
- Further Reading ... 242

7. Jan Scholten's Group Analysis Greg Cope ... 243
- Jan Scholten ... 247
- Group Analysis ... 249
- Reverse Law of Similars ... 251
- Homeopathy and the Minerals ... 251
- Homeopathy and the Elements ... 255
- The Plant Kingdom ... 260
- Prescribing Techniques ... 261
- Case example ... 263
- References ... 269
- Further Reading ... 270

8. Eizayaga Ben Gadd ... 271
- Introduction ... 275
- About Eizayaga ... 278
- Treating the Patient versus Treating the Disease ... 279
- Different Types of Similitude ... 280
- Totality of Symptoms ... 282
- Classification of Symptoms ... 284
- Classification of Diseases ... 285
- Layers ... 287
- Lesion Layer ... 287
- Fundamental Layer ... 289
- Constitutional Layer ... 290
- Miasmatic Layer ... 293
- Prescribing ... 294
- Posology ... 295
- Repertory ... 296

- Criticisms of Eizayaga's Approach — 297
- Case Example — 298
- Conclusion — 303
- References and Further Reading — 304

9. Keynote Prescribing — 307

- Definitions — 309
- Keynote Materia Medica's — 310
- Why Keynote Prescribing at All? — 311
- Misapplication — 313
- History and Development of Keynote Prescribing — 314
- The Components of the Method — 316
  - Totality Again — 316
- Red-line Symptoms — 317
- Will Taylor and Meg Ryan - Practical Keynote Prescribing — 318
- What are the Characteristic Features of a Keynote? — 320
- The 'Three-legged Stool' Approach to Keynotes — 321
- Storming the Fortress / Achieving Break-through at the Weak Spots — 322
- 'Minimum Syndrome of Maximum Value' — 323
- Experts at Work - a Few More Examples — 324
- Analogous Parts — 328
- Ruling Features of the Case Reflect the 'Genius' of the Remedy — 328
- Other Leading Proponents — 332
- Advantages of Keynote Prescribing — 339
- Disadvantages of Keynote Prescribing — 342
- Further Reading — 344

10. Isopathy — 345

- Definitions — 348
- Introduction — 348
- Practicalities — 350

• Context	351
• Isopathy and Pre-Homeopathic History	352
• Advocates	357
• The Response to Isopathy	361
• Collet and Others	364
• The Controversy	365
• Refining the Method	379
• Advantages and Some Extraordinary Examples	380
• Conclusion	385
• Further Reading	385
• Appendix	387

11. Tautopathy — 397

• Definition	400
• What Exactly Is the Method?	400
• Why Do We Need It?	402
• Review of the Literature	404
• Application of Tautopathy	417
• The Pill, Naprosyn and Cortisone and Vaccinations	418
• Intercurrent Prescribing	419
• Case Examples - Patel	420
• Who Uses It Today and Research	422
• Limitations	423
• Provings and Tautopathy	423
• Further Reading	424
• Appendix	425

12. Organ Prescribing, Organopathy and Burnett — 429

• Introduction	432
• Background	432
• Affinity, Organ Prescribing, Organopathy, Supporting the Organs	434
• Specificity of Seat	435

- Locality ... 439
- The Limitations of the 'Totality of Symptoms' ... 443
- Drilling Deeper: Burnett's Influences ... 446
- Rademacher and the Organ Remedies ... 447
- Burnett's Cases ... 449
- Burnett's Use of Potency ... 454
- The Organ Remedies ... 455
- Random Gems from Burnett, Rademacher and Others ... 456
- Nosodes ... 459
- For and Against ... 460
- Computers and Burnett ... 462
- Burnett's Works ... 462
- Conclusion ... 463
- Further Reading ... 466

13. Polypharmacy, Complexes and Combinations ... 467
- Definitions ... 469
- Literature and Opinion ... 469
- Controversy, Mongrelism, Multilation and Perversion ... 470
- The Double Remedy Experiments of 1833 ... 472
- The Technique Itself ... 487
- Why NO! Opinions Past and Present ... 489
- Contemporary Opposition ... 501
- Why Yes! Opinions - Past and Present ... 509
- Some Commonly Used Combinations ... 510
- When Is it Best to Use Polypharmacy? ... 514
- Further Reading ... 516

14. Conclusion ... 519
- Method and Totality ... 519
- If You Meet Hahnemann on the Road, Kill Him ... 526
- The Influence of Hahnemann ... 527

- The Implications of Individualism in Homeopathy 532
- Teachers in Contemporary Homeopathy 537
- Method or No Method 539
- Implications for Practice 543

References *545*
Index *559*

Introduction to Method

Chapter 1

Introduction

Contents

- Why this Book
- Literature Review
- Watson's Methodologies
- Mathur's Principles
- Nomenclature, Methods and Methodology
- The Different Methods and their Classification
- Method at the Coalface of Homeopathy – A Personal Story
- Flexibility with Principle
- Culture Football and Buddhism
- What Authors Say and What They Do

In this chapter you will:

1. Learn why there is a need for a contemporary text-book on homeopathic method
2. Familiarise yourselves with the literature that is already published
3. Grasp why there are different opinions and traditions of homeopathic method

Chapter 1

Introduction

Homeopathy, utterly bewildering and nonsensical to the majority inhabiting the 21st century, asking 21st century questions, breathing positivist air, is somehow the most effective source of clarity and healing to others. To those who philosophically come from an extremely relevant but different parallel paradigm, it makes perfect sense. Homeopaths perceive things constructively, their reality is subjective, and to them there is no real objective separation of the observed from the observer. They look for pattern, structure and process. They define the fundamentals of health, disease, cure and the nature of the problem differently than others. Above all, they seek to create change by using an ancient principle of similars as opposed to the equally ancient principle of creating change through opposite force.

Homeopaths are passionate about their profession, and they are fiercely individualistic. It is this individualism that attracts people to homeopathy, but is also one of its Achilles heels. Individualism celebrates difference. But in an evidence-based world that celebrates same-ness, normal-ness and bland-ness, in a world where clinical decisions are as much dominated by lawyers, insurance salesmen and compliance officers as doctors and nurses, homeopathy and homeopaths have to be prepared to swim upstream, and against the flow.

Homeopathy is perhaps the most radical of complementary and alternative medicines. I often ask the enrolment advisers who work at Endeavour College of Natural Health, the multi-disciplinary college in Australia in which I work and run its homeopathic department, what it is like to try and sell homeopathy as opposed to massage or herbal medicine. They shake their heads. Homeopathy is a hard sell in the 21st century. Even the word itself is problematic. Homo-what? Not only are the fundamental principles challenging and new to most people, but the fact that it is practiced in such a wide variety of ways adds to the complexity of the situation, and the difficulty we all have in getting a clear message across to a willing public. There is no shortage of potential CAM clients.

Why This Book

To the immense frustration of homeopathic researchers, patients and educators, there is no one-way, best and obvious practice in which homeopathic clinicians do their work. Homeopathy is just ... homeopathy, right? In the 21st century, shouldn't we be able to say, this is what we do and this is who we are. These are our tools and this is our scope? But actually it's a very complex situation. Homeopaths use different methods to get their results, not just one. This is the bottom line. This in itself would not be such a problem if they then did not have an opinion about other people's methods.

Introduction

On a road trip to a symposium in Cambridge in 2010, I asked Dr Frederik Schroyens about it. His response was with a metaphor. There are different ways to build a house: brick by brick, using mud, with wood or with stone. The important thing is that it is sound. The method itself is not crucial as long as it is sound, watertight, and earthquake resistant. In the writing of this book, I have asked many homeopaths around the world to explain their methods. One said, "I match the person's symptoms to the proving, this is the homeopathic method." But it wasn't the method of the next person I asked.

While the underpinning principles, sometimes called laws of homeopathy are clear, and explored by some of the giants of homeopathic literature, and further in volume four in the series, *Foundations of Homeopathic Philosophy and Theory*, individual interpretation of those principles and the needs of the immediate patient and the specific clinical setting lead to an overwhelming difference in the delivery of homeopathic medicine.

Quite simply, the practice of homeopathy is different in Germany, India, the US, the UK, Ghana, Argentina, New Zealand, and Canada. More importantly it is different in different parts of those places. One homeopath prescribes predominantly in one way in one part of the city, and another homeopath, perhaps just down the street prescribes in a different way. The reality of homeopathic practice is that of course all homeopaths each have their own style. It is often said that no two homeopaths think, reason, or prescribe in the same way.

In volume one of this series, I articulated, described and explained the homeopathic landscape of case taking. It explored the instructions from the very beginnings in the 1790s about case taking and attempted to make clear why since that time homeopathy has evolved in the way that it has and why it is the way it is now. In the same way, this volume will explore the landscape of homeopathic method. To those people outside of the profession, it comes as some surprise that homeopaths, even after 200 years, do not seem to have professional agreement about the best way to evaluate a set of facts after a case taking and proceed with a prescription. This lack of agreement has slowed down the profession in gaining general acceptance in many arenas, most notably clinical research. There are different schools of homeopathic thought and reasoning. When it comes to acute and chronic case evaluation, the different schools have different ideas. This can become an area of confusion for students at the undergraduate level.

As a consequence, a primary driver for this book is to attempt to highlight and overcome the perceived problem that the public, students and practitioners of homeopathy have about the inability to develop consistency across the profession and have a similar approach to case taking and homeopathic prescribing. In other professions, even professions close to homeopathic medicine, a group of osteopaths, physiotherapists or herbalists are likely to come up with a similar or the same treatment strategy given a similar set of facts. We don't see that so much with homeopathy. Observers are immediately suspicious, especially in such an unequivocally evidence-based world. But homeopaths are happily individualistic, and are used to justifying their prescriptions and treatment plans and strategies with a staggering array of statements such as, 'that this is just what I do,' or 'there are no right answers.'

Most experienced homeopaths will tell a similar story. In order to maximize one's success and get better positive results in clinical practice, one cannot rely on one style or one method entirely. Flexibility and elasticity are qualities that are required. Like a monoculture that is susceptible to attack and requires an extreme amount of chemical protection to ensure its survival, one-dimensional homeopathic practice, even when practiced well or even brilliantly, will only be successful in a certain number of cases. Evidence suggests that thriving practice and successful prescriptions require flexibility of method, and equal flexibility in good measure as a part of their psychographic make up. This flexibility allows homeopaths to know when to stop one line of thinking or treatment, and move to another strategy.

Literature Review

Given this situation, it is a surprise that there has not been more literature on the subject. There are essentially no books or articles on homeopathic method other than those by Watson, Tyler and Mathur. Mathur published his *Principles of Prescribing* in 1975. While not widely known, it takes readers through the prescribing style of the '*pioneers*' of homeopathy. Interestingly it starts with specifics, prophylaxis and then moves to other styles of prescribing, miasmatic, nosodes and more. It is an excellent read. With cases from Lippe, Clarke, Kent, Hahnemann and a myriad of others each style is given a pragmatic emphasis. Interestingly, the motive was to identify and document the changes from *Hahnemannian* homeopathy to *Scientific* homeopathy. Tyler in *Different ways of Finding the Remedy* explored different methods also.

In homeopathy, the Remedy is the thing. Potencies, administration-the questions that divide us, are matters of personal experience. People have done brilliant work using widely different range of potencies and administration, provided that they had found the remedy. Without that the magic refuses to work. We are here to consider different ways of finding the remedy, because the essential thing, for a homoeopathic prescription (and on this we all agree), is a like remedy for a like abnormal condition (Tyler 1927).

Watson's Methodologies

Ian Watson's small but important book appeared in 1991. Students immediately latched on to its pragmatic and useful message. Undergraduate students tend to become overwhelmed with the different styles of their tutors, clinical supervisors and lecturers. Anecdotal evidence suggests this lack of best practice is one of the most significant reasons that students stop studying homeopathy and move on. For other students, this variety of methods doesn't seem to be an issue. Some are able to integrate these different options and see it as an opportunity rather than a lack of clarity.

Nevertheless, at some point in the life cycle of a homeopathic student, they become aware of what they do not know. This awareness is a difficult moment in the training. The initial excitement of starting something new and radical has worn off, and students become aware of such things as the number of remedies they still have to learn; the medical sciences they still have to master; importantly realizing that to master one system is fine, but that mastery of that system will not guarantee universal success in every clinical situation. Of course, students deal with this reality in different ways. Some study harder. But many have reported that it was Ian Watson's book that was the key to realizing that there were different styles of practice and how they all fitted together. Furthermore, it is often reported that his useful classification, simple descriptions and easy style make the book so useful and so pragmatically important. It has been reported many a time that finding Watson's book was that 'aha' moment in the training.

Watson's 100 pages were accessible and immediately practical. The chapters, arranged alphabetically, aetiologies, arborivital medicine, constitutional prescribing, genus epidemicus, isopathy, layers, miasmatic prescribing, organ remedies, physical generals, polypharmacy, repertorisation, specifics, symptom similarity, tautopathy, therapeutics, 15 in all, give a basic introduction and capture the core issues of these different methods of prescribing homeopathy. The introduction best captures the need for a book on method.

An average group of doctors eavesdropping on a conversation amongst an average group of homeopaths have much in common with a Martian who accidentally picks up the cricket commentary. One of my goals for homoeopathy is that it may be picked up and used by anyone in a way that is more or less can measure it with their current level of understanding and expertise.

Prevalent amongst many of the current teachers and practitioners homeopathy is a desire to teach homeopathy at its highest (and most difficult) level. Whilst I share this desire, my belief is that adhering to this goal exclusively is a positive hindrance to the widespread development of homeopathy. The majority of those who could be using homeopathy right away are deterred or prevented from doing so by the formidable effort and shifts in understanding that seemed to be required.

It is with this in mind that I have written this book. My hope is that anyone with an interest in homeopathy and familiarity with its basic principles will be stimulated to learn one or more of its many applications and, more importantly, to apply what they have learnt when they are healing the sick.

The major purpose of this book then, is to expose the reader to a wide cross-section of the many diverse ways in which the principle of similars may be applied in practice. My intention is not to produce confusion for those for whom homeopathy is a simple and straightforward affair. Rather I would hope that to encourage practitioners and students at all levels will feel encouraged to widen the scope of their prescribing beyond their own and, hopefully my own, present limitations (Watson 1991).

These points are well made. One of the roles that I have had in the last two years is to run a large, multi-campus department of homeopathy. I have been responsible and accountable for curriculum, quality, assessment and pedagogy. I have been in many uncomfortable situations where experts in the design of education curriculum are bewildered by what homeopathic educators try to do when writing and constructing curricula.

An educationalist approaches design of a curriculum from the perspective of starting with simple concepts so that students are encouraged to *understand*, and *explain*, and the curriculum can be leveraged to appropriately *assess* those students in the *foundation* years. Then, the level of complexity of concepts and ideas gradually increases step by step to ensure that students are able to:

- *integrate* that information before they leave their course, whether a diploma, an advanced diploma or degree
- *apply* those ideas, theories and techniques with competence and confidence.

Homeopaths often have it upside down and back to front. Virtually, all if not every homeopathic course on the planet starts the lecturing, teaching and learning of homeopathy from Hahnemann, and from the principal of similars, an extremely new idea for most and one that in any system or taxonomy is a complex idea. Then on top of that, students explore the infinitesimal dose, totality and minimum dose, all of which have various levels of interpretation and disagreement. Using say, Bloom's taxonomy, these require higher cognitive skills right up front. Then bizarrely, the final years of study are loaded up with remembering the indications of small remedies that will hardly ever be used. In the context of what Watson is saying, the level of homeopathic information pitched to students is still not right and as educators we have to do better.

In addition, many colleges attempt from the very beginning, from first year to teach Sensation Method homeopathy or advanced Kentian homeopathy as best practice. These advanced approaches, often taught poorly, only succeed in confusing and disenchanting many students along the way. Watson (1991) manages to thread the needle of reducing many complex ideas to their essential parts. Students who are in the middle of this process of learning homeopathy in an extremely complex way are appreciative and generally love Watson's book, for its size, its tone and its intention.

Beyond the works of Watson, Tyler (1927) and Mathur (1975), there is little else. Authors such as P Sankaran (1996), Close (1924), Kent (1900) and Vithoulkas (1980) describe keynote or constitutional prescribing in some way but nothing else is devoted to strategies of clinical evaluation, or comparing them. This is not to say that homeopathic experts around the world don't discuss these issues. Simon Taffler, Kim Elia, Richard Pitt, David Levy, myself and others have all discussed in conferences or papers different methods. But there are no other articles or textbooks examining method in a comparative way. It is up to the homeopath to go to the individual casebooks and other published material of authors such as Burnett or Kent to understand their method.

But other than that, everyone seems to have their own style, their own way. This book about homeopathic technique and method is therefore necessary from a landscape perspective, describing each method and commenting upon it in a non-judgmental and critical way.

Since Watson's book was published in 1991, homeopathy has experienced a seismic change with the dual influences of Scholten and Sankaran. Both of these authors essentially published since Watson's work became available and the consequences are incalculable. These are not slight variations on Hahnemann's method but represent a challenge to homeopathic thinking and prescribing to its very core. Watson's book needs to be updated on that point alone and a dedicated method textbook is warranted.

Nomenclature, Method and Methodology

There is also a question on the simple use of the word 'methodology'. For years my friend and colleague David Levy has been at pains to point out that technically the word 'methodology' is used to describe an overarching approach to the study of methods, e.g. grounded theory methodology, phenomenology, critical social studies, feminist studies etc. These are methodologies that can be applied to the study of methods, including homeopathic methods of case taking, analysis etc. The implication is that the correct term is 'method' and not 'methodologies'.

While discussing terminology, it is actually quite artificial to talk about Hahnemannian homeopathy or Burnett's organopathy. We do it lazily and simplistically. I only do it in the context of this book in an attempt to assist students, graduates and experienced homeopaths in identifying the lineage of what they are doing. Of course, it was only Hahnemann that practiced Hahnemannian homeopathy. But plenty of practitioners, daily prescribe in this style and follow to the letter the instructions of the founder. This is notably the case in Germany with both medical homeopaths and Heilpraktiker. But in addition to that many homeopaths do much more. So when I speak of Sequential homeopathy or Kentian homeopathy, it is to acknowledge that there is a set of guidelines advocated, and a new or different interpretation of some of the fundamentals of homeopathy (perhaps totality for example) that allows such an interpretation to make sense.

It is also important to remember that it is impossible to speak about the differences in homeopathic method without speaking about the individuals that devised them, discussing some history and perhaps controversies. In looking through the literature, there are at least twenty different identifiable methods and very likely more. Most of these methods have some time devoted to them in this work.

The Different Methods and Their Classification

At the beginning of this work it was decided to classify the different homeopathic methods and styles historically, that is Hahnemann through to Sankaran and beyond, from the beginning to the present. But then not everyone is historically minded. Homeopathic method could just as well be classified alphabetically. I also considered this classification. There was also the possibility of classifying methods according to cultural reference points - English homeopathy, Indian homeopathy, as well as French and German perspectives. This approach was dismissed because homeopathy is prescribed differently in each of these countries even though there may well be trends in a certain direction. I further considered basing the book on the historical figures that devised or championed a particular method.

In the end, I chose a classification based on my own understanding of the *totality of symptoms*. To my mind, this concept is what fundamentally distinguishes between different styles of prescribing for the most part. At least half of the methods described in this book are complete systems in themselves. Other methods are really there to support and augment, or even use as a last resort in those clinical situations where there is no identifiable or meaningful totality of symptoms in the case. And this is where these methods are so valuable. In other words, I have ordered this discussion of homeopathic method according to how that method interprets the Hahnemannian concept of totality. The actual chapters are arranged largest to smallest because I see all of these styles of prescribing as having their place. There is one exception. I have started with Hahnemann to provide context and facilitate the flow through the book. Moreover, I have invited some experts to contribute their understanding to the work rather than relying solely on my own research or opinion.

Method at the Coalface of Homeopathy - A Personal Story

I have told this story in a number of seminars and conferences with mixed reception. My own introduction to the practice of homeopathy was coloured by a change of country. I learned my homeopathy in the UK in the early 1990s. Like most students, I was completely caught up in assignments, assessments, trying to earn a living and pay the bills. There was one thing that I was confident about, and that was that I was learning homeopathy and that I was going to be good. Looking back, one of the striking things about observing homeopathic practice and very good homeopaths in their own clinics during that time was that they took good long cases focused on the presenting symptom, and then in the course of a consultation really started to extract and explore the threads that ran through the case. Sometimes they looked to the constitution and prescribed. A lot of the prescriptions were based on some of those stolen essences from Vithoulkas. I remember watching some astonishing results that served to give me step-by-step confidence that not only was homeopathy extremely effective but ultimately reinforced in me that I would be able to do it.

One thing led to another, and I found myself in Australia having already begun a practice in the UK. I immediately found that the skills I needed to attract clients, and talk with them seemed to be redundant in the middle of Sydney. Most of my clients seem to be unimpressed with the idea that a consultation might take longer than an hour. They also looked at me strangely and with some suspicion if I asked them about anything other than their presenting symptom. I remember some raised eyebrows when I asked about recurring dreams, when symptoms began, what their childhood may have been like - all of the things which in the English homeopathic context seemed so normal and homeopathic. In the mid-90s environment of the inner west of Sydney, these questions seemed out of place. *Natrum muriaticum* had been a staple prescription in the UK, and I think it was about three years of prescribing in Sydney before I found myself using that remedy, ironically to an Englishwoman who was depressed and homesick.

What slowly dawned on me over a period of time was that I felt unprepared for the realities of practice in Sydney and was being confronted with them every day. My understanding of homeopathic principles, philosophy and theory was solid but I must have been sleeping through my lectures on therapeutics, or perhaps there were none. People came to see me asking for relief for their headaches. My style of prescribing and my approach in taking their cases was to look for the reason that they had their headaches in the first place. While for the most part many good-natured clients indulged me, there were also many that left disappointed.

Introduction

In one memorable situation, I remember watching a client get out of a taxi before coming to see me in my clinic. He reached into his pocket to pay the taxi driver and all of this change spilled into the street. He was so flustered and in such a hurry, and so late to see me that he left his coins rolling around in the gutter and ran into the building. This is a far cry from the clients that I first saw in practice in the UK. In the suburbs of Bristol, Bath or the more rural folk of Devon, there were very different agendas, lifestyles, and ultimately levels of health. This point is crucial because vitality levels in rural and regional clients is very often significantly higher than in adrenally challenged and exhausted city clients. (I have heard my Indian colleagues completely disagree with me however when talking about the levels of health and vitality of their clients in Mumbai, Delhi and Kolkata). Quite simply the style of homeopathy has to be different.

The upshot of that experience was that over a period of time I realized that the style of homeopathy that I had learnt (which I thought was homeopathy and which I now call post-Kentian) was useful for about 40% of my cases in that city clinic context. And I realized in quick time that it was up to me to go back to the books to deal with some of the other presentations that appeared in the clinic. Not all will agree with me because there is the reality that a very good Kentian or Bönninghausen prescriber will be able to deal with a vast majority of cases. What I noticed in my own practice was that by drilling both down and sideways, I was able to increase my effectiveness as a practitioner when incorporating different styles of prescribing.

An honest audit of my own casework reveals many inconsistencies over the years. Some cases I started with isopathy, other cases I attempted numerous totality prescriptions over considerable months before changing my strategy. But on talking with many experienced homeopaths, there are similar stories. Many make it up as they go along. A primary purpose of this book therefore is to create simplicity. So often in the course of the last decade of teaching homeopathy and running clinical training subjects in colleges and universities, it has been obvious that students need to unlearn much of what they have learnt because they have simply misunderstood information they have been given or have been unduly influenced by individual lecturers over emphasis on a particular point or style.

For complete disclosure, my clinical style of prescribing could best be summed up as an attempt to understand the totality of symptoms of the disease in a person in order to select a remedy. Remedy selection and understanding the totality of symptoms represents the technical part of homeopathy. However, to ensure that the remedy's work is maximised, patients are engaged as deeply as possible in the therapeutic relationship. Therefore it is not constitutional prescribing, but rather the application of a Bönninghausen and Hahnemannian approach in a contemporary context, with heavy emphasis on the therapeutic relationship between the practitioner and the patient.

I went into some depth on this issue in my first book of the series. One of the major conflicts in homeopathy is about whether we are treating broad-brush stroke totality of the person or the totality of symptoms of the diseased individual.

Personally, I have had very little success with essence-style prescribing and prescriptions for symptoms based on the constitution of the client. I have had two notable exceptions but only with two remedies. I have had innumerable patients, too many to consider, who have really been *phosphoric* in the broadest definition of the word, and have responded very well simply with a single dose of *Phosphorus*. It just works. It's brilliant. It's such an amazing remedy and in a phosphoric type, it doesn't matter what the presenting symptom seemed to be because it just seems to work. But beyond that I'm simply not very good at it. I learned materia medica from Misha Norland in the early 1990s and this synthetic style of looking at the broadest and deepest themes, underpinned my study of remedies. I later consolidated my method of learning materia medica with Jeremy Sherr who emphasised other aspects of a remedy profile.

Not all cases are cured by the same style of prescribing. Not all cases are the same. Practitioners do their work in different parts of the city, town and country. Some have wealthy, some have poor, some have radical, and some have edgy clients. The method used, and ultimately the medicine and treatment plan given, will depend on who takes and evaluates the case.

Flexibility with Principle

Ultimately the principle involved here is flexibility. But flexibility without principle can be misguided. I am not advocating that superficial understanding of these methods is a way to maximize success in the clinic. They must be studied in depth and the further reading and references provided in each of the chapters need to be explored.

Culture, Football and Buddhism

To the outsider's eye, homeopathic medicine seems strange. There is an intriguing mixture of emphasis on the natural as well as the scientific, listening to clients and prescribing for clients. In lectures over the last decade, I have often looked for a good analogy for the reasons homeopaths differ in their prescribing. I have already explained why they differ in their case-taking styles. From an historical or anthropological perspective, homeopathy began in Germany, and very quickly spread, due to its immediate and dramatic successes to France, then Italy, and Britain. By the mid 1800s, it was well entrenched in the USA, South America and India.

Bizarrely, in this way, it is not too dissimilar to the spread of football. This global phenomenon started in England, but these days it is expressed so differently in different countries, Brazil (samba, the beautiful game, passionate, creative, intuitive), Holland (total football), Germany (efficient, effective) Africa (spontaneous) etc. It is different in every culture even though it started the same. An examination of the history of Buddhism demonstrates a similar phenomenon. It started in India and because of that success and utility soon spread to Sri Lanka and the rest of south-east Asia, to Tibet through China and Japan. In each place it adopted some of the existing pre-cultural aspects of the spiritual practices of those places, which is why Tibetan Buddhism has such a startlingly different set of practices to Zen Buddhism as it is practiced in Korea. It moved slowly over the generations northwards out of India and into the Tibetan plateau where it encountered the traditional and more primitive style Bon set of practices. Today, in Japan there is still a Bon holiday. Over countless generations they merged, morphed, developed so that today both can be seen. Homeopathy is no different. Therefore, a book on homeopathic method is also a celebration of the global medicine that it is. Germans play football differently than the Swiss, differently than the New Zealanders, Canadians and Cubans.

It is not about everyone doing the same homeopathy. We can sustain difference in the profession as long as there is rigour. What we cannot have is laziness. That is inexcusable. And we cannot have ineffectiveness. Therefore, students need to know when to apply these different methods, when to use them and when not to.

This work on method is therefore based on the assumption that Hahnemannian homeopathy serves as the building block, the cornerstone and the foundation. While Hahnemann's is a style of homeopathy that is still practised today (and many educators and clinicians would prefer that this remains as fundamental in the practice of homeopathy), others such as Kent in the 19th century and Whitmont in the 20th century steered homeopathy in a different direction. Realizing that the emotional world of the patient was important to consider in the evaluation of a case, they encouraged that the practitioner emphasized different aspects of the case. Further, in the 21st century, Sensation Method developed as a possible way to evaluate the patient's symptoms and situation. What is more, there are now pseudoscientific augmentations such as the use of colour, the use of kinesiology to facilitate practice and improve results. Quite clearly many homeopaths have moved on from Hahnemann. To some, homeopathy that focuses on the symptoms of the patient, the story of the patient is now limited in the 21st century context. It is argued that homeopathy has moved on and there are more sophisticated ways of understanding patients and by borrowing from other professions and traditions, we are able to practice homeopathy more deeply and effectively.

What Authors Say, What They Do, and Change over Time

It must also be remembered that authors' ideas change over time as they learn, adapt, and move on. Often you will hear someone in homeopathic circles say, 'Kent thought this', and 'Bönninghausen did that'. This is of course nonsense. Just because someone writes something doesn't mean it gets locked into to some sort of time warp. We know this is the case with Sankaran's work. Since the *Spirit of Homeopathy* in 1991 he has changed his mind, evolved, moved on, and gone back. Of course that does not mean that all his early works are redundant and should be forgotten. It means that he wrote something once, and does another thing today. We also know this to be the case with Hahnemann. He changed his mind. Often! After all we have his casebooks to review, and it is possible to look at the publications of his philosophical and theoretical works, such as the *Chronic Diseases* or the *Organon of Medicine*, and compare them to what he was doing in his casework at the time. We also know this to be the case with Kent. His philosophy book contains ideas and opinions that are simply the opposite of what we see in his case books and published case material.

What is bemusing to homeopathic students, and eventually becomes clear to all practicing homeopaths, is that the differences in style of prescribing come down to a few very fundamental issues. It is ultimately the individual interpretation of the basic principles of totality, peculiarity, what health is, what cure is, and what disease is that demarcates practitioners and their prescriptions. While examining the different methods of prescribing in this book, I will argue that it is a different understanding of the healthy person that drives why Hahnemannian homeopathy and Kentian homeopathy is fundamentally different. It is exactly the reason why the Sensation Method is different and requires a different method than Sequential Method.

It is my sincere desire that this book serves as a vehicle to help homeopaths, be they experienced or new, gain a clearer understanding of what it is that they are doing when they are prescribing, and why they are prescribing the way that they are. Through this clarity, it is my hope that homeopaths will denigrate their colleagues much less. Understanding why prescriptions differ between homeopaths can be attributed to these different understandings of the fundamental principles of health, cure, disease, peculiarity etc. It is not because they are 'wrong'. This egotistical dismissal of other experienced homeopathic findings and results demonstrates nothing other than small mindedness and immaturity.

To the clinical researchers reading, this book might help explain why they receive opposition to a clinical trial or research design in which they are involved. To the interested patients of homeopathy, this book might explain why their homeopaths do what they do. To the experienced homeopaths, this book might be useful to assist in gaining a deeper understanding of unfamiliar methods, or explain why patients of homeopaths using these unfamiliar methods have been prescribed certain remedies. To homeopathic students, this work will assist in untangling the intriguing spaghetti with which they find themselves wrestling.

Just as in the first book of the series on case taking, there is a very simple message. It doesn't matter what sort of a case taker or prescriber you are. As you move into your practice, start to find your feet, and get a number of clients under your belt, it is crucially important to reflect on what is going on, to take stock and work out what sort of a case taker you are. Be aware of the lineage from which the case taking comes and attempt to leverage and maximise what you can from it.

This method book delivers a similar message. There is no right way. There has never been just one way. Anyone that tells you anything else is simply egotistical. That is not to say that there is not an appropriate way to begin one's study, and a very good way to begin one's practice, and to get 100, 200, 1000 cases in your filing cabinet before beginning to tinker with new styles and approaches and methods. There is no one right way to practice homeopathy in every clinical situation. Just as osteopaths will draw on a range of techniques that they learned to employ in individual cases at one time, homeopaths should likewise retain flexibility as appropriately. In one patient with specific types of information, the homeopath could be looking at a broad totality approach. With another client, the homeopath will be searching for sensation, and applying kingdom, or group strategies. If other attempts at creating change have not been successful, it may be entirely appropriate to use isopathy or some other strategy.

To acknowledge that there are different methods, homeopaths, graduates and students would do well to read some history, read the original works of the great homeopaths of the past, read, learn, read more and learn more again. In this book, I've attempted to not only rely on my interpretation of some other works of the great homeopaths over the last 200 years, but also look at some of the interpretations of those homeopaths and lecturers around the world who really have made a name for themselves in a particular style of prescribing.

Over the years I have received plenty of assistance from friends and colleagues, and in particular some conversations have been pivotal in my understanding. Not that I profess to be right. Nevertheless, I will take this opportunity to thank Ben Gadd, Rachel Roberts, Kate Chatfield, Dale Emerson, Dr Frederik Schroyens, Richard Pitt, and Simon Taffler.

Chapter 2

Hahnemann, Bönninghausen and the Totality of Characteristic Symptoms of the Disease

Contents

- Totality of the Characteristic Symptoms of the Disease
- Samuel Hahnemann
- Hahnemann in Paris
- His Cases and How He Practiced
- Cases Illustrative of Homeopathic Practice
- Underpinnings of Hahnemannian Homeopathy
- Peculiarity
- Totality
- Causation
- Health
- Disease
- Cure
- von Bönninghausen
- Complete Symptom
- The Therapeutic Pocketbook
- Cases

- Disadvantages of the Method
- Advantages of the Method
- Method in Epidemic Diseases
- Further Reading

In this chapter you will:

1. Reflect on the different interpretations of the 'totality of symptoms' and the implications of this
2. Explore the simplicity of the Hahnemannian method
3. Familiarise yourself with a selection of his cases and how he practiced
4. Learn about the application and refinement of the method by von Bönninghausen

Chapter 2

Hahnemann, Bönninghausen and the Totality of Characteristic Symptoms of the Disease

Totality of the Characteristic Symptoms of the Disease

An article appeared in an Australian homeopathic journal in the 1990s. It had an immediate impact on the way that homeopathy is prescribed in some parts of Australia. D'Aran eloquently discussed the difference between prescribing on the totality of the person and treating the totality of the diseased person, and argued that Hahnemann's homeopathy was very clear in treating the disease. The article was written as a reaction to poorly practiced Kentian homeopathy that he observed in Australia at the time, and also as a word of caution to the wave of new ideas and homeopathic theories going around at that time. That article represented a fundamental difference to the way in which homeopathy is presented, practiced, and taught in Australia. By contrast, lecturers in other parts of the world say, and students repeat and believe that homeopathy treats the whole person.

It made a very basic point that this is a difference between the schools of homeopathy. One side argues that there is the system of homeopathy that attempts in multiple conversations, and using many remedies, to cure the chronic disease as practiced and advocated by Hahnemann. The other side counters that homeopathy is characterized by searching for the golden thread, the essence of the fundamental problem, and looking for that one perfect holy grail of a medicine that will unravel the patient's symptoms which are but a manifestation of the fundamental disturbance. D'Aran argued then and still does that the simplicity of homeopathy was lost and contaminated by later developments. Aphorism six of the *Organon*, he argued, confirms that the job of the homeopath is to look for the deviations of the former healthy state of the now diseased individual. These signs represent the disease. In other words, the simple job of the homeopath in the case-taking process is to identify the presenting symptoms and then trace those symptoms back until the patient was last healthy. This is a good place to begin our exploration of method. Since it is very difficult to distinguish and disentangle the method employed by Hahnemann and his case-taking style, a useful adjunct to reading this chapter would be to look at Gray's (2010) chapter on Hahnemann's case taking.

In Watson's *Methodologies* (1991), there is a specific chapter on physical generals, in which he implies that there is a specific method devoted to these physical generals. He called this method a variation on constitutional treatment, differing only in that physical general symptoms are highest in the hierarchy of symptoms above mental and emotional and physical particular symptoms (Watson 1991). By physical general, he meant any physical symptom or modality that refers to the patient as a whole and not just one part.

To my mind, this perspective is not entirely accurate because Hahnemann was the first to create, and Bönninghausen perfected and systematized, a method of homeopathy where all symptoms were essentially considered equal, and it mattered not whereabouts they were on the body or in the body, but rather how characteristic or complete they were. Only strange symptoms were to be emphasised.

I have included in this book a more than cursory biography of Hahnemann for the simple reason that in order to understand his ideas and style of prescribing, it is important to know about the man, what he did, where he went, and how things changed over time. To so many people, there is surprise that homeopathy comes from the Western medical tradition, from a scientific tradition, and not, as many people think, from any esoteric stream.

Samuel Hahnemann 1755-1843

Hahnemann was the third child in the family of three boys and two girls. His birthplace was Meissen, which is now in modern Germany, but back then was Saxony. His father was a porcelain printer by profession and the young Hahnemann was educated by his father in what can only be considered to be a strict educational regime. By the age of 12 he was tutoring in Greek. It is frustrating that there are so many gaps in the historical record about his youth and adolescence that might offer insight into some of his later attitudes, discoveries and behaviours. His birthplace,

> Some 27km northwest of Dresden, at the heart of a rich wine-growing region, Meissen is a compact, perfectly preserved old town. Crowning a rocky ridge above it is the Albrechtsburg palace, which in 1710 became the cradle of European porcelain manufacturing. The world-famous Meissen china, easily recognised by its trademark insignia of blue crossed swords, is still the main reason the town is such a favourite with coach tourists. Fortunately, the Altstadt's cobbled lanes, dreamy nooks and idyllic courtyards make getting away from the shuffling crowds a snap (Lonely Planet 2011a).

In the autumn of 2010, I went to Cöthen, Meissen, Leipzig and Dresden to try and get a feel from the perspective of the 21st century for what it was like 250 years ago. Dresden of course is featured in the Kurt Vonnegut's book and movie Slaughterhouse 5. In my mind I had visualised the cobbles, classical music, mud in the streets and shops full of China. The guidebook says of Dresden,

> There are few city silhouettes more striking than Dresden's. The classic view from the Elbe's northern bank takes in a playful phalanx of delicate spires, soaring towers and dominant domes belonging to palaces, churches and stately buildings (Lonely Planet 2011b).

There is all of that, as well as a bunch of roundabouts and convenience stores, spectacular wurst and excellent beer.

We know a lot about Samuel Hahnemann, but there is also a lot that we have no idea about. He studied medicine at the University of Leipzig. With one exception when he made a trip to Vienna, he never left Germany until his 80th year. In 1779, he completed his medical studies at Erlangen. He moved to Dessau in 1781 and met his first wife Johanna there. Hahnemann supplemented his income working as a medical officer by translating books especially in chemistry, and as his family grew over the next 20 years he moved multiple times. Eventually abandoning medical practice in 1789, he moved to Leipzig and began translating full time, and it was here in 1790 while translating Cullen's *Materia Medica* that he began his first experiments with homeopathy. For more on Hahnemann's life, times and travels, read Winston's (1999) *Faces of Homeopathy*.

In 1790 while translating Cullen he made his startling decision to start experimenting on himself with Peruvian bark, eventually leading to his discovery and publication of the idea of similars. This new take on an old idea led to innumerable further provings that were conducted over the next few years on himself, family and his friends. In 1792, Hahnemann was invited to move from Leipzig to Georgenthal by the local duke, to set up an asylum for the insane in the wing of his castle. 'Our Duke will soon hand over his hunting castle in Georgenthal and have it furnished' (Haehl 1922). Here he cured the Hanoverian police minister, Klockenbring (his only patient), who was insane.

It was also during this time that Hahnemann discovered the prophylactic use of *Belladonna* in scarlet fever. Based on his observations of a family, the children of which had scarlet fever, he published his article using *Belladonna* as a prophylactic. Controversy, professional jealousy and suspicion followed him and his successors. The physicians and apothecaries of

Königslutter rallied to have him removed from the city, and in 1793 he was forced to move on. He and his family were accompanied to the edge of the town by many of the patients whom he had cured. It was during his journey the wagon carrying his family and his possessions was overturned and his infant son was killed.

Further moves followed, and in 1796 Hahnemann found himself in Königslutter. During this time, he published several essays, which included:

- *Friend of Health - on hygiene.*
- *Essay on a New Principle for Ascertaining the Remedial Powers of Medicinal Substances.* It was in this essay that Hahnemann claimed that medicines should be employed on the basis of similars.
- *Are the Obstacles to the Attainment of Simplicity and Certainty in Practical Medicine Insurmountable?* This article was written against the idea of mixing medicines.

By the very end of the 1790s, he began to fully practise medicine again. And he was writing prolifically. In 1801 he wrote the essay, *Cure and prevention of Scarlet Fever*. Soon came the book *Medicine of Experience* (1806), an exposition of his whole doctrine, and a precursor to the *Organon* that was written in Torgau.

It is to our great fortune that Francis Treuertz's recent *Genius of Homeopathy* (2011) fills in significant gaps, with an excellent historical dig into one of the most important periods of Hahnemann's life. His letters highlighting the communications between patients and himself in the 10 years from 1793 to 1805 make for surprising reading and crystallise the degree to which he changed his mind over time. What is clear is that Hahnemann absolutely took on the role of what we would consider today to be a naturopath. Advice about nutrition, exercise, sleep and water are at the centre of every communication as well as taking a dose or two of a medicine. There was advice on what to wear, the type of clothes and massage. While he clearly made a policy decision later in the 1830s to stop the practice there is clear evidence of more than one homeopathic intervention being used at one time, remedies being used for constipation in the afternoon and other symptoms in the morning. The nutritional advice was of its time, goose fat, sausages, Hungarian wine and beer find pride of place and are advocated enthusiastically. And there are also big surprises. Over and over in these 10 years Hahnemann advocated the use of electricity as a therapeutic tool. We see it all in Hahnemann during this time, in fact all of the problems that beset the profession today. Like many contemporary homeopaths he was always complaining about money. There were never enough thalers or groschen. Furthermore, there was some hubris. 'Put your trust in only God and me,' said Hahnemann in 1794. 'You have not acted well to consult another doctor, I don't care who he may be.... and without boasting I may say to you that you would long ago have been in your grave if I had not studied your really uncommon and ticklish constitution.' He wasn't even shy of writing letters to the editor addressed to everybody demanding that he be paid properly and that people sent stamped addressed reply paid envelopes when they wrote to him. It also seems that a lot of people sent him lottery tickets as payment. Who knew?

In 1810, 201 years ago and when Hahnemann was 55 years old, the first edition of the *Organon* was published. There were immediate attacks on this work, including the most vociferous by Professor Hecker of Berlin. Hahnemann, for once preferring silent contempt, left it to Frederick Hahnemann to undertake the defence of his father. Soon, after so many years of moving, and after so many years of defending himself, Hahnemann succeeded in getting his first university job. He applied for a position in the faculty of medicine at Leipzig University to give lectures on homeopathy. Reasonably enough, he was requested to deliver a thesis to the faculty, and it was at this time that he wrote his paper drawing on sources from four languages on the drug *Veratrum album*. It was so well received he immediately began work. He then lectured twice a week and developed a following amongst many of the students. But he was never one to act diplomatically, and this time of his life is as much punctuated with academic successes as furious, unyielding rants against the excesses of conventional medicine and growing opposition. He was bitter in his condemnation of medicine as it was practiced and the 60 year-old Hahnemann was uncompromising in his attitudes.

Between 1810 and 1821, he wrote articles on the treatment of burns, the second edition of the *Organon of Medicine*, *Aesclulapius in the Balance*, a criticism of medicine and *Materia Medica Pura* (1811), the first collection of drug provings on the healthy body. His time there had coincided with Napoleons march across Prussia and Saxony and the siege of the city, yet it was not that, but the opposition to his ideas and medicine that determined he move on.

Throughout this time he was attracting significant negative press, most notably in medical journals, and so he began publishing in more general interest magazines for the public where he had easily his greatest support. It was not a bad strategy and one that has significance today in the 21st century. Punch magazine for example, and other similar publications to whom we wrote were the 19th century version of Twitter. Another publication soon followed, *On the Value of the Speculative Systems of Medicine* but following too much harassment Hahnemann decided to leave Leipzig. Eventually it was a combination of opposition at the University of Leipzig, plus the fact that he was unable to manufacture, prescribe and dispense his own medicines because of the monopolies of the city apothecaries, meant he was again forced to leave.

1821 saw him back in the city of Cöthen, and once again as a successful practice flourished, he became surrounded by patients, advocates and followers of the new discipline of homeopathy. I find that of significant historical interest and a little ironic that he conducted a large amount of prescribing through the mail. It was here that the third, fourth, and fifth editions of the *Organon* were published, as well as the second and third editions of *Materia Medica Pura*.

In 1827, he invited his two oldest and most esteemed disciples to Cöthen, Stapf and Gross, to talk about his theory of chronic diseases and his discovery of a completely new series of remedies for their cure. The following year, the 1st and 2nd volumes of *Chronic Diseases, their peculiar nature and homeopathic treatment* appeared. This work was not received well by all of his followers. Some perceived it as the truth while others saw significant holes in it, did not understand fully, and were not satisfied. Once again Hahnemann was subjected to ridicule. Many articles and letters went to and fro between these factions.

Success is a double-edged sword, and there is no doubt that the elderly Hahnemann was as satisfied as he was mortified by some of the practices of those describing themselves as homeopaths (Winston 1999). Opposition aside, in 1829 a large number of students and admirers gathered at Cöthen to celebrate the 50th anniversary of his medical degree. The Central Society of German Homoeopaths was also founded. The success of homeopathy began to spread to Europe and America, which of course only increased the attacks by opponents. During this time Hahnemann wrote a pamphlet entitled *Allopathy; a warning to all sick persons*.

After a life of some considerable hardship, in 1830 Hahnemann's wife died. She is a fairly invisible shadow in his life, and significant historical work needs to be done to unearth her role in the life of Hahnemann. Thereafter he was looked after by his daughters.

Part of the reason for the quick spread of homeopathy had been due to the 1831 cholera epidemics in Germany and greater Europe. Hahnemann quickly speculated the remedies which should prove specific for it, in each of its stages and printed information which he forwarded to homeopaths all over the country for its treatment and prophylaxis. He completed this legwork before he had even seen or treated a single case. He simply read carefully about all of its symptoms. His treatment for cholera was *Camphor* in the first stage, *Cuprum* in the second stage, then *Bryonia* and *Rhus tox* alternating as the symptoms moved from one to the other. The contemporary Australian homeopath and academic Dr Isaac Golden reminds us that Hahnemann was an absolute advocate of prophylaxis. And wrote as early as 1801,

... a medicine which causes symptoms so similar to those of the invasion of scarlet fever, as belladonna does, must be one of the best preventative remedies for this children's pestilence. It should however be put to the test with candour, carefulness and impartiality – not cursorily or hurriedly, not with the design of deprecating the originator of it at the expense of truth.

But if its efficacious prophylactic power has incurred or may still incur opposition from prejudiced, ill-disposed, weak minded and cursory observers, I may be allowed to appeal against their conduct to the more matured investigation of the clear sighted, dispassionate portion of the public, and to trust to time for a just verdict. I should esteem myself happy if I should see, some years hence, this scourge of mankind in any measure diminished by my labours" (Hahnemann 1801).

And then comes one of the more delightful episodes in the entire history of homeopathy, the Hollywood ending of Hahnemann and his second wife. In 1834, Melanie d'Hervilly, a Frenchwoman came to Cöthen for treatment and to study homeopathy. She clearly captivated Hahnemann, now 80. Rumour has it that she did not leave the house until three days after she entered for her consultation, and they soon married to much consternation. With significant opposition and suspicion from his colleagues and friends, they soon left for Paris where she obtained authorization for him to practice. There was a lot of criticism of the marriage. Accusations of gold digging followed her throughout her life with Hahnemann in the historical record.

We see an extraordinary change in Hahnemann at this time from the hermetic, academic, unsocial life of study, contemplation and seclusion of domestic retirement in Cöthen, to Paris where he entertained, frequented the Opera, and saw patients not only in his home, but also at their own houses. His work was still prolific. He published a 2nd edition of *Chronic Diseases* and prepared (but did not publish) his 6th edition of the *Organon* before his death. He also set up a free clinic for the poor. Hahnemann wrote few letters during this period though he had been a prolific writer. Haehl questions whether he received all of his mail, suggesting that Melanie may have intercepted it.

Hahnemann in Paris

It is worth reflecting on Hahnemann in Paris. Napoleon was fresh in the memory. But life in Paris was a long way from the hardship and constant moving of living in Germany. Initially they took an apartment on the left bank at 26 Rue des Saints Pères, south of the Seine opposite the Ecole des Beaux Arts. Some weeks later, they moved to 7 Rue de Madame, further south and on the western side of the Luxembourg Gardens, a great place for a walk and a pipe. In a letter in January 1836 to his German friends, he describes this house as '...free from noisy streets, our large windows overlook a pretty garden... with backdoor opening into the Park of Luxembourg...a large garden with trees, which is an hour's walk in extent.' (Haehl 1922). In 1837, Hahnemann and Melanie moved house again, this time to 1 Rue de Milan in the 9th arondissment. This is a short east-west street joining the Rue de Clichy with the Rue d'Amsterdam, very close to the Gare St Lazare and to the north and west of central Paris. Number 1 is at the eastern or Rue de Clichy end of the street. Not so much today, but back then it was a very noisy and bustling area with fewer trees and less fresh air than they had enjoyed at their former residence. It was at this house that he stayed until his death. It was also to here that the many students, doctors and famous and celebrated visitors came to seek him out for tuition, treatment and advice, such as Paganini (who he only treated once because Paganini hit on Melanie). Hahnemann was utterly enamoured with Melanie. In a letter (Haehl 1922) to Hering he wrote,

> I am now in Paris where I shall probably settle. My second incomparable wife, Marie Melanie d'Hervilly, who is a model of scientific and artistic acheivments and industry, and who is endowed with a noble heart and clear intelligence, loves me immeasurably, and makes a heaven of earth. In her youth she was very much esteemed and valued by the intellectual society here, we were married at Cothen on January 18th 1835 and have been living in Paris since 25th June 1835. She has already acquired much skill in our divine science of healing, through her diligence and has already achieved many brilliant cures in chronic diseases among poor patients. All this has made me ten years younger and never during the last forty years have I enjoyed such uninterrupted good health as since re-marrying. My Melanie senses all my wishes and requirements without awaiting a hint from me...she is an angel in human form.

Furthermore, it was also here that the main founders of English homeopathy in the 1830's Quin, Everest, Leaf and Paul Curie came. Hahnemann clearly enjoyed his time in Paris, being as fluent in French as he was in Italian, English and Spanish. He was celebrated in the most fashionable European city of the day.

Hahnemann died on 2 July 1843 of bronchial catarrh to which he had been prone. Controversially, Melanie kept his body there before burial until the 11 July. He was buried in Montmartre cemetery to the north of Paris in grave number 8, (and in 1878 Melanie was buried in grave 9). It is said that in driving rain, and with virtually no one there, Hahnemann was buried as Melanie had not informed anyone of his death.

At the insistence of international homeopaths, in 1898 it was agreed that his grave should be opened so that his remains could be identified and then moved to the more prestigious Père Lachaise cemetery in the east of Paris. On May 24 1898, the two graves were opened and the remains identified from a large lock of Melanie's hair around his neck and from his engraved wedding ring. Hahnemann was moved across the city to his grander and more appropriate tomb.

Like all people he changed over time. We simply do not know the degree to which he distanced himself from his early writings. All we do know is that in his unpublished 6th edition of the *Organon* which finally saw the light of day in 1921, he describes it as 'the most perfect method'. I have not talked about the changes in the 6th edition from the 5th in this work because they are covered in *Case Management*, Vol 3 of this series. For specific details on Hahnemann's life and where he lived, go no further than the *Faces of Homoeopathy* (Winston 1999).

His Cases / How He Practiced

While we cannot be sure, (we were not there), some significant remnants survive the ages and give us clues about how Hahnemann practiced on a daily basis. We know, for example, that when he lived in Paris (Winston 1999), his wife Melanie took the notes while he took the case, often not even bothering to look at the patient while he smoked a pipe. In addition, Handley's excellent books on Hahnemann (1997) and Melanie (1990) deserve thorough reading.

Cases Illustrative of Homeopathic Practice

Many persons of my acquaintance but half converted to homoeopathy have begged of me from time to time to publish still more exact directions as to how this doctrine may be actually applied in practice, and how we are to proceed. I am astonished that after the very peculiar directions contained in the *Organon of Medicine* more special instruction can be wished for. I am also asked, "How are we to examine the disease in every particular case?" As if special enough directions were not to be found in the book just mentioned.

As in homoeopathy the treatment is not directed towards any supposed or illusory internal causes of disease, nor yet towards any names of diseases invented by man which do not exist in nature, and as every case of non-miasmatic disease is a distinct individuality, independent, peculiar, differing in nature from all others, never compounded of a hypothetical arrangement of symptoms, so no particular directions can be laid down for them except that the physician, in order to effect a cure, must oppose to every aggregate of morbid symptoms in a case a group of similar medicinal symptoms as exact as it is to be met with in any single known medicine, for this doctrine cannot admit of more than a single medicinal substance (whose effects have been accurately tested) to be given at once (see *Organon of Medicine*, § 271, 272).

Now we can neither enumerate all the possible aggregates of symptoms of all concrete cases of disease, nor indicate a priori the homoeopathic medicines for these (a priori undefinable) possibilities. For every individual given case (and every case is an individuality, differing from all others) the homoeopathic medical practitioner must himself find them, and for this end he must be acquainted with the medicines that have till now been investigated in respect of their positive action, or consult them for every case of disease; but besides this he must do his endeavour to prove on himself or on other healthy individuals medicines that have not yet been investigated as regards the morbid alterations they are capable of producing, in order thereby to increase our store of known remedial agents, so that the choice of a remedy for every one of the infinite variety of cases of disease (for the combatting of which we can never possess enough of suitable tools and weapons) may become all the more easy and accurate.

That man is far from being animated with the true spirit of the homoeopathic system, is no true disciple of this beneficent doctrine, who makes the slightest objections to institute on himself careful experiments for the investigation of the peculiar effects of the medicines which have remained unknown for 2500 years, without which investigation (and unless their pure pathogenetic action on the healthy individual has previously been ascertained) all treatment of disease must continue to be not only a foolish, but even a criminal operation, a dangerous attack upon human life.

It is somewhat too much to expect us to work merely for the benefit of such self-interested individuals as will contribute nothing to the complete and indispensable building up of the indispensable edifice, who only seek to make money by what has been discovered and investigated by the labours of others, and to furnish themselves with the means of squandering the income derived from the capital of science, to the accumulation of which they do not evince the slightest inclination to contribute.

All who feel a true desire to assist in elucidating the peculiar effects of medicines-our sole instruments, the knowledge of which has for so many centuries remained uninvestigated, and which is yet so indispensable for enabling us to cure the sick, will find the directions how these pure experiments with medicines should be conducted in the *Organon of Medicine*,

In addition to what has been there stated I shall only add, that as the experimenter cannot, any more than any other human being, be absolutely and perfectly healthy, he must, should slight ailments to which he was liable appear during these provings of the powers of medicines, place these between brackets, thereby indicating that they are not confirmed, or dubious. But this will not often happen, seeing that during the action upon a previously healthy person of a sufficiently strong dose of the medicine, he is under the influence of the medicine alone, and it is seldom that any other symptom can shew itself during the first days but what must be the effect of the medicine. Further, that in order to investigate the symptoms of medicines for chronic diseases, for example, in order to develop the cutaneous diseases, abnormal growths and so forth, to be expected from the medicine, we must not be contented with taking one or two doses of it only, but we must continue its use for several days, to the amount of two adequate doses daily, that is to say, of sufficient size to cause us to perceive its action, whilst at the same time we continue to observe the diet and regimen indicated in the work alluded to.

The mode of preparing the medicinal substances for use in homoeopathic treatment will be found in the Organon of medicine, § 267-271, and also in the Chronic diseases. I would only observe here, that for the proving of medicines on healthy individuals, dilutions and dynamizations are to be employed as high as are used for the treatment of disease, namely, globules moistened with the decillionth development of power. The request of some friends, halting half-way on the road to this method of treatment, to detail some examples of this treatment, is difficult to comply with, and no great advantage can attend a compliance with it. Every cured case of disease shews only how that case has been treated. The internal process of the treatment depends always on those principles which are already known, and they cannot be rendered concrete and definitely fixed for each individual case, nor can they become at all more distinct from the history of a single cure than they previously were when these principles were enunciated. Every case of non-miasmatic disease is peculiar and special, and it is the special in it that distinguishes it from every other case, that pertains to it alone, but that cannot serve as a guide to the treatment of other cases. Now if it is wished to describe a complicated case of disease consisting of many symptoms, in such a pragmatical manner that the reasons that influence us in the choice of the remedy shall be clearly revealed, this demands details laborious at once for the recorder and for the reader.

In order, however, to comply with the desires of my friends in this also, I may here detail two of the slightest cases of homoeopathic treatment.

Pain: Bryonia alba Case:

Sch-, a washerwoman, somewhat above 40 years old, had been more than three weeks unable to pursue her avocations, when she consulted me on the 1st September, 1815. 1. On any movement, especially at every step, and worst on making a false step, she has a shoot in the scrobiculus cordis, that comes, as she avers, every time from the left side. 2. When she lies she feels quite well, then she has no pain anywhere, neither in the side nor in the scrobiculus. 3. She cannot sleep after three o'clock in the morning. 4. She relishes her food, but when she has ate a little she feels sick. 5. Then the water collects in her mouth and runs out of it, like the water-brash. 6. She has frequently empty eructations after every meal. 7. Her temper is passionate, disposed to anger. 8. Whenever the pain is severe she is covered with perspiration. 9. The catamenia were quite regular a fortnight since. In other respects her health is good.

Now, as regards Symptom 1, belladonna, china, and rhus toxicodendron cause shootings in the scrobiculus, but none of them only on motion, as is the case here. Pulsatilla (see Symp. 387) certainly causes shootings in the scrobiculus on making a false step, but only as a rare alternating action, and has neither the same digestive derangements as occur here at 4 compared with 5 and 6, nor the same state of the disposition. Bryonia alone has among its chief alternating actions, as the whole list of its symptoms demonstrates, pains from movement and especially shooting pains, as also stitches beneath the sternum (in the scrobiculus) on raising the arm (448), and on making a false step it occasions shooting in other parts (520, 574). The negative symptom 2 met with here answers especially to bryonia (558?); few medicines (with the exception, perhaps, of nux vomica and rhus toxicodendron in their alternating action-neither of which, however, are suitable for the other symptoms) shew a complete relief to pains during rest and when lying; bryonia does, however, in an especial manner (558, and many other bryonia-symptoms). Symptom 3 is met with in several medicines, and also in bryonia (694). Symptom 4 is certainly, as far as regards "sickness after eating," met with in several other medicines (ignatia, nux vomica, mercurius, ferrum, belladonna, pulsatilla, cantharis), but neither so constantly and usually, nor with relish for food, as in bryonia (279). As regards Symptom 5 several medicines certainly cause a flow of saliva like water-brash, just as well as bryonia (282); the others, however, do not produce the remaining symptoms in a very similar manner. Hence bryonia is to be preferred to them in this point. Empty eructation (of wind only) after eating (Symptom 6) is found in few medicines, and in none so constantly, so usually, and to such a great degree, as in bryonia (255, 239). To 7. One of the chief symptoms in diseases (see Organon of Medicine, § 213) is the "state of the disposition," and as bryonia (778) causes this symptom also in an exactly similar manner bryonia is for all these reasons to be preferred in this case to all other medicines as the homoeopathic remedy. Now, as this woman was very robust, and the force of the disease must accordingly have been very considerable, to prevent her by its pain from doing any work, and as her vital forces, as has been observed, were not consensually affected, I gave her one of the strongest homoeopathic doses, a full drop of the pure juice of bryonia root, 1 to be taken immediately, and bade her come to me again in 48 hours. I told my friend E., who was present, that within that time the woman would be quite cured, but he, being but half a convert to homoeopathy, expressed his doubts about it. Two days afterwards he came again to ascertain the result, but the woman did not return then, and, in fact, never came back again. I could only allay the impatience of my friend by telling him her name and that of the village where she lived, about three miles off, and advising him to seek her out and ascertain for himself how she was. This he did, and her answer was: "What was the use of my going back? The very next day I was quite well, and could again commence my washing, and the day following I was as well as I am still. I am extremely obliged to the doctor, but the like of us have no time to leave off our work; and for three weeks previously my illness prevented me earning anything."

Vertigo, vomiting: Pulsatilla pratensis Case:

W-e, a weakly, pale man of 42 years, who was constantly kept by his business at his desk, came to me on the 27th December, 1815, having been already ill five days. 1. The first evening he became, without manifest cause, sick and giddy, with much eructation. 2. The following night (about 2 a. m.) sour vomiting. 3. The subsequent nights severe eructation. 4. To-day also sick eructation of fetid and sourish taste. 5. He felt as if the food lay crude and undigested in his stomach. 6. In his head he felt vacant, hollow and confused, and as if sensitive therein. 7. The least noise was painful to him. 8. He is of a mild, soft, patient disposition. Here I may observe:-

To 1. That several medicines cause vertigo with nausea, as well as pulsatilla (3), which produces its vertigo in the evening also (7), a circumstance that has been observed from very few others. To 2. Stramonium and nux vomica cause vomiting of sour and sour-smelling mucus, but, as far as is known, not at night. Valerian and cocculus cause vomiting at night, but not of sour stuff. Iron alone causes vomiting at night (61, 62), and can also, cause sour vomiting (66), but not the other symptoms observed here. Pulsatilla, however, causes not only sour vomiting in the evening (349, 356) and nocturnal vomiting in general, but also the other symptoms of this case not found among those of iron. To 3. Nocturnal eructations is peculiar to pulsatilla (296, 297). To 4. Feted, putrid (249) and sour eructations (301, 302) are peculiar to pulsatilla. To 5. The sensation of indigestion of the food in the stomach is produced by few medicines, and by none in such a perfect and striking manner as by pulsatilla (321, 322, 327). To 6. With the exception of ignatia (2) which, however, cannot produce the other ailments, the same state is only produced by pulsatilla (39 compared with 40, 81). To 7. Pulsatilla produces the same state (995), and it also causes over-sensitiveness of other organs of the senses, for example, of the sight (107). And although intolerance of noise is also met with in nux vomica, ignatia, and aconite, yet these medicines are not homoeopathic to the other symptoms and still less do they possess symptom 8, the mild character of the disposition, which, as stated in the preface to pulsatilla, is particularly indicative of this plant. This patient, therefore, could not be cured by anything in a more easy, certain and permanent manner than by pulsatilla, which was accordingly given to him immediately, but on account of his weakly and delicate state only in a very minute dose, i.e., half-a-drop of the quadrillionth of a strong drop of pulsatilla. This was done in the evening. The next day he was free from all ailments, his digestion was restored, and a week thereafter, as I was told by him, he remained free from complaint and quite well. The investigation in such a slight case of disease, and the choice of the homoeopathic remedy for it, is very speedily effected by the practitioner who has had only a little experience in it, and who either has the symptoms of the medicine in his memory, or who knows where to find them readily; but to give in writing all the reasons pro and con (which would be perceived by the mind in a few seconds) gives rise, as we see, to tedious prolixity. For the convenience of treatment, we require merely to indicate for each symptom all the medicines which can produce the same symptoms by a few letters (e.g., Ferr., Chin., Rheum, Puls.), and also to bear in mind the circumstances under which they occur, that have a determining influence on our choice and in the same way with all the other symptoms, by what medicine each is excited, and from the list so prepared we shall be able to perceive which of the medicines homoeopathically covers the most of the symptoms present, especially the most peculiar and characteristic ones,-and this is the remedy sought for.

Some other cases

Insanity:

Belladonna Case: Julie M. a country girl; 14 years old; not yet menstruated. 12th September, 1842. A month previously she had slept in the sun. Four days after this sleeping in the sun, the frightful idea took possession of her that she saw a wolf, and six days thereafter she felt as if she had received a great blow on the head. She now spoke irrationally; became as if mad; wept much; had sometimes difficulty in breathing; spat white mucus; could not tell any of her sensations. She got Belladonna, 2 weakened dynamization, in seven tablespoonfuls of water; of this, after it was shaken, a tablespoonful in a glass of water, and after stirring this, one teaspoonful to be taken in the morning. 16th.-Somewhat quieter; she can blow her nose, which she was unable to do during her madness; she still talks as much nonsense, but does not make so many grimaces while talking. She wept much last night. Good motion. Tolerable sleep. She is still very restless, but was more so before the Belladonna. The white of the eye full of red vessels. She seems to have a pain in the nape of the neck. From the glass in which one tablespoonful was stirred, one teaspoonful is to be taken and stirred in a second glassful of water, and of this from two to four teaspoonfuls (increasing the dose daily by one teaspoonful) are to be taken in the morning. 20th. Much better;

speaks more rationally; works a little; recognises and names me; and wishes to kiss a lady present. She now begins to shew her amorous propensities; is easily put in a passion, and takes things in bad part; sleeps well; weeps very often; becomes angry about a trifle; eats more than usual; when she comes to her senses she likes to play, but only just as a little child would.

Belladonna, a globule of a higher potency: seven tablespoonfuls shaken in two glasses, 6 teaspoonfuls from the second glass early in the morning. 1 28th. On the 22d, 23d and 24, very much excited day and night; great lasciviousness in her actions and words; she pulls up her clothes and seeks to touch the genitals of others; she readily gets into a rage and beats every one. Hyoscyamus X , seven tablespoonfuls, andc., one tablespoonful in one tumblerful of water; in the morning a teaspoonful. 5th October. For five days she would eat nothing; complains of belly-ache; for the last few days less malicious and less lascivious; stools rather loose; itching all over the body, especially on her genitals; sleep, good. Sacch. Lactis for seven days, in seven tablespoonfuls, andc. 10th. On the 7th, fit of excessive anger; she sought to strike every one. The next day, the 8th, attack of fright and fear, almost like the commencement of her illness (fear of an imaginary wolf;) fear lest she should be burnt. Since then she has become quiet, and talks rationally and nothing indecent for the last two days. Sacch. Lactis, andc. 14th.-Quite good and sensible. 18th. The same, but severe headache; inclination to sleep by day; not so cheerful. New sulphur (new dynamization of the smallest material portion) one globule in three tumblers; in the morning one teaspoonful. 22d.-Very well; very little headache. Sulphur, the next dynamization in two tumblers. She went on with the sulphur occasionally until November, at which time she was and still remains a healthy, rational, amiable girl.

Hemorrhoids, sore throat:

Mercurius solubilis Case: O-t, an actor, 33 years old, married. 14th January, 1843. For several years he had been frequently subject to sore throat, as also now for a month past. The previous sore throat had lasted six weeks. On swallowing his saliva, a pricking sensation; feeling of contraction and excoriation. When he has not the sore throat he suffers from a pressure in the anus, with violent excoriative pains; the anus is then inflamed, swollen and constricted; it is only with a great effort that he can then pass his faeces, when the swollen haemorrhoidal vessels protude.

On the 15th January, he took, in the morning before breakfast a teaspoonful of a solution of one globule of belladonna X then the lowest dynamization, dissolved in seven tablespoonfuls of water, of which a tablespoonful was well stirred up in a tumblerful of water.15th.-In the evening aggravation of the sore throat. 16th.- Sore throat gone, but the affection of the anus returned as above described; an open fissure with excoriative pain, inflammation, swelling, throbbing pain and constriction; also in the evening a painful motion.

He confessed having had a chancre eight years previously, which had been, as usual, destroyed by caustics, after which all the above affections had appeared. 18th.-Merc. viv. one globule of the lowest new dynamization I, (which contains a vastly smaller amount of matter than the usual kind), prepared in the same manner, and to be taken in the same way as the belladonna (the bottle being shaken each time), one spoonful in a tumberful of water well stirred. 20th. Almost no sore throat. Anus better, but he still feels there excoriation pain after a motion; he has however no more throbbing, no more swelling of the anus, and no inflammation; anus less contracted. One globule of merc. viv.

(2|0) the second dynamization of the same kind; prepared in the same way, and taken in the morning. 25th.-Throat almost quite well; but in the anus, raw pain and severe shootings; great pain in the anus after a motion; still some contraction of it and heat. 30th.- In the afternoon, the last dose (one teaspoonful). On the 28th the anus was better; sore throat returned; pretty severe excoriation pain in the throat. One globule in milk-sugar for seven days; prepared and taken in the same manner. 7th February.-Severe ulcerative pain in the throat. Bellyache, but good stools; several in succession, with great thirst In the anus all is right. Sulphur 2|0 in seven tablespoonfuls, as above. 13th.-Had ulcerative pain in the throat, especially on swallowing his saliva, of which he has now a large quantity, especially copious on the 11th and 12th. Severe contraction of the anus, especially since yesterday. He now smelt here merc., and got to take as before merc. v. 2|0, one globule in seven tablespoonfuls of water, and half a spoonful of brandy. 20th.-Throat better since the 18th; he has suffered much with the anus; the motion causes pain when it is passing; less thirst. Milk-sugar in seven tablespoonfuls. 3d March.-No more sore throat. On going to stool a bloodless haemorrhoidal knot comes down (formerly this was accompanied with burning and raw pain), now with merely itching on the spot. To smell acid. nitri. and then to have milk-sugar in serve. Almost no more pain after a motion; yesterday some blood along with the motion (an old symptom). Throat well; only a little sensitive when drinking cold water. Olfaction of acid. nitri. (olfaction is performed by opening small bottle containing an ounce of alcohol or brandy where one globule is dissolved, and smelt for an instant or two. He remained permanently cured. (Hahnemann 1843).

Underpinnings of Hahnemannian Homeopathy

Much is revealed in these cases and casebooks. There are no hour-long consultations, no in-depth analysis of the psyche. These sound like 20-minute consultations, half an hour at most. What we see in Hahnemann's casework is a simplicity that is so easy to replicate and teach. By emphasising the components of the case and searching for a complete symptom, Hahnemann's homeopathy is characterised by sensation, location, modalities, concomitants, cause, as well as the name of the complaint or condition. As argued in *Case Taking* (Gray 2010), the simplicity of this method married to searching for simple and easily identified aspects of the case, the totality of symptoms, strange rare and peculiar symptoms, constitutes effective and achievable health management in virtually every patient.

Peculiarity

Peculiarity was strongly emphasised and demonstrated in these examples. He focused on looking at the individual, strange, rare and peculiar symptoms of the patient's condition or disease. This point is worth emphasising. It was a symptom such as 'burning pain better for hot water,' that was a strange, rare and peculiar symptom in Hahnemann's context. In addition, the modalities in this regard were clearly important, as were the concomitant symptoms. Some have misinterpreted peculiarity to mean he was asking about strange aspects of the person, which is a liberal interpretation. From this perspective, symptoms only become strange or rare or peculiar in the context of the individual. Homeopaths looking at the same case may see something that the patient says as peculiar when another homeopath will not because of their different life experiences or opinions. Strangeness, rare-ness and peculiarness are clearly subjective. Singing in the street would be strange if the patient were a bank manager, but common if the patient were drunk (Watson 1991). In chronic diseases, the strange symptoms often go undetected, unnoticed because of the innumerable ways in which the patient has normalized their health.

Totality

This is where it gets interesting because examining the *Organon* in detail demonstrates that Hahnemann was far from precise when defining *Totality*. Take for example aphorism 6, in which Hahnemann clearly says that the job of the homeopath is to seek the totality of the characteristic symptoms from when the patient was last healthy. Left undefined is what he meant by 'characteristic' and what he meant by 'healthy'. As alluded to previously, totality has different interpretations in homeopathic medicine, and it is these fundamental points that distinguish the different methods. The concept of totality of symptoms is so useful in homeopathy and so annoying all at once. The idea itself will be explored in a subsequent volume in the series, but it must be pointed out at the outset, it is the skilled understanding of the totality of symptoms in the case that essentially determines the appropriate method to use in curing the case. Homeopaths prescribe different remedies to the same patient because they identify a different totality of symptoms

Causation

What is also revealed in these case-books is that the cause was usually of some physical origin, nothing deeply psychological as suggested by some. The exciting cause could be something as mundane as a fall, an injury, winter, or working in cold conditions.

Health

Hahnemann's case-books also reveal a degree of a mixed message. We have on the one hand the pragmatism of his case-books, his precise, practical and effective acute and chronic case work. But we can also see how this differs from the philosophy, dogmatism, inspiration and aspiration of the *Organon of Medicine*. We must explore these discrepancies in some depth because they create considerable confusion in homeopaths and homeopathic students.

It is in aphorisms 9, 10 and 11 Hahnemann gives us some glimpses into his perspectives and understanding on health and disease. It is here that Hahnemann clearly states that the healthy person has a free flow of energy in, through and around them. He is clear in his opinion, the dynamis rules with unbounded sway. This vital force, dynamis, the vital principle, animates the body and keeps the structure, the skin bag of the body in good order. This good order allows the wearer of the body to use it for our highest purposes.

Aphorism §9

In the healthy condition of man, the spiritual vital force (autocracy), the dynamis that animates the material body (organism), rules with unbounded sway, and retains all the parts of the organism in admirable, harmonious, vital operation, as regards both sensations and functions, so that our indwelling, reason-gifted mind can freely employ this living, healthy instrument for the higher purposes of our existence.

A quick discussion cannot do this aphorism justice. In the *Dynamis* postgraduate course in homeopathy, Jeremy Sherr spends two or three years essentially examining this one issue. Just what is the healthy person? A couple of generations of homeopaths have been inspired by this broadest possible definition of health, and from this perspective it is easy to see that some homeopaths are happy to work with their patients above and beyond their presenting symptoms or physical ailments. If *Health* constitutes that a person is in great physical and vital operation, as well as also living one's life purpose and the life dream, then it is easy to see how a practitioner could work with many clients for a considerable amount of time. The fingernail biting gets cured, the anxiety gets better, the exploration of early mother issues is improved, dealing with the boss of the insurance company takes another block of time before getting on to the issues of why we are here and what is our purpose in life. Such an elegant philosophy of health and ultimately disease that is articulated by Hahnemann fits well in the 21st century. But this reveals a strange paradox for us. This is not what he did in his own practice. There was a sore knee. He gave *Bryonia* and the knee and the patient was 'cured'. A migraine got better, the person's arthritis was cured. Without doubt, he engaged with clients in the treatment of their chronic diseases that lasted for a number of years. This idea that Hahnemann was the founder of some new-age movement is projected on Hahnemann by many contemporary homeopaths, and is clearly not accurate. To idealise and project on to the past is incorrect at best, and hubris at worst. He was a doctor who found a better and gentler way of curing patients, symptoms, and diseases than was available at the time.

Disease

Aphorism §15

The affection of the morbidly deranged, spirit-like dynamis (vital force) that animates our body in the invisible interior, and the totality of the outwardly cognizable symptoms produced by it in the organism and representing the existing malady, constitute a whole; they are one and the same. The organism is indeed the material instrument of the life, but it is not conceivable without the animation imparted to it by the instinctively perceiving and regulating dynamis, just as the vital force is not conceivable without the organism, consequently the two together constitute a unity, although in thought our mind separates this unity into two distinct conceptions for the sake of easy comprehension.

Hahnemann argued that disease is interior and invisible, and as a consequence we have to rely on the outward signs of the internal imbalance in order to know the disease. These external signs of the internal imbalance tell the physician which medicine is required. For Hahnemann, disease was a disturbance of the vital force interior and invisible, which can only be known through these externalised symptoms. Symptoms were thus the externalised language of disease.

Cure

Very often in teaching homeopathic students and demonstrating a case, perhaps on paper or by video or DVD, there is an inevitable question. 'So what happened'? 'How did the patient do'? A patient may well have presented with asthma that was the reason for coming. However in the course of case taking, the patient may well have talked about the relationship issues, what's going on with boyfriends, mothers, stresses at work, and the amount of coffee drunk every hour.

Students for some reason are often not satisfied with the answer. The problem the patient had, the asthma 'got better' But what about the boyfriend? 'Were the issues with the mother resolved'? These are inevitable questions, and very often a wave of disappointment spreads across the face of the student when you say, 'well I have no idea about the mother or the boyfriend, and I don't know if they still drink coffee because after two sessions of homeopathy the asthma was gone and they no longer returned.' Such disappointment or unrealistic expectations about what is cure, reflects a different interpretation of what cure actually is.

But for Hahnemann cure was both an event and a process. In aphorisms 1, 2, 3 9, 10 and 11, he gives immense clarity on his overall understanding of cure. Cure was a process, gentle rapid and permanent removal and annihilation of the disease. What we are left with then is both the pragmatism of his case books, the do-it-yourself manual articulated by the *Organon of Medicine*, and the inspiration he provides in those initial aphorisms.

von Bönninghausen 1785-1864

To discuss the application of Hahnemann's homeopathy,

it is useful to get familiar with one of its clearest and best practitioners. Clemens Maria von Bönninghausen was born in the Dutch province of Oberyssel, and he became a doctor in criminal and civil law. In addition, this was somehow married to a love of botany and agricultural methods, which over time brought him into contact with several botanists who also coincidentally shared a homeopathic interest. It was in 1827 when he contracted tuberculosis and received *Pulsatilla* that he was converted to homeopathy at the age of 43. He began studying and writing immediately, and many of his works were written in the first couple of years after his introduction to homeopathy.

Little distinguishes Bönninghausen's and Hahnemann's homeopathy. However in many instances Bönninghausen describes and articulates the process even better. He focused on the disease and the totality of symptoms of the diseased person.

Complete Symptom

Central to the method is determining a complete symptom in precisely defined complaints. It is often forgotten that in the thinking of Bönninghausen, a *symptom* is a finding. A *Complete Symptom* therefore comprises something;

- objective e.g., ulcer
- subjective e.g., sensation (burning pain)
- a location e.g., left leg
- a modification (modality) e.g., feels better with applying heat to the painful part.

In other words, a complete symptom for Bönninghausen consisted of a sufficiently qualified complaint defined by a,

- Complaint (objective/subjective) which was fully qualified by its specific,
- Location and,
- Modalities.

Importantly, the complaint does not necessarily need a pathological label.

To be technically correct, it is important to remember that locations and modalities are not symptoms in themselves, but rather defining components of a symptom which serve to render it complete. Thus they are distinguishing *features* rather than symptoms. As Bönninghausen said:

- What (Complaint/sensation)
- Where (Location)
- How (Modifications)

As a consequence, practitioners are fully justified in creating a genuine and legitimate homeopathic diagnosis. For example, an '*Arsenicum album* ulcer' is the homeopathic diagnosis. A *Sanguinaria* headache is the homeopathic diagnosis because we have identified the complaint, located it and individualised it with a modality (D'Aran 2008).

Other points to consider are:

- Only distinguishing complaints need be considered according to clarity and completeness.
- A case of disease may therefore be individualised through its group of significant complaints in unique combination.

- Once a case is complete, then its corresponding remedy can be identified.
- When the medicine is identified, the homeopathic diagnosis is complete.

If each complaint has no clear relationship or shared modality, then the most disturbing or important complete symptom must be prescribed on. Then as each complaint improves, the next will present itself in its own completeness and so on until all complaints are resolved and homeostasis is regained. This is from Aphorism 209 where Hahnemann talks about multiple conversations being required to cure a case and using multiple remedies.

Aphorism §209

After this is done, the physician should endeavor in repeated conversations with the patient to trace the picture of his disease as completely as possible, according to the directions given above, in order to be able to elucidate the most striking and peculiar (characteristic) symptoms, in accordance with which he selects the first anti-psoric or other remedy having the greatest symptomatic resemblance, for the commencement of the treatment, and so forth (Hahnemann 1922).

The Therapeutic Pocketbook

Bönninghausen published the first repertory, the *Repertory of the Anti-psoric Remedies*, with a preface by Hahnemann in 1832. It sold very quickly, prompting a second edition in 1833 which was retitled, *Systematic Alphabetical Repertory of Homoeopathic Remedies First Part*, again with an introduction by Hahnemann. This was followed later by the *Repertory of Medicines which are not anti-psoric* or *Systematic Alphabetical Repertory of Homoeopathic Remedies Second Part* in 1835. Later still, a *Therapeutic Pocketbook for Homeopathic Physicians* was published providing the critical tool for implementing the method. Out of respect for his work and clinical expertise Hahnemann wrote 'if I should be ill myself unable to help myself I would not entrust myself to any other physician' (Howard 2003).

Cases

This case from my own clinic is still one of my personal favourites and highlights the system and method. I like it because it highlights the differences in method between Kent with the simplicity of Hahnemann/Bönninghausen's approach. I initially tried the Kentian approach unsuccessfully three times in dealing with this case. The presenting symptom was back pain in a male age 23.

>I have a problem in my back, left side, dull uncomfortable pain. It throbs. It can last for 1 day or 2 ½ days. It starts on the left side of my back and works its way round to my abdomen, takes 12 hours-ish to get there. Tender. It's better from bending over and curling up. It weakens me. I throw up from it. Not often, but I have to go to bed. And I need a hot water bottle which makes it better.
>
>First time was in Canada May 95. I was hospitalised. So intense, in the ambulance, I threw up, they discharged me. Told me it was nothing. That was the worst time. There have been a couple of instances since then. Every two months or so I get it. comes on with or without stress. When I am stressed it jumps on me. I stopped meat and it didn't come on for a while. Then it

did. Came on from a bowl of cereal with milk. I am suspicious of milk, had it for the last 2 days.

Dull pain thumping on the left side. Sharp pain on the right side or middle. When I piss during an episode I feel as if it is going to hurt, but there is no pain.

During an episode my pooh is pretty runny. I refuse to go to any GPs or anything, refuse painkillers, aspirin, had it checked out and they could find nothing.

At this stage, I was confused. The man had a back pain but it sounded very much like a kidney stone. Furthermore there are some digestive aspects to the case. I decided to ask him about when it began, the cause.

It was a very very depressing part of my life. I didn't like me. I was escalating downwards. Lots of negativity around this area (points to his groin). I suppressed my emotions for 10 years. You could say, so to speak that I have a base chakra situation. It started when I was running away from my problems and jumping into the fire from the frying pan.

I really pushed on this point to understand what he was talking about. What is a base chakra situation? Eventually he told me that he was confused about his sexual identity, didn't know if he was gay or straight, and it was a terrible problem to him. He'd been unable to speak to his parents about it, or anyone for a decade. The consultation goes on for another hour and a half but essentially that was the story. I definitely got caught up in the story. The post-modern, Jungian half-trained psychotherapist in me was sitting bolt upright.

On evaluation, the affinities, the self-esteem, the shamefulness, the sexuality, plus the symptoms led to a prescription of *Thuja* 30c. It did nothing, and the pain came back some days later. I was stunned because I was so confident in my prescription so I gave him a dose of 200. Still nothing. I gave him *Lachesis* 200. I was disappointed when again there was absolutely no response to the remedy. He was getting very impatient with me after two or three weeks of this and that prescribing and no result. There was no doubt that the case comprised confusion and his suppression of sexuality, trying to hide the shameful part of himself. I had convinced myself that the central focus of this case was his suppressed homosexuality. This had to be at the centre of the case. Clearly it was the cause of all of his problems – creating this 'base chakra situation'. In addition to that, and what confirmed those prescriptions for me was that he was withholding and secretive in his delivery of the symptoms, often hiding them in practiced psychobabble.

Eventually and thankfully I changed my approach. I grilled him about the exact symptoms but essentially got nothing new. I had a clear location, and sensations. Subjective and objective. Pain in the area of the left kidney going to the abdomen and the bladder. When he has the pain, he feels as if he will urinate blood, bends him over, every 2 months. Sharp pain extending. Next there is a clear modality. The one thing I was startled to hear him say was that he was only 23 years old. I was convinced he was a decade older than that as his face was quite worn. I used the *Therapeutic Pocketbook*:

1. What was his complaint? Pain, sharp and extending
2. What was the location? Left side of the back
3. What were the modalities? Better for curling, bending,

4. The concomitant, he looked much older than he was, which I interpreted as old age premature.

Applying this simple formula to an overwhelming case full of complex psycho-dynamics led to a prescription of *Berberis*. In fact, reworking this case highlighted to me that in a case with 35 clear physical symptoms, 33 of which were in the remedy *Berberis*, no other remedy came close. *Lycopodium* was a distant second. I gave *Berberis* in a 200th potency.

What happened subsequently was a good lesson for me also. I didn't see him again, and at the time I put the experience down to poor homeopathy, bad prescribing, and a multitude of other self-deprecating conclusions. About 18 months later, I was walking back to the clinic from lunch and I saw him on the other side of the road, and he saw me. He came across the road and I berated him, 'you never showed up for your last appointment.' He looked at me quizzically and said, as I've now heard 100 times since then, 'why would I bother to spend $100 to come and tell you that I don't have any pain.' In other words because of his absence I'd assumed failure. He told me that he never had a subsequent episode. Further similar cases can be read in Watson (1991 pages 64-66).

Disadvantages of the Method

There are limitations and criticisms of the method. Certainly there are some issues in using it, but from a pragmatic and practical perspective, they are not overwhelming. This system becomes more complex when:

1. The mental state or symptoms dominate and there is little to characterise them. Becoming familiar with the

different way Bönninghausen structures his repertory and places his mind symptoms is the key to overcoming this issue. Mostly they are used as concomitants to the main complaint. This style of prescribing is perfect where there are mental symptoms in the case, or if the mental state in the case is vague, unclear and cloudy but when there are other clear characteristics. In such a case, there is actually no need to go there, there is no need to speculate about the mind, the mentals, the mental state. Where cases are one sided, incomplete or confused, this technique is brilliant and achieves meaningful results.

2. Proving symptoms are fragmented. This is an interesting point. Bönninghausen broke down and deconstructed proving symptoms differently than Kent. When you understand these differences, the limitations are not insurmountable.
3. Over-generalisation with loss of individuality when characteristics are not carefully obtained. The method is, like all homeopathy, harder with few characterising symptoms representing the disease.
4. There are only 120 or so remedies, the ones that were known and understood well in 1846, there is no *Lachesis, Medorrhinum* or other clinical necessities.

There is a variation in the method as advocated by Boger. His concept of totality, and hence his *Synoptic Key* (1915), was based on perceiving the *pathogenesis of symptoms over time* as the *genius* of the remedy, as well as the patient's disease. Pathogenesis means the pathological changes that occur as disease progresses, in changing signs and symptoms. Boger gave very clear instructions on the areas that were needed for a pathogenetic totality. His *Synoptic Key* describes the genius of remedies in a similar format.

A. Modalities
B. Mental state
C. Sensations
D. Objective Observations
E. Location

It has to be said that many homeopaths have criticised Boger's interpretations and tinkering with Bönninghausen's work. Not only did he add more remedies, he also altered the underlying structure and pedagogy of Bönninghausen's method. The attempts at 'improving' upon it have usually meant that the book loses its integrity, and the accuracy and the work of Boger and others cannot completely be relied on (Dimitriadis 2007). Further limitations have been reported in that the method requires:

1. medical or paramedical training
2. in depth understanding of miasms.

Again these perceived limitations are hardly overwhelming.

Advantages of the Method

Limitations acknowledged, there are strong clinical advantages. Bönninghausen's method follows inductive logic, and is very reliable. In skilled hands, and with the right tools, this method very often results in an effective remedy selection within 15 minutes in skilled hands and with the right tools. In addition, the Concordances help in prescribing the next related remedy for cure.

In Watson's (1991) chapter on Physical Generals he talked about Bönninghausen and drawing attention to the importance of the general symptoms over particulars in the construction of his *Therapeutic Pocketbook* to reflect this approach. He writes that one of the clear advantages of this method is that it relies far less on any psychological and speculative interpretation on behalf of the practitioner to arrive at an indicated remedy. Because homeopaths are not trained in counselling or psychoanalysis, it makes perfect sense to rely on the body and symptoms as the language of the body to indicate the remedy as opposed to any guesswork. So often the physical body guides the practitioner to the medicine. As Watson alludes to, this is one of the beauties of homeopathy there is no need to be dogmatically stuck to one route when the patient is telling you blatantly that another more reliable path is available to you (Watson 1991).

Another clear advantage of this method is that the remedies which are less fully developed in the context of materia medica simply come out of any well-worked repertorisation. Smaller remedies come to the fore and beg to be prescribed. Focusing on the modalities, the sensations, the locations, the causations, and understanding the nature of the complaint and exploring those in a clear way also encourages the patient to be confident in your skills. All these aspects of the case are equally important and when characteristic they are explored and equally emphasised. Later, the food cravings, menstruation, sexual desire and function are particularly important to explore, ask about, and any other characteristic information should be delved into. The method advocated by Hahnemann and Bönninghausen, (remember a lawyer by profession and skilled in botanical taxonomy) is so easily replicable. Every symptom is a manifestation of the disorder of the diseased person, and each symptom comes from the same source, and therefore leads back to that source.

Method in Epidemic Diseases

There is a variation that is important when it comes to treating epidemic diseases. Epidemics in the Hahnemannian context are different from both individual acute diseases, manifesting in just one person, and sporadic diseases affecting a few people in one population. Epidemics need to be approached in a different way. Genus Epidemicus instructions from Hahnemann suggests that during a true epidemic of acute disease a majority of cases will respond to the same medicine, provided the medicine is similar to the characteristic symptoms of the epidemic.

§101

It may easily happen that in the first case of an epidemic disease that presents itself to the physician's notice he does not at once obtain a knowledge of its complete picture, as it is only by a close observation of several cases of every such collective disease that he can become conversant with the totality of its signs and symptoms. The carefully observing physician can, however, from the examination of even the first and second patients, often arrive so nearly at a knowledge of the true state as to have in his mind a characteristic portrait of it, and even to succeed in finding a suitable, homoeopathically adapted remedy for it.

§102

In the course of writing down the symptoms of several cases

of this kind the sketch of the disease picture becomes ever more and more complete, not more spun out and verbose, but more significant (more characteristic), and including more of the peculiarities of this collective disease; on the one hand, the general symptoms (e.g., loss of appetite, sleeplessness, etc.) become precisely defined as to their peculiarities; and on the other, the more marked and special symptoms which are peculiar to but few diseases and of rarer occurrence, at least in the same combination, become prominent and constitute what is characteristic of this malady. All those affected with the disease prevailing at a given time have certainly contracted it from one and the same source and hence are suffering from the same disease; but the whole extent of such an epidemic disease and the totality of its symptoms (the knowledge whereof, which is essential for enabling us to choose the most suitable homoeopathic remedy for this array of symptoms, is obtained by a complete survey of the morbid picture) cannot be learned from one single patient, but is only to be perfectly deduced (abstracted) and ascertained from the sufferings of several patients of different constitutions (Hahnemann 1922)

This treatment strategy at first seems out of step with what we know of the Hahnemannian method. Yet its success year after year during the winter when our practices fill up with colds, coughs and flu has proved so reliable. Phone calls and e-mails to friends and colleagues to confirm the kinds of cases they are getting, the types of symptoms they are seeing, and which remedies are being used with some success, goes part of a way to determine likely medicines that best fit the *genus epidemicus* of the immediate epidemic disease. One or two remedies usually cover this large totality, and it is from the choice of these few remedies selected for the whole of that disease the individual patient gets treated. For years Paul Herscu has argued that with worldwide epidemics a reality, the homeopathic community needs to develop more sophisticated communication channels for the next big global epidemic or pandemic.

In summary, where possible look for complete symptoms.

- **Location, Complaint, Modality** (LOCOMO) in the Dimitriadis system of the Bönninghausen method
- **Sensation Location Modality Causations** in the Hering system
- **CLAMS** (Concomitants, Location, Aetiology, Modality, Sensation) in the Watson system

Practically every patient is able to describe a symptom, find a sensation, point to a location and articulate a modality. From that information, from that completeness, the job of the homeopath is to construct or build a repertorial picture. The best tool for this type of case is in the *Therapeutic Pocketbook*.

There is no doubt that there is an elegant simplicity to this method, the homeopathic process of matching the symptom picture of a patient to the known symptom profile of a remedy as understood through its proving and materia medica profile. This can be relied on as the bread-and-butter of homeopathic prescribing on a daily basis. Thriving practice can easily be accomplished by doing this well. But of course it does not work nor is it appropriate in every case. There are complex psychodynamics, deepening and worsening pathological processes, poor lifestyles and other obstacles to take into account when prescribing. Homeopathy is of course as much about managing people and managing symptoms as it is about symptom removal.

Further Reading

- Bönninghausen — *Therapeutic Pocketbook*
- Boger — *Boenninghausen's Characteristics in Repertory*
- Lippe — *Keynotes of the Homoeopathic Materia Medica*
- Dimitriadis — *The Bönninghausen Repertory: Therapeutic Pocket Book Method*
- Dimitriadis — *Homoeopathic Diagnosis*
- Haehl — *Samuel Hahnemann His Life and Works*
- Hahnemann — *Cure and Prevention of Scarlet Fever*
- Hahnemann — *Organon of Medicine*
- Winston — *Faces of Homeopathy*
- Gray — *Case Taking*
- D'Aran — *Totality of the Whole Person or Totality of the Whole Diseased Person*

Chapter 3

Kent and the Totality of the Characteristics of the Person

Contents

- The Person not the Disease
- Totality of the Characteristics of the Person
- James Tyler Kent
- Kent's Legacy
- Swedenborg
- What Is Disease?
- Kentianism
- Other Influences
- Kent's Case Work
- Waiting and Waiting
- Subtle Changes
- Spiritualism and its Role in Homeopathy's Decline
- Kent's Method and Repertorisation
- Cases
- Further Reading

In this chapter you will:

1. *Identify how Kentian homeopathy differs from its Hahnemannian roots*
2. *Learn about the influence of Swedenborg*
3. *Familiarise yourself with Kent's case work and consider if it reflects his philosophical and theoretical position*
4. *Grasp the critique of Kent and his influence in the progression of homeopathic thought and practice.*

Chapter 3

Kent and the Totality of the Characteristics of the Person

If the primitive substance is normal, that which it creates is normal. Disease, which flows into the body, comes from within by influx through the primitive substance. Kent

Can man meditate and become an Atheist? A man who cannot believe in God cannot become a Homoeopath. Kent

The Person not the Disease

The fundamental difference between the two traditional broad schools of homeopathy is the interpretation of totality. Hahnemann made it clear that the job of the homeopath was to look for the symptoms of the patient representing the disease from when the patient was last healthy. The Kentian, and post-Kentian proponents of homeopathy, have a very different view, whether they know it or not. With stronger emphasis on the emotional and mental aspects of the case, looking at the essence of the fundamental problem, the golden thread that runs through the case, symptoms are seen as the language of disharmony. Rather than being distracted by the outside with symptoms that represent the disease, these practitioners perceive that it is far better to attempt to create meaningful and lasting change with a prescription that gets to the very centre of the problem. This seductive idea is often borne out in practice. When done well, the results can be fantastic.

Some of the consequences of these ideas however are that we see bewildered, confused, and unconfident homeopathic students who are desperately interpreting their cases and getting average results and sometimes no results when they step out into practice. When this method is performed poorly, students and practitioners identify aspects of personality that have nothing to do with the disease. A disappointing consequence of this poor application is that many homeopaths feel the unnecessary duel dramas of anxiety and guilt that they are not curing their patients in the unrealistic and dramatic way in which they have idealised. And patients are none too happy either. This is not to say that some cases do not require deep questioning and evaluation that takes into account all the very mental and emotional components of the case.

Totality of the Characteristics of the Person

I have often wondered how it transpired that homeopathy started in the pursuit of curing the symptoms of the patient, but ended up in the 20th and 21st century (especially in the US, UK, Australia and New Zealand) as being articulated as a healing modality that cures the person. Recently I was in the US lecturing and I finally worked it out. It comes down to legalities. After the Flexner Report in the early years of the 20th century, homeopathy was legally under threat and smart and flexible homeopaths realised that if they pitched their work as 'constitutional' or 'whole person' orientated, this was a way to ensure they would not be sued as practicing medicine without a license. It was a pragmatic solution. After a while, they started to believe their own media message, and with the influx of more psychologically presenting patients as the century progresses, the reorientation became concretised.

In a biomedical world, homeopaths have to wrestle with this conundrum. Hahnemann says, and virtually all homeopaths agree, symptoms are the outward signs of the internal and invisible disease. But then what? Hahnemann then seems to say that these symptoms are to be identified because they represent the disease. The job of a homeopath is to find these symptoms through good case taking, then remove them using the technical tools of the repertory, materia medica, the proving record and the selection of a homeopathic remedy that also has these signs and symptoms, and that this will relieve the suffering of the patient. A more metaphysical interpretation is that because those symptoms are merely the outward manifestation of the internal imbalance, one's prescription of the infinitesimal dose should be pitched to that one specific internal disturbance. And in the Kentian tradition of course, this translates to a higher potency and perhaps just one dose.

To complicate matters, some homeopaths are biased toward this style of prescribing, and advocate getting to the centre to be more profound. These homeopaths perceive any other style of case taking as suppression on the vital force of the patient, driving the disease inward, and worse, making the patient sicker. Removing the symptoms deprives the organism the opportunity to reveal to the homeopath the totality of symptoms, and therefore the medicine they need.

So on the one hand, we have the school of homeopaths that saw then and see now Kent's work as advanced, even classical, see it as getting better results, deeper cures and anything else is seen as pathological and suppressive. On the other side, we see those who argue the method involves too much speculation. Homeopaths make the mistake of knowing they should be prescribing for the totality but then choose all the symptoms they can see, rather than those which are characteristic, or strange, rare and peculiar. It is argued on this side that going for large totalities messes up our cases and makes our practices less busy. It is hard, we do not always get it right, it is less mathematical, and not as certain.

James Tyler Kent (1849-1916)

With the two schools identified, it must be acknowledged that homeopathy took a turn in the 1880s under the influence of Kent. He completed his medical degree at the Eclectic Medical Institute in Cincinnati, Ohio in 1871. According to Pierre Schmidt, his entire medical study apparently lasted 4 months. He began a medical practice in St Louis, Missouri in 1874 and taught anatomy at the American Medical College. This was the 1870s, the civil war was just finished, and north and south were putting back the pieces of their country. In Europe, Monet was painting, Garibaldi was walking, and Bismarck was unifying Germany. Disraeli and Gladstone were yelling at each other in the House of Commons.

Kent's first wife, Ellen, died in 1872, at the age of 19 years.

He moved to Missouri as he had some family there and married his second wife Lucy. He became a professor (of anatomy at first), though there was no pay for the title and it did not hold the prestige it would today. His first publication, *Sexual Neuroses* came out in 1879. In 1880 (some argue 1878), Lucy became ill and was cured by a Dr Phelan, who had studied homeopathy with Hering. Intrigued, Kent left the Eclectic School to take up the study of homeopathy officially, though he had done some earlier reading on the subject. He became professor of materia medica at the Homoeopathic Medical College in Missouri, one of the oldest in the US. In those early days, Kent used Bönninghausen's *Therapeutic Pocketbook* as his repertory. Later he accepted a position of professor of anatomy at the Homoeopathic Medical College of St Louis in 1881, becoming professor of materia medica in 1883.

In 1890, he founded the Post-Graduate School of Homoeopathics in Philadelphia, and by this time the influence of the Swedenborg Church was diffusing into in his lecturing work and writings. The school and its free clinic flourished. By the time it closed in 1900, it had seen over 40,000 patients, and trained many physicians, all of whom became the leaders in the homeopathic movement and kept homeopathy alive in the United States and the United Kingdom through the first half of the 20th century.

Lucy died in October 1895 and Kent married Clara Louise in 1896. She was already a physician herself. It is said that she had consulted many famous homeopathic physicians and each of them had prescribed her *Lachesis*. Kent studied her case carefully and concluded that she was presenting with a proving of *Lachesis* that had become iatrogenic, lasting many years. Kent predicted she would have *Lachesis* symptoms all her life. Together with others they established the Bryn Athyn Chapter of the New Church of Emmanuel Swedenborg, whose theology influenced the work of Kent and his *Lectures on Homoeopathic Philosophy* particularly.

Kent believed that both Hahnemann's and Swedenborg's teachings corresponded perfectly. Swedenborg's influence was immense, for instance, Kent's adoption of the psyche in three levels: the loves and hates (Swedenborg's Soul), the rational mind (Swedenborg's Reason and Intellect) and the memory (also Swedenborg's Memory). Kent's lectures on the Organon are deeply infused with the religious philosophy he practised and believed. Through his students' insistence, these lectures were later published as the *Lectures on Homoeopathic Philosophy* (1900), a fascinating fusion of Hahnemann and Swedenborg's ideas. In 1900, Kent and Clara moved to Evanston Chicago where they lived near the Farringtons (Harvey and Ernest) and other followers of Swedenborg. Kent practised in a busy street just off Michigan Ave. He lectured at the Dunham Medical College. Carol Dunham himself lived in New York and had been a student of Bönninghausen in Germany. Kent then lectured at the Hahnemann Medical College in Chicago, and also the Hering College. In November 1910, Kent founded the Society of Homoeopathicians, and also edited the new *Homoeopathician* Journal. Kent died on June 5th 1916 of chronic glomerulo nephritis aged 67. He was buried in Stephensville, Montana.

Kent's Legacy

The legacy of Kent is incalculable. Generations of homeopaths have been taught by his students, in the same tradition and with his attitudes and values. But his star is not shining as brightly in the last decade or so as academics have explored the influence of Swedenborg on homeopathy. Whilst Kent went on to become a homeopathic household name after his death, and his influence extinguished Hughes interpretations of homeopathic philosophy in the trans-Atlantic battle for supremacy in the mid 1800s, a revision of his role is being re-emphasised in homeopathic history. Klaus-Hening Gypser in particular has maintained his life and work have been mythologised unnecessarily. Acknowledging his influence as a popular teacher and a brilliant practitioner, the value and consequences of his influence have been questioned. To my mind, it is entirely appropriate to review and argue the role of significant historical figures. It is all part of academic rigor and robust enquiry. Swedenborg's huge influence on modern homeopathy deserves exploration. However, and bizarrely, the debate has rather settled on the role of Kent in homeopathy due to questions about his parentage. The 'evidence' is that Kent was born the son of Stephen and Caroline Kent. However, on his death certificate different names are given, which has given rise to speculation about his parentage. This, plus the fact that he was married three times but had no children, has implied for some that he was either infertile, or knew of his uncertain parentage and so avoided having children who might have been genetically unfit. In addition, some commentators have argued that because he was schooled out of Woodhull, apparently this suggests the Puritans in his county knew of his incestuous birth and sent him away. Nevertheless, after Hahnemann, Kent has had the largest influence as a theoretician, a practitioner, a writer and as a teacher on homeopathy. His influence has been especially strong on American, Indian and British homeopathy while the western European homeopaths seem to have been largely untouched by his influence, except in Switzerland and the influence of Pierre Schmidt.

Swedenborg

In 1840, there were 850 Swedenborgians in America. By 1870, there were 18,700. The New Church had a high proportion of doctors in its total membership. 'Nearly all rejected allopathy for some other medical system, and most of those who rebelled chose homeopathy, and many ministers not only endorsed it but were physicians themselves (Treuherz 1984).

Francis Treuherz has explored the influence of Kent in depth.

> As a follower of the Christian mystical sect of Immanuel Swedenborg, Kent delivered a blend of Hahnemann's Organon and miasm theory, spiritual forces and an early pre-Freudian psychology. The human being was comprised of will, understanding and intellect. Kent approached his philosophy with typical vigour. He viewed all Hahnemann's works and especially The Organon with a fundamentalist zeal, seeking to amplify and reinterpret every word of the Master, much like a theology scholar or biblical commentator. His Lectures On Philosophy, for example, is almost a Swedenborgian commentary to the Organon. This has alientated some. To him these were precious and immutable homoeopathic truths that it is sacrilege even to question, let alone dilute, negotiate or compromise. He even goes as far as saying:
>
> 'Can man meditate and become an Atheist? A man who

cannot believe in God cannot become a Homoeopath.'[Kent, 1926, Aphorisms]

It is especially in Kent's rather arrogant use of language, which hits us when reading his works, which really illustrates this fundamentalism and the precious certainty of his approach to homoeopathy. The following quote from many possible ones, clearly demonstrates this:

'...beware of the opinions of men of science. Hahnemann has given us principles...it is law that governs the world and not matters of opinion or hypotheses. We must begin by having a respect for law, for we have no starting point unless we base our propositions on law.' [Kent, 1900, Lectures, p.18]

Kent infers that homoeopaths must base their whole approach upon the hard dogmatism of these ideas, which he elevates to the status of certitudes, and not upon the ever-shifting ideas of 'mere men'. He is claiming a great authority and power behind such 'immutable principles', a power which like some divine form, stands 'above and behind us' and which we dare not abrogate or dilute for fear of our Soul's damnation.

As an attitude, this is so indistinguishable from that of fundamentalist religion, that it is clearly apparent how this form of homoeopathy possessed, and generated for itself, so many problems with creative and imaginative people who much prefer to experiment and find truths out for themselves, e.g. Samuel Hahnemann. This whole approach denies anyone the privilege or luxury of that kind of freedom. Total and unquestioning devotion to a given creed seems to be the basis of Kentianism, not reason or real-world experiment. As to whether Kent was truly a Hahnemannian homoeopath, see Hehr, 1995 and Cassam, 1999.

It is especially when he lapses into the moral sphere of homoeopathy that his deep dogmatism shows itself. When he is speaking purely about homoeopathy, which is rare, he does well, but as soon as he enters human affairs, a certain clearly-recognisable 'Bible-punching' tone seems to shines through. As the following quotes clearly demonstrate:

> 'It is law that governs the world and not matters of opinion or hypothesis. We must begin by having a respect for law...' [Kent, 1900, p.18]

> 'This means law, it means fixed principles, it means a law as certain as that of gravitation...our principles have never changed, they have always been the same and will remain the same...' [Kent, 1900, p.28]

> 'Had Psora never been established as a miasm upon the human race, the other two chronic diseases would have been impossible and susceptibility to acute diseases would have been impossible...' [ibid. p.126]

Kent would have no dealings with allopaths nor with low-dilutionists, who were dismissed as 'mongrel, milk-and-water half-homoeopaths'. Homoeopathy was seen very dogmatically by them as pure classical homoeopathy as 'laid down in tablets of stone by the master' or nothing. This narrow, simplistic and somewhat inflexible view of homoeopathy had split American homoeopathy right down the middle, causing a very acrimonious clash of ideologies. It is generally conceded that this bitter wrangling contributed significantly to the precipitous decline of homoeopathy in the USA during the first half of this century.

To Swedenborg, the realms of nature, and particularly the body and mind of man, were theatres of divine activity...A 'universal analogy' existed between the various realms of creation. The physical world was symbolical of the spiritual world and this, in turn, of God. He conceived a resonant system of hierarchies of God, universe and man. He became a theologian and established the Church of the New Jerusalem.

A Supreme Divine purpose reigned throughout creation. The life of the universe, whether physical, mental or spiritual was the activity of Divine Love. The physical universe is given its true place in the economy of creation, the womb of man's most enduring and real life. Briefly, Swedenborg was heretical to mainstream Christianity because he espoused that personal liberation could be won easily from an all-loving God and that 'original sin' was non-existent.

> '...he dispensed with the idea of original sin'

As with Paracelsus and later Theosophists, the link with homoeopathy is to be found in the vast hierarchies of form and spirit that he conceived as existing between God, mind and matter, and penetrating throughout the universe. Kent linked all of this to the process of potentisation, the vital force and the miasms of Hahnemann, seeing them both as philosophies that fully confirm each other and which for him, married together splendidly, into a new organic creation. The following quotes from his Aphorisms more than amply illustrate this point:

> 'Radiant substances have degrees within degrees, in series too numerous for the finite mind to grasp.'

> 'The lower potency corresponds to a series of outer degrees, less fine and less interior than the higher.'

> 'When it has passed to simple substance, the Radiant form of matter, it has infinite degrees. To express the degrees from

the Outermost to the Innermost, we might say a grain of Silica is the Outermost; the Innermost is The Creator.'

'There are degrees of fineness of the Vital Force. We may think of internal man as possessing infinite degrees and of external man as possessing finite degrees.'

'There are degrees within degrees to infinity.'

'Low potencies can cure acute diseases because acute diseases act upon the outermost degree of the Simple Substance and the body. In chronic disease the trouble is deeper seated, and the degrees are finer, hence the remedy must be reduced to finer or higher degrees so as to be similar to the degrees of chronic disease (Treuherz 1984).

What Is Disease?

Commentators emphasise the influence of the philosophy of Kent, as well as focus on the philosophy of Swedenborg, because it is the only way to understand why the practical application of homeopathy using Kent or using Hahnemann yielded different results. At the core of this discussion is a different understanding of what constituted *disease*. In chapter one of his philosophy book (1900), Kent argued that to understand disease we must understand the human being, and particularly just what constituted the healthy human being. For Kent, allopathic medicine ignored the vital principle and dealt only with pathology and ultimates, which denied the existence of any principals. And because allopathic medicine focused on ultimates and the results of disease, there was no need for understanding anything to do with the cause of disease, and no understanding of true physiology that, as Hahnemann argued, is the vital principal.

Kent and the Totality of the Characteristics of the Person

To Kent, the role of homeopaths included examining the entire life and being of the patient to understand the true nature of the disease of the patient, to find the seed of the disease or the cause, to understand how it evolved over the life of the patient, and to prescribe the remedy accordingly. Kent was utterly uninterested in the results of disease but instead, in the disease itself. He argued the organs do not constitute the human being ... the human being is prior to the organs. The disturbance of the human being comes prior to the disturbance of the organs. Kent is saying 'what caused the liver, or the spleen, or the pancreas to become disturbed?' Fundamentally, what it always comes back to is a disturbance of the will or the understanding. These are always prior and primary to the organs and tissues in the material body of the human being. Kent argued that if the will and the understanding are in order - then we have a healthy human being. This in itself is not so hard to digest. But what happens next is harder to swallow. Kent was extremely moralistic. Your liver or spleen or pancreas would not have become disturbed if you were living the right way, leading a good life. It is ultimately poor decisions, and immoral behaviour therefore that leads to disease. The mind is first at all times. If we are to treat the sick, then we must treat the person with the illness - not the house of the person with the illness.

So for Kent, underpinnings of the practical application of homeopathic medicine, the nature of disease was a disturbance of the will and the understanding. We can perceive this by understanding the totality of symptoms and through fully taking the case, and we can cure a sick person by understanding and perceiving the nature of disease - the state of health of the human being.

As a consequence, we have inherited a situation in the 21st century where the major division in approach in homeopathic medicine is due to an earnest attempt by Kent to protect Hahnemannian thought and homeopathy from allopaths. But he did it through the lens of his religious beliefs, and in the process altered those homeopathic principles. In addition, his earnestness often became dogmatism.

Kentianism

The aphorisms and precepts of Kent contained in his *Lesser Writings* don't hold back:

> Forty eight pages of proverb (in the biblical sense), sententiousness self-righteous (like Samuel Johnson), and uncalled-for homily (like Polonius), sometimes couched in a manner which assumes obeisance superiority. There is something in the transmission of ideas in homeopathy which demands reverence to the authority of a great predecessor, a Master, a Guru, a Prophet. This is of relevance elsewhere to a discussion of the reliability of the evidence of provings. In this case, it appears likely from the introduction to the book that the collection was made posthumously. Kent has had a share of reverence; the Thorson's reprint of Philosophy, contains no less than nine eulogies (Treuherz 1984).
>
> > 'All hail James Tyler Kent, to all endeared when as their chief his pupils proudly claim in ages yet unborn shall be revered'
> >
> > 'can anyone say Kent is dead!' Kent is laid away amid the snow-capped mountains of Montana! Kent never died! The earthly shrine of his immortal mind returns to dust amid the western mountains - Kent still lives....'

The aphorisms begin with a quotation from Swedenborg and include many references to his terminology, such as:

> If the primitive substance is normal, that which it creates is normal. Disease, which flows into the body, comes from within by influx through the primitive substance.
>
> We have in the image of the disease an exact representation of the image of a remedy. Do all things come by chance? Can man meditate and become an atheist? A man who cannot believe in God cannot become a homoeopath.
>
> There are degrees of fineness of the Vital Force. We may think of internal man as possessing finite degrees and of external man as possessing finite degrees.
>
> What reason has man to say that Energy of Force is first? Energy is not energy per se but a powerful substance. The very Esse of God is a scientific study.
>
> Eternal Principles themselves are authority. The Law of Similars is a Divine Law. So soon as you have accepted the Law of Similars, so soon have you accepted Providence, which is law and order.
>
> You must see and feel the internal nature of your patient as the artist sees and feels the picture he is painting. He feels it. Study to feel the economy, the life, the soul.
>
> You cannot divorce Medicine and Theology. Man exists all the way down, from his innermost spiritual, to his outermost Natural (Treuherz 1984).

It makes for great reading. Some practitioners and students alike are utterly inspired by it, and others less so.

But it must be acknowledged that Kent created the first

coherent, persuasive and highly influential philosophy, identifiably different to Hahnemann. This philosophy has largely gone unchallenged within homeopathy since its inception, formulated as a synthesis of Swedenborgian mysticism, and the more romantic portions of Hahnemann's Organon and the Miasm Theory of The Chronic Diseases.

Treuherz, (1984) argued that Kent's homeopathy seemed rooted in a rather dogmatic and puritanical attitude and came from a pedantically scholastic and uncritical reverence for everything Hahnemann wrote.

Kentianism, then, was metaphysical, dogmatic, puritanical and millennial. Homoeopaths who failed to achieve results with the high dilutions lacked intellectual skill and rigour, as well as the moral fibre for the arduous task of identifying the simillimum. In short, so far as Kentians were concerned, the faithless were responsible for the corruption and decline of the movement (Treuherz, 1984).

He continues;

Blind uncritical adoption of Kent's homoeopathic ideas, and elevating those ideas to classical, is deductive and didactic and denies that the facts of the outer world are in any sense superior to, or an arbiter for, theoretical 'principles'. In that sense it seems stubbornly medieval in its extreme deductivism. It turns its back completely on the empirical approach of scientific rationalism and thus on allopathy.

This stubborn determination to studiously ignore the rest of medicine and the 'ideological push' of the last 200 years makes it appear to the modern eye, as reactionary, hard-line and hard to digest.

Experience has a place in science, but only a confirmatory place. It can only confirm that which has been discovered through principle or law guiding in the proper direction. Experience leads to no discoveries, but when man is fully indoctrinated in principle that which he observes by experience may confirm the things that are consistent with law (Treuherz, 1984).

This position is strongly dogmatic and arguably fundamentalist. Ironically, it is not that different to the scientism (Milgrom 2008, 2010) we see so readily published in the media and in the poorly argued articles by the opponents of homeopathy today (Ernst 2002, Shang et al 2005, Baum and Ernst 2009). Science, like homeopathy, is rooted in observations and experiments in the outer world, not in the enforcement of dogmas.

Kent seems to stress the philosophy and principles of homeopathy over and above the simple fact that it is primarily a system of therapeutics in which the progress of the patient is always far more important than the religious beliefs of the practitioner.

Kent's Other Influences on Homeopathy

Repertory

One of his greatest contributions to the profession of homeopathy and its teachings was his completely unique style of repertory. Although others exist, Kent's famous repertory, is still the popular choice, and has been described as more complete, systematic and precise with more well-described symptoms.

Types

Kent is also known for developing *pictures* of constitutional types of patients. A well-known example would be his description of *Sulphur* as *'the ragged philosopher.'* There are many works based on Kent's principles, including a book by one of his pupils, Margaret Tyler. Tyler further developed this idea of *pictures* into the book *Homoeopathic Drug Pictures*. It was believed that a useful way of identifying materia medica profiles was to anthropomorphize them; a *Pulsatilla* type looked like...etc.

Books

In addition to *The Repertory*, Kent compiled the *Homoeopathic Materia Medica* and *Lectures on Homoeopathic Philosophy*. His other works were later collated into *Minor Writings* and *Lesser Writings*.

Potency and Remedies

Initially Kent had practiced using tinctures and lower potencies. As his experience grew, he began using higher potencies more. He then prescribed mainly high potencies produced by German manufacturers except those of Swann and Fincke. Apparently he later discarded these as he was not satisfied with their manufacturing process. At the height of his practice around the turn of the century, Kent and his students were reported by Pierre Schmidt to be treating thousands of patients annually. Overwhelmingly the majority of prescriptions from Kent involved a single remedy, in a single dose, and usually in a high potency. It is worth noting that by the time that Kent became prominent in homeopathy, a high potency was no longer what Hahnemann considered a high potency. Hahnemann considered a 30c to be an extremely high potency. At the time that Kent was writing, a high potency might be considered a CM in the centesimal scale.

Waiting and Waiting

A key component of Kent's prescribing method was to wait until the response to the prescription had clearly ceased before repeating or re-prescribing. This approach will be fully explored in the next volume in the series on case management. It is important to highlight that this point is clearly at odds with Hahnemann's best practice as described in the fifth and sixth editions of the *Organon* involving frequently repeated doses and numerous consultations. Many patients and many homeopaths even today still mistakenly assume that best practice and homeopathy involves one dose and wait.

Kent's Hierarchy

Kent understood disease to be a physical manifestation of something much greater, which he described as a disturbance of the will and the understanding. Consequently skin eruptions, alopecia, asthma, warts on the hands are therefore from a direct cause; lack of flow between, or communication between the many and the one, earth and heaven, the individual and God.

In the whole non-dual undivided universe, simple substance flows downward, into, and through the human being. The *vice regent of the soul*, simple substance, is endowed with formative intelligence. Closer to its source, it is so fine and refined that nothing earthly can make any impact upon it, but as it gets to the more grounded and material parts of the human being, it becomes coarser and less refined and able to be manipulated and affected by medicines.

A symptom manifesting on the material body, the results of disease, can be easily affected by crude allopathic or herbal medicine; but not to cure fully and not permanently. If the question is asked, 'why is this person ill?' then the reason for that is clearly not to be found in the material body and the answer lies further up the hierarchy, in the realm of the mind and simple substance. If the cause of disease is not material, the medicine required to cure, to reconnect the material to the divine, needs to be immaterial also. An infinitesimal medicine, one in a high potency is needed. There are degrees of fineness of vibration and the medicine needed to affect the material body must be orientated and calibrated to the disconnection and the disturbance. For the most part, if the cause of the problem is as Kent argued due to disturbance of the will and the understanding, then a very high potency of that homeopathic simillimum is necessary to create the change and make those re-connections.

The Mind

From the emphasis discussed in the previous section, it is little surprise that for Kent the Mind came first. In his *Lectures on Homeopathic Philosophy* (1900), first came the emotional and mental symptoms pertaining to what can described as the will and the understanding, the intellect being the next important, followed by those of the memory. He considered the following as high-grade symptoms:

1. Symptoms depicting the emotional state: loves, hates, desires and aversions
2. Symptoms of intellect (comprehension)
3. Symptoms affecting the memory
4. Fears, impulsive behaviours, suicidal impulses and thoughts

He argued common mental symptoms were of little use in individualising the case because they indicated a large group of remedies. The peculiar, queer, rare and strange symptoms were still of prime importance, although the emphasis was still geared to the mind. Important, but lower on the hierarchy, were the physical general symptoms in the case. Sensations and complaints, conditions of aggravation and amelioration, and modalities were sometimes useful but, as Kent argued, less important. The characteristic particulars were sometimes of importance in the final stage of differentiation between medicines out of the few that possibly resembled the image of the patient. But that image was usually revealed through the mental picture as opposed to the particulars on the physical plane. Lastly physical particulars and the disease symptoms manifesting in the case, the headache, the migraine, the pain in the stomach were last and often irrelevant. Wherever possible, the remedy prescribed needed to bear as much similarity to the mental and emotional symptoms and the state since this was perceived as being fundamentally causative in the case.

To some therefore, Kent was the man that took homeopathy forward with uncompromising and fundamental principle and the dogmatic voice of reason. Ultimately, in order to understand Kent's prescribing, one has to deeply examine his philosophy. Many readers of *Lecturers on Homoeopathic Philosophy* have assumed that that was the way he practiced at all times. His case-books clearly question that assumption. His *Minor Writings* and *Lesser Writings* contain extremely pragmatic prescriptions and excellent results. So what about his casework? Were his cases, case evaluation, case analysis, and case taking reflective of these puritanical, moralistic, and dogmatic attitudes?

Kent's Case Work

Mrs. K., aged 40, a midwife. She complained of the abdomen; she believed she had a tumor. Severe knife-cutting pain in the region of uterus running up to left mamma; pains, undefined, running up and through pelvis, worse lying down, aching up and through the pelvis, worse lying down, aching in the sacrum, dragging down in the uterine region as if the uterus would escape. Empty, "all-gone" feeling in the stomach. Greenish-yellow leucorrhoea, with itching in labia and mons veneris; intense sexual desire. The os uteri was said to be ulcerated and eroded, and it was sensitive to touch. The contact of the finger with cervix brought on the sharp pain that she described as running to the left mamma. The uterus was enlarged and indurated. She had been the mother of several children; had had several abortions, and was accustomed to hard work. She had been treated locally by a specialist of acknowledged ability, and she had taken many remedies of his selection as well as from her own medicine case, all very low. Her catamenia quite normal. To take up the important and guiding features of this case we must compare several remedies, but principally Murex and Sepia. The cutting pain in the uterus has been found under Curare. Murex and Sepia, but Murex is the only one producing a cutting pain in the uterus going to the left mamma. The "all-gone" empty feeling in the stomach is characteristic of Murex., Phos. and Sepia. Throbbing in the uterus, belongs only to Murex. The dragging down is common to both Murex and Sepia, but the sexual teasing only to Murex. Both have a yellowish green leucorrhoea. Pain in sacrum is common to Murex, Sepia and many others. "Enlargement of bowels" is found in Allen under Murex, not mentioned in Minton's Uterine Therapeutics. The pains in Murex go upward and through, worse while lying down. In Sepia the patient is better lying down, and the pains go around. Murex 200, one dose was given. She was much worse for several days. Then improvement went on for two weeks. The remedy was again repeated. One year later she complained of a return of her symptoms. One dose was followed by relief, since which time she has made no complaint, but praises the individualizing method.

M. A. W., aet. 30, asks treatment for abdominal tumor, which is large enough to give her the appearance of being about eight months pregnant. She is a house maid, and her friends will not go out with her fearing that people will think they are associating with an unmarried pregnant woman. She had consulted two surgeons who refused to operate because of the rigidity and extensive adhesions, and also because of the sickly aspect of the girl. The face was indeed waxy and sickly looking. These surgeons told her she would die from the tumor. The tumor was first noticed five years ago. It became prominent on the right side of the uterus and extended up to the pelvis; was said to be movable until two years ago. The uterus is now immovable and the tumor which hangs over the right side of the pelvis is very hard, as large as a child's head, and cannot be made to move in any direction. June 1st, 1888. -Pain in the pelvis now and then. Swelling in the pit of the stomach not due to the tumor. Swelling of the feet, indenting on pressure. Constant congestive headaches which she could give no description of, only "it aches all over." Eats but little, and what she eats causes nausea. Constipation; no desire for stool; takes physic, hence no modalities of value. Goes two or three weeks without a stool. Always feels a constriction about the waist, which most likely is due to pressure of tumor, hence it is not a valuable symptom. Sensation of great fullness after eating, and she mentions above that she eats but little. Menses fairly regular "with cramps." She has not drank water for eight years, as it makes her sick. Feet burn so that she must take off her slippers to cool them. Starts in sleep, and when awake starts at the slightest noise. Restless sleep. Pain in left side of abdomen. Teeth decayed when young. They are dark and bad looking. Wants hot things; cannot take cold things into the stomach. Pain in the stomach after cold things. Pain and nausea after water, cold or warm. Pain in left groin. She had this pain before the tumor was felt. Lyc. cm; one dose, and Sac-Lac. morning and night, dry on the tongue. July 23rd.-The remedy increased the symptoms so much that she was alarmed and would not return for many weeks, but now is so much better in a general way that she returns to report and ask for more medicine. Upon close questioning it was found that for a week or more her symptoms were on the increase. Her stomach symptoms at first grew worse, then improved and now are worse again. Lyc. mm. She got one dose and s. l. Aug 2nd-Reports that all the symptoms are better, and she is feeling greatly improved. Aug. 31st.-Pain in pit of stomach. Pain in forehead, vertex and temples. Bowels no better. If she drinks water she feels so full and gets cramps. Sleepless; starts suddenly. S. L. No change in tumor. Sept. 15th.-

Feet do not swell now. She vomits and has a pain in stomach after eating or drinking. Lyc. mm. Oct. 28th.-Symptoms all passed away, except that she has a pain in right side, in the tumor. Nov. 27th.-No symptoms. Calls at intervals but gets only s. l. Jan. 23rd, 1889. -Symptoms returning, especially the stomach symptoms. Lyc. MM. June 3rd.-She has been improving steadily and was free from symptoms. Bowels move every three or four days. Stool normal. Feels more swollen than for some time. Uncomfortable. Bad feelings return. Pain in right groin. Feet swollen. Headache in forehead and eyes. Pain in lumbar region. Lyc. mm. Feet burn. August 15th.-Symptoms have been gone since here last, but now all are coming back. Lyc. 2mm. December 31st.-She has reported several times, but there were no symptoms. Bowels regular. She can eat and drink anything. She looks well. She says the last powders have made her well. The tumor is what most readers will ask about, but has not been mentioned, as the tumor was not treated. The patient was cured and the tumor at last report was small; the uterus was movable and with it the small tumor also moved. She did not mind the tumor as she was so well and shapely.

Irritable, weak-minded, worse from mental exertion. The head topples over because the neck is emaciated; the face is wrinkled and has a sickly look; the temples are marked by distended veins. The face looks old, the infant looks like a little old person. (Also, Bar-c., Iodine, Natr-m., Op., Sulph.) (If from syphilis, Aur-mur.) The whole body is emaciated and wrinkled; the emaciation spreads from the lower limbs upward (which is the reverse of Lyc. and Natr-m.) Enlarged glands, especially in the emaciated abdomen. Diseases change from place to place (metastasis). Mumps go to the mammae or to the testes, Rheumatism leaves the joints and endocarditis appears with profuse sweat; cannot lie down for the dyspnoea; sinking as if dying, pulse feeble. Rheumatism comes on when a diarrhoea has ceased too suddenly. Piles which get worse as the rheumatism abates. Bleeding from the piles in amenorrhoea. (Graph.) Hydrocele in boys. Distended abdomen. (Ars., Bar-c., Calc., Iodine, Lyc., Puls., Sulph.) Piercing pains in the heart. Piercing in the ovaries, mostly the left. Wakes in a fright and trembles, is covered with cold sweat. The extremities are numb and tingle as if thawing, after having been frozen. High fever after the rheumatism has gone to the heart. The wasting child has hectic fever with a ravenous appetite. Lives well yet emaciates. (Also Iodine, Natr-m.) Abrotanum attacks the white fibrous tissues, the joints, pleura, peritoneum, etc. Gouty nodosities in the wrist and fingers. Rheumatism goes to the heart, compare with Cactus, Dig., Kalm., Lach., Naja., Spig., Spong. The grand features of this remedy are metastasis; marasmus spreading upward.

Mrs. P. suffered from gouty deposits about the finger joints, which were very painful during cold, stormy weather. The joints and nodes were sore and hot at such times. The nodes ceased to be painful and sudden hoarseness came; ulcers in the larynx followed; great dryness in the nose and painful dry throat; sticking in the cardiac region. She lost flesh but the appetite kept good. Calc-phos. had been prescribed by her former attendant. After duly considering the case, Abrot. 45m. was given. She suffered for many days after this dose with a most copious discharge from her nose and bronchial tubes; expectoration was copious, thick, yellow. Hoarseness ceased at once. In a month she ceased coughing; the finger joints became painful and swollen considerably. In three months she had no pain and the nodes were scarcely perceptible. She is now perfectly well and has been so one year. She had only one dose of the remedy, as the case was doing well enough, i. e., as the symptoms were taking the right course to recovery in the proper way. She suffered much pain on the road to recovery but I know of only one way to cure these cases, and that is to let the remedy alone when the symptoms are taking the proper course.

Mrs. T. had suffered from chronic rheumatism of the left ankle and knee for several years. She rubbed the limb with a strong liniment and the rheumatism was speedily cured. But it was not long before she needed a physician. I saw her friends surrounding her bed, she was covered with a profuse, cold sweat, sitting propped up on pillows. Her friends said she was dying, and I thought so too. She had a small, quick pulse; there was pain at the heart and auscultation over heart, revealed the usual story, which is too well known to all, as there are many such cases. She was six months pregnant. Gave her Abrot., and she slowly recovered. The little one now bears my Christian name in honor of the great cure. She has recovered, perfectly free from rheumatism, and the lad is now several years old. These two cases show what Abrotanum can do when properly indicated. It is a powerful remedy and must not be repeated. It acts many weeks, in waves or cycles; it is too seldom used.

Abscess on side of face: Tarentula cubensis: A middle-aged gentleman had an abscess on the side of the face just in front of the ear. Suppuration was advanced and the fluctuation was marked. Silicea had done some good as it had controlled the pain. The cavity was aspirated by a surgeon several times but it continued to refill. After three weeks there was no abatement of the difficulty. The integument took on a new feature, becoming bluish, mottled with great burning and sharp cutting pains. The hardness was extending and the opening gave out a bloody thin excoriating fluid of foul smell. He was chilly and nauseated and had symptoms of pyaemia. After one dose of Tarantula cubensis 12x an immediate change for the better took place, no more pus formed and he was well in ten days. The discolored localization became a bright red and then faded to the natural color. The nausea and general pyaemic symptoms were greatly relieved within twelve hours. No more medicine.

Subtle Changes

While we are unable to critique Kent's use of this prescribing method, we certainly have significant feedback on anecdotal evidence of the success of the 21st century context. Today proponents of this style of prescribing tend to encourage the patient to return at monthly or even six weekly intervals. Often very subtle changes are seen to take place over this prolonged period of time. It is not uncommon for a patient to be given no medicine, and many months after the original dose has been given (Watson 1991, Vithoulkas 1980).

It is crucial therefore to constantly explain to patients just what the process involves, especially those new to homeopathy who are not accustomed to receiving no medication after having talked for an hour or more to a practitioner. Many homeopaths choose to prescribe placebo in this situation with dubious ethical and legal consequences. Still worse, if the original prescription was inaccurate, weeks or months go by before a new and more accurate medicine is given. In the 20th century, influential homeopaths such as Roberts, Tyler, Blackie, Wright-Hubbard, Schmidt, Paschero, Ghegas, Coulter and Vithoulkas, amongst others, have based their work writings and prescribing on the work of Kent.

Case Examples

Female age 36. I moved to Australia 18 months ago. I am facing some old ghosts of when I was here 10 years ago. I am here indefinitely. I am home sick. I have a house in the UK. I am used to having my family around in a caring environment, I have been feeling the separation from my family a great deal. I am on antidepressants. Aurorex 2 x day. My mother visited and I could not stop crying. Feeling the separation from my mother. Went back to England at Easter. There was a terrible pull.

I then got over it a bit. All this grief. My characteristic response to everything is tears. I feel childish and incapable. I am no good at anger. I hold a lot in and it bursts out as tears.

I am so worn out with my daughter's constant activity. And my husband is someone who is like my daughter. He is fine when everything is going his way and it is ugly when I oppose him. He is in love with Australia and he doesn't understand how I feel about England.

I bury a lot of my feelings. Tears are babyish. They are beyond my control. I have this awful silent response to things. I feel a release but then I feel bad because it is beyond my control. I suppose I am male dominated and I certainly had a controlling father, but tears are a weak response. God I have to grow up. Sigh.

When did it begin? Ten years ago. My husband and I met when I was 16. We split up. I came to Australia. I thought I had met a man but he was married. We had a fling. I loved him. My husband knew all about this and he came and saved me. He came out to Australia. He tried to persuade me to go back to England. But I had fallen in love with my boss, I was offered a permanent job in Australia working with this man. I decided to stay. I went back to England to tie up all of my lose ends. I stayed with my husband just to save money but knew something happened. I was pregnant 6 weeks later.

There is something in Australia that makes me see things differently, therefore I am having to face these demons. There is this man I thought I was in love with and he is still in Sydney. I first met him in England. My husband and I had split up. He was a free Australian spirit, surfer, married with a child. I worked with him and we had this affair. It was hell. We all lived in shared house. There was so much deception. I had to pretend. It was such a huge mess. Even then I thought it was too far from my family. Then I went back to London. It was so far from family so I got close to my family. But in fact I am still not happy being close to them.

Now on OCP Microgynae. On pill since 19. When I went on the pill I got very, very tearful. Started period at 15 years old. After daughter was born I stopped the pill. Menses were irregular and the advice was take the pill or life long HRT. This was in 1995.

This is one of those cases. A patient wants to talk. While there is a presenting symptom, it is an emotional one. She is stuck, melancholic and depressed. It's not a difficult case. The symptoms, the process she is in, all correspond to a large totality prescription of *Natrum Mur*.

RX: *Natrum mur* 30c, 5 days.

Follow-up One: Everything is good. I don't trust it yet but it is good. I was grotty after the remedy. Then I was positive and optimistic and I felt less trapped. I was in and out of bed. I have much more energy and I am not so cautious or analytical or hesitant. I do not weigh up every situation before I speak any more. I feel much less abandoned. It is the same with the relationship. Normally I would have been put off by him in an argument. This time I was able to go forward. Actually it's incredible. I haven't felt tearful at all. Before the remedy I had so many fears. I had an awful sensitivity to the news. Before for me everything was all overwhelming. Craving Mayonnaise. I eat spoonfuls out of the jar. It is a joy in my life. *Natrum Mur* 30c, 5 days.

Remedies over the next months

July	*Nat Mur* 30 5 days
August	*Nat Mur* 30 5 days
September	*Nat Mur* 30 5 days
October	*Nat Mur* 30 5 days
November	*Nat Mur* 200 one dose

Strategy

Initially she was on Aurorix 400 mg per day. From the outset, the strategy with the first remedy was to reduce the Aurorix to 300 mg. She did. Soon she was taking 4 half tablets, twice per day, which was then reduced to 3 half tablets per day. By September, she was reducing the Aurorix 200 mg. Two half tablets a day, by October 100 mg half a day, and soon after she was off her medication.

Further Reading

- Kent — *Materia Medica*
- Kent — *Lectures on Homoeopathic Philosophy*
- Kent — *Lesser Writings*
- Tyler — *Different Ways of Finding the Remedy*
- Watson — *Guide to the Methodologies of Homeopathy*
- Dimitriadis — *Homoeopathic Diagnosis*
- Treuherz — *The Origins of Kent's Homoeopathy*

Chapter 4

Constitution and Constitutional Prescribing

Contents

- Introduction
- The Confusion
- The Prescribing Style in a Nutshell
- Massive Totality
- Definitions of Constitution
- Advocates of Constitutional Prescribing
- What Is Constitution
- Von Gravogl's Hydrogenoid, Oxygenoid, Carbo-nitrogenoid Constitutions
- Clarke's Constitutions
- Lesser's Attitude
- Vannier's Constitution and Types
- Mappa Mundi Type and Temperament
- Little
- Benefits and Disadvantages
- Conclusions

In this chapter you will:

1. Explore the various interpretations and definitions of 'constitution'
2. Learn how the concepts of constitution, constitutional type and constitutional prescribing are all different
3. Identify the historical advocates of this approach
4. Develop the skills to seach, find and comprehend the debate about the use of this method.

Chapter 4

Constitution and Constitutional Prescribing

The constitutional medicine is a picture of the sum total of the strengths and weaknesses of the person, mentally, emotionally and physically. It is in the early undiagnosable stages of illness that we must find the constitutional medicines. Margery Blackie

These are....developed 'pictures' of the medicines, 'constitutional types' as they became known, from the patients emotional symptoms ... identifying for example, 'Sulphur' patients, who were scruffy and lazy, 'ragged philosophers' as he termed them. Miranda Castro

Introduction

In this chapter, I have relied on a number of sources. First, the excellent work in multiple articles by David Little (1996-2007 at *www.simillimum.com* and *www.wholehealthnow.com*), Clarke (1925), and also I have taken into account the typology work of Vanier, Lesser and Ian Watson (1991). I have deliberately kept this chapter separate to the work on Kent. Many might argue they are one in the same. But to my mind, a significant distinction needs to be maintained.

The Confusion

There is little in homeopathy more misunderstood than the term constitution. Also (and mistakenly) sometimes known as Kentian Homeopathy, Classical Homeopathy, Centralist Prescribing or Essence Prescribing, it has involved taking the whole person into account as far as possible and treating the person simultaneously on all levels- physical, mental and emotional. But this has virtually nothing to do with the term constitution. To quote Little,

> There are some who are averse to the use of the word "constitution" in any manner. They are even more averse to the term "constitutional remedy". This term was introduced by Kent to indicate a chronic or anti-miasmatic medicine that affects the whole patient. This term was complementary to the 'acute remedy', which was more suitable for the transitory, local phenomena associated with acute crisis. Kent's constitutional medicine had nothing to do with giving remedies by classical constitutions or temperaments. It was simply the remedy that was most suited to treat chronic diseases and miasms. Actually, Kent spoke out against the use of classical constitutions and temperaments in homeopathy in his *Lesser Writings* (Little Hahnemann on Constitution and Temperament 2011).

To further obfuscate, homeopathic students will have read authors that said this …

> Let us take the example of Calc. carb. When it is found that the patient is fair, fatty, flabby, easily fatigued and tired on walking, chilly with much sweating, cold extremities, sour smell of body, a tendency to grow fat, catch cold very easily, and has scrofulous, rachitic diathesis with remarkable psoric and sycotic features, we prescribe Calc. carb., whatever may be the complaints. Because during proving, above types manifested a large number of

symptoms with greater intensity. Similarly for curative purpose when this drug is applied, this group of patients responds very quickly and positively' (Mohanty 1983).

This perspective seems to directly contrast or even oppose the fundamental principles of matching symptoms from a proving to the diseased symptoms of a patient. As a consequence for both students and practitioners, not to mention patients, there is considerable confusion about what to do. What is more, students might find a rubric that looks like this...

"Fibre, lax., constitutions-agar., bar-c., bor., CALC., calc-p., Caps., cinnam., hep., KALI-C., MAG-C., MERC., OP., PHOS., SABAD., Sil., spong."

What on earth does this rubric mean? We need to understand the mis-use and mis-understanding of the word 'Constitutional'. It is important to realise that the concept of constitution is not a Hahnemannian approach, even though he did mention the constitution in his writing. It is important to grasp the concept accurately, and also to see how it is fraught with problems, speculation, practitioner ego/healer judgments, and sometimes even delusions on behalf of the practitioner. We also need to reflect on its value.

To further the confusion, many patients come to the homeopath for 'constitutional treatment'. They want to improve their overall health rather than wait until illness occurs. So to a degree, the general public have identified and integrated the ideas of homeopathy as capable of boosting weak constitution and decreasing susceptibility to disease. Members of the public in some countries seeking constitutional treatment expect that the homeopath will be interested in and get an understanding of the whole person. In fact, this is a by-product of a well-taken case.

The Prescribing Style in a Nutshell

Blackie (1986) nails the issues when she said,

> The constitutional medicine is a picture of the sum total of the strengths and weaknesses of the person, mentally, emotionally and physically. It is in the early undiagnosable stages of illness that we must find the constitutional medicines.

This is a style of prescribing for healthy people, or those in the early undiagnosed and sub-clinical phase of chronic disease. But some prominent authors have seen it differently and perhaps unwittingly added to the confusion by advocating that people who are ill need a *constitutional remedy*, a remedy not based on the Hahnemannian concept of a remedy chosen on the externalised symptoms of the internally deranged *wessen*, but on a metaphor, that by lobbing a pebble in to the middle of a diseased persons pond, the ripples that are created by that perfect intervention will reach the edge and organize all the individual symptoms in the path. Treat the *person* not the *disease* say some. Therefore the emphasis turns to learning everything there is to know about a person.

In homeopathy, the term constitution seems to be used most frequently when referring to *constitutional prescribing* to indicate the consideration of a wider, broader deeper totality than that called for by an acute episode. It is also used to differentiate between *types* of patients by describing them according to various systems of classification, and in determining common and characteristic symptoms of disease.

The perceived benefits of this essence prescribing and its clinical application seem to be:

1. In cases when patients offers their symptoms in a more complete and descriptive way

Constitution and Constitutional Prescribing

2. In cases where clear pathologic symptoms in the body level are missing
3. In reinforcement of a deep understanding of the patient and a wide and deep case-taking
4. For students, as an easier way to learn a whole contextual remedy picture.

This last point is a good one. Without doubt it is certainly more interesting and keeps students awake in the classroom. But what is the ultimate cost to homeopathy? What are the benefits of knowing a few lines of essence at the expense of knowing actual proving symptoms? On the other hand, the perceived limitations may well be:

1. What to do when the patient offers no essence or descriptive symptoms or one-sided pathology on the physical level
2. In emergency cases or acute illness
3. Beginners of homeopathy clinging to the essence picture and not recognizing it when it appears differently in the patient
4. For the most part, there is no essence in small remedies. In addition the question arises whether only one essence exists for every remedy, and if it can be transferred to other countries with different social, cultural, religious, gender, etc. context. In other words, just who determines what an essence is? Does it change as time passes through the decades? Just what does a worn out washerwoman actually look like in the 21st century? What does a ragged philosopher do for a living in contemporary London or Mumbai?
5. Caricatures of remedy pictures emerge based on essence. In Priestman's (1988) *Introduction to Borland's Homœopathy in Practice*, she states,

> It has been found that certain medicines are indicated very frequently, and that many people exhibit symptoms which correspond to the symptom picture or 'drug' picture of each of these medicines. ... Unfortunately, over the years, it has become a common habit for homeopathic doctors to speak of the medicines as if they were the patients and vice versa.

This is also a well-made point. The lazy description of a *Pulsatilla* or a *Sulphur* makes professional homeopaths seem like not very competent psychics, and reduces our credibility as a profession.

The Disadvantages of Constitutional Prescribing

> *Know your drugs by their peculiarities just as you recognize your friends not by the number of limbs but by their idiosyncrasies* (Tyler in Clarke 1925).

> *Type and temperament do not rule out a remedy if other indications correspond. If present, however, they are a valuable confirmation. Do not think that remedies particularly adapted to women are never indicated in the male sex. Sepia, for example, is frequently called for in men* (Clarke 1925).

What seems clear from the literature and from my own personal experience in practice is that if *Constitutional Prescribing* is done well then perhaps a number of cases may be improved. Done poorly, it leads to bland prescriptions of polycrests. It leads to inane conversations about a *Pulsatilla* person, a *Sulphur* person that bear no relationship to clinical reality. Germain Greer must need *Sepia*, Peter Jackson must need *Sulphur*, Nicole Kidman must need *Phosphorus*, Paris Hilton must need ... Constitutional prescribing seems to suggest that homeopaths are able to, like astrologers, have some sort of solution for the psychological, physical and emotional make up of a person. Constitutional prescribing seems to suggest that a single remedy that works every time in all situations. It is a lovely fantasy but a fantasy nonetheless. As mentioned, it flies in the face of homeopathy's origins and Hahnemann's directions.

Kent, Watson and Constitution

In his textbook Watson devotes a chapter to constitutional prescribing and focuses to a large extent on Kent. He sees constitutional prescribing as synonymous with what he calls Kentian and classical homeopathy. Mathur's (1975) brilliant chapter on *Constitutional Symptoms* does the same. Watson is correct on a number of points but on this one I am not so sure that he is right. I will attempt to untangle some of the confusion. To my mind, what Watson calls constitutional prescribing is not constitutional prescribing. Towards the end of this chapter, I will define constitutional prescribing as something else completely. Somehow in the 100 or so years from Kent to the present, significant confusion has arisen. If anything is to be learned from the previous chapter on Kent, although Kent wrote about constitution, his style of prescribing illustrated in his case-books was significantly different. In my opinion, Watson's chapter on constitutional prescribing misuses the term constitution; the chapter could well be titled Kentian homeopathy. Even on that count, I have misgivings because as I have argued in the previous chapter, there is a serious disconnect between what Kent did in his own practice, what he wrote in his books, what he said in his lectures, and what people said he said 80 or 100 years later. This is not to say that Mathur and Watson are entirely off the mark. Both their chapters are rich and full of stunning cases. Yet their description of constitutional prescribing is in fact Kentian. This is the point. Mathur (1975) writes,

> Dr Kent was of the opinion that it is the sick individual as a whole that needs to be cured rather than the totality of symptoms or the pathological condition of the diseased organs of the patient.

In his book, Watson accurately argues that the style of prescribing was the cornerstone of many successful homeopathic practices. In the 1980s and 90s in the US and the UK, this was without doubt the case. He then goes on to describe how, at the same time, this method is the most difficult and challenging of all homeopathic approaches. This represents a difficult duality for homeopaths because it is seductive on the one hand, and complex on the other. It is like golf. The promise of that sweetly hit ball that sails directly towards the pin as if some extraordinary force just happens to use your body to propel the ball the way you wanted it to go. Of course, it never happens like that, the next time or the next time, or the next time. Watson rightly describes the seductive nature of this style of prescribing because when it works, it really works. The results can seem to be miraculous. In itself, this is no problem because we also have miraculous results in surgery, osteopathy and accounting. The problem is that the method is not entirely replicable. This method allows such an individual degree of artistry to be brought into play to get the results being reported. In other words, all results derive from artistic, individualistic application and can't be repeated. The brilliant, individual homeopath is able to create an astonishing response due to individual, artistic interpretation. Furthermore, as Watson rightly points out, the emphasis is usually on the psychological components of the remedies and the patients, and seems to fit in with a new age philosophy that almost dovetails into the work of Deepak Chopra or Louise Hay (Watson 1991).

Massive Totality

It seems that most constitutional prescribing, from this perspective, is perceived as attempting to understand the essence, the gestalt of the disease, or another way of describing it might well be looking at the largest possible totality of symptoms of the person. The method involves taking the whole person into account as far as this is possible and treating the person on all levels - physical, mental and emotional. The expression, treat the person not the disease, comes from this line of thinking. I remember when I was a student loving the fact that in the UK, the *Society of Homoeopaths* advertising brochure included the (paraphrased) message, 'sweeping the doorstep when the snow is falling is a waste of time. It is not the snow that is the problem it is the winter'. This seemed to encapsulate the idea perfectly. It is easy to make the leap from looking at the broadest brush strokes of a person's health, life and make up to really relying on those key aspects of the psychological make-up. Who is this person? It is not too long a bow even to argue a case that Hahnemann also emphasised these aspects because in the *Organon* from aphorisms 210 to 213, he drew attention to the importance of the mental and emotional state of the patient when seeking to find a remedy. It is there in black and white.

Limitations

In the 1980s and 1990s, Watson rightly pointed out that

Kentian homeopathy was so widely taught in practice that many were misled into believing that it was the only way to practice homeopathy. Without a doubt, the constitutional approach has its place, where the patient is healthy, with sub clinical symptoms, and it can be extremely useful in chronic functional disorders where there are well-marked mental and emotional as well as general symptoms. This includes a wide demographic of patients who may present with allergies, irritable bowel syndrome, digestive problems, insomnia, migraines, menstrual and menopausal symptoms, in chronic conditions or syndromes where from a purely medical perspective there is no organic cause to be found. But it is less useful in advanced serious diseases or in those situations where patients are heavily medicated or use recreational drugs and alcohol. This is not to say that results cannot be obtained, but it is skilful work.

To the great detriment of the profession of homeopathy as a whole, many new graduates start off in practice attempting to prescribe using this seductive but difficult method, get bland results, and get dispirited and disheartened. Worse, many sometimes may feel that they are letting the patient or themselves and even homeopathy down by abandoning the best and highest ideal in favour of a specific treatment, therapeutic treatments or even a referral to another practitioner or discipline. Ultimately, this method requires putting all of the eggs in one basket. It is to aim for the centre, to hope for the best, to go for gold, to go for glory. During poorly done 'constitutional' homeopathy, it is almost as if the homeopath forgot to ask the crucial question, 'when were you last healthy, what are you like when you are healthy?' Suddenly in the case, there are 200 pieces of information instead of 10 clear characteristics.

In addition, the reality is that the response to the single dose of a high potency remedy can be easily disturbed and anti-doted by lifestyle, or by an anti-doting substance such as coffee, toothpaste or allopathic drugs. I am constantly astonished how many patients ask if they are allowed to use toothpaste when undergoing homeopathic treatment. Where does is this idea come from? Patients using this style of homeopathy have to be self disciplined, motivated and compliant, and that may well be the case in some islands in the Mediterranean Sea, in Kolkata, in Yorkshire or Cornwall but not in Sydney, New York City, Toronto, or Rio de Janeiro. A colleague of mine in Brisbane, Peter Berryman put it beautifully. 'How many times have I underwhelmed my patients over the years using one dose of medicine that was at best a guess?' He advocates, and taught me the value of prescribing until there is a response before stopping and observing. It was his teaching, in conjunction with reading and re-reading the *Organon* and *Chronic Diseases* by Hahnemann, which encouraged me to rethink what I thought I knew about homeopathy in this regard.

What is more, the business model for this style of prescribing is full of flaws, and many homeopaths have given up and moved away from homeopathy because they were only able to see their clients according to this perceived best practice, every six weeks. To sustain a practice, and earn a living from that practice, requires a massive number of clients. How much is it possible to charge a patient for a consultation, perhaps the third, when no medicine is given? That is awkward in the 21st century. This, as opposed to how Hahnemann prescribed or how homeopathy is prescribed in India, Germany, France and many other places around the world.

Another significant limitation is that the case taking and analysis can be very time consuming, and requires a high level of skill and perception by the practitioner to get consistently successful results. This limitation has the dual consequences of putting homeopathy out of the reach of would-be practitioners, enforcing the mistaken view that successful practitioners are somehow mystically brilliant. More importantly, it persuades a vast number of practically orientated homeopaths and doctors who could well use great homeopathic interventions in their cases to move on and find something else to do because they see that this style of prescribing is so difficult and requires an enormous amount of time. As Watson (1991) argues, if doctors and other health professionals attracted to homeopathy were first taught how to use other methods of homeopathy effectively, therapeutics, specifics, Bönninghausen technique, then perhaps they would be able to incorporate these methods into their practices much more easily before moving on to the more difficult techniques.

A further significant limitation of this style of prescribing is that it lends itself to the prescribing of a handful of remedies at worst, and a couple of dozen at best. These have been worked up into fully developed psychological profiles in the work of say Philip Bailey's *Homoeopathic Psychology*, Sankaran's *Soul of Remedies*, Vithoulkas' *Stolen Essences*, Laylor's *Homeopathic Psychiatry*, Whitmont's *Psyche and Substance*. In actual fact, having 100 well-developed remedies from this constitutional perspective limits practice to those more well-known polycrests. In this regard, it is the same as Herscu's excellent ideas on cycles and segments. The actual application of the method is limited by having so few developed remedy profiles.

Definitions of Constitution

Little argues that Hahnemann certainly made it clear that deep-acting homeopathic remedies affected the whole patient through the medium of the vital force. In this sense, chronic medicines are certainly "constitutional remedies" (Little 2011).

Vithoulkas (1980) in the *Science of Homeopathy* describes the constitution as the genetic inheritance template modified by our environment. He further describes it as a person's fundamental structure. A strong constitution is one that can withstand considerable pressure without falling ill. A weakened constitution in contrast has increased susceptibility to illness. My favourite example of this is the founder of modern Germany, Bismarck. It was estimated that he had smoked 185,000 cigars, and drunk 95,000 bottles of champagne during his life. That is a Rolls-Royce constitution.

Be that as it may, in the literature, the definitions of constitution are inconsistent:

Term	Definition	Source
Constitutional	Something that affects "the whole constitution" and is not "local". Something that is constitutional pertains to the "whole constitution".	Taber's Medical Dictionary
Constitution	The aggregate of person's physical and psychological characteristics.	Webster's Dictionary 1999
Constitutional	Belonging to or inherent in the character or makeup of a person's body or mind: a constitutional weakness for sweets.	Webster's Dictionary 1999

Constitution	The ensemble of characters of the individual, performed from the very beginning of the biological existence and transmutable as such to offsprings, which includes: (a) General appearance (psychosomatic make-up of individuals), (b) Temperament (ensemble of the possibilities in the physical, psychological, biological and dynamic spheres of the individual, (c) Diathesis., (d) Miasmatic background. Diathesis. This is an exaggerated constitutional type which predisposes individuals to disease if any adverse input is faced. Constitution. It is the natural condition of body and mind which includes general appearance (psychosomatic make-up of the individual), temperament (ensemble of the possibilities in the physical, psychological, biological and dynamic spheres of the individual), diathesis (this is an exaggerated constitutional type which predisposes one to disease if any adverse input is faced), and miasmatic background. A remedy can be prescribed on constitution-implied totality safely. Examples: Abrotanum: Constitution 1. Appearance: Marasmus of lower extremities (Apis. mel., Arg. nit., Ars. alb., Calc. carb., Plumb, Sanic., Upper - Plumb., Iod., Lyco.). 2. Temperament : (a) Ill-natured (b) Inhuman. Likes to do something cruel. 3. Miasm : Psoric and sycotic. 4. Diathesis : Tubercular. Aconite: Constitution 1. Appearance: It is adapted to young robust persons having dark hairs and eyes with rigid muscle fibres, full of plethoric habits, who lead sedentary life. 2. Temperament : Sanguine. 3. Miasm : Psoric and sycotic. 4. Diathesis : Tubercular.	Mohanty 1983

| Constitution | Constitution: is that aggregate of hereditary characters, influenced more or less by environment, which determines the individual's reaction, successful or unsuccessful, to the stress of environment. | Close 1924 |

From these definitions, especially when couched in this type of language, it is easy to see how homeopathic treatment and homeopathic medicines are perceived to treat a type of person or a constitution.

Etymology of the Word 'Constitution' in the Context of Homeopathy

David Little (2011) comes to the rescue to clarify the meaning of constitution in the context of homeopathy.

> In the German text Hahnemann used the term, beschaffenheit (make up), which is usually translated into English as the word "constitution". This, however, does not reflect all the usages of the German term. This term can be used in a variety of ways that have nothing to do with the human constitution. The root word "schaffen" means "to do, to make, to work". Beschaffen is a verb that means, "to procure, make something available", and as an adjective it means, "constituted". The English word, constitution, comes from the Latin root, constituere, which means constitutes: to set up, to establish, to form or make up, to appoint to give being to. Beschaffenheit is usually translated as constitution in relationship to the Latin root "constiture" in homoeopathic works. *Chambers Dictionary* defines constitution as: the natural condition of the body or mind; disposition. In this sense constitutional means; inherent in the natural frame, or inherent nature. The *W. Turner's Dictionary*, published in Leipzig in the 1830s, defines

the German term, Beschaffenheit, as nature, quality, temper, condition, constitution, disposition and circumstance. Therefore, the term Beschaffenheit may include any circumstance, condition or quality related to the physical constitution and mental temperament as well as dispositions. This shows how the term was used in Hahnemann's lifetime. Modern German may not clearly convey this meaning. The homeopathic usage is related directly to the practice of medicine not the common usage of a layperson on the street. The term constitution is used at least 16 times in *The Chronic Diseases*. Pages 30, 34, 35, 48, 75, 90, 98, 99, 101, 103, 142, 143, 145, 181, 242, 243, etc.

The term "beschaffenheit" may have the following meanings in German.

1. A quality of someone or something that is inherent or a characteristic trait that serves to define or describe its possessor.
2. The make-up or way something is composed or arranged, its constitution, composition, construction or nature.
3. A medical term for inherent traits and qualities of the human being [constitution; make-up and qualities of the body and/or soul].

The meaning of Beschaffenheit in English depends on the context in which it is used. For example, in aphorism 5 we find the term "die erkennbare Leibes-Beschaffenheit", which means ascertainable or recognisable bodily make-up. This term "Leib" is not commonly used in modern German but in older times it meant the body with special emphasis on the abdomen. This area is a key centre for storage of vitality in the organism. The vitalists and Mesmerists considered the vital energy to have two major centres of force. These are the energy of the spirit in the brain and pineal gland and the reserves of vital power stored in the abdomen. This reference to the objective make-up of the 'centre of the body' refers to the nature of physical constitution and vitality of the individual that is being investigated (Little Hahnemann on Constitution and Temperament 2011).

Advocates of Constitutional Prescribing

Numerous examples exist in the homeopathic literature from Hahnemann that refer to constitution and constitutional prescribing. In the *Dictionary of Organon* (Joardar 2002) writes,

Constitutional diagnosis; To assess the peculiarities of an individual during his or her healthy state. The peculiarities of each individual are put together and assessed in three ways. These are:

- Actual constitutional diagnosis
- Developmental constitutional diagnosis
- Environmental constitutional diagnosis

The actual constitutional diagnosis is done by observing the peculiarities of the individual during his healthy state, to be compared with the pathologic state. Only then, 'the physician clearly perceives what is to be cured in disease that is to say, in every individual case, of disease' (Sec 3 of Organon). The developmental constitutional diagnosis is done by examining and finding out the various etiological factors 'the most significant points in the whole history of the chronic disease' (Sec 5 of Organon). The environmental constitutional diagnosis is the assessment of the modalities, or the individual's characteristic conditions, which means how does the environment, including time, place and circumstances affect this person. Constitutional medicine: Any and every antipsoric medicines are constitutional medicines. A constitutional medicine corrects the constitutional defects, inherent and acquired. A constitutional medicine acts best only after other miasmatic effects are removed or brought to latent state. Antipsoric drug: Hahnemann's antipsoric drugs are nothing but constitutional drugs... (Joardar 2002).

On the constitutional approach, Kanjilal in *Writings on Homoeopathy* argues,

Constitution is a term which covers vast dimensions in width, depth and intricacy. It has two fundamental factors (a) the endogenous and (b) the exogenous. The endogenous factors are innate in the organism incurred from the heredity through the genes. They endow the organism with various forms of proneness, tendencies, susceptibilities, immunities which are technically known as analogues. The exogenous factors are incurred gradually and steadily since birth, from the various intimate details of the environmental factors. Ultimately, these exogenous factors may become so much intimately mingled up or even compounded with the endogenous factors, that they both together may give a new type of constitution to the particular individual- totally distinct from the progenitors and even others of the same species. From this approach we shall find that each individual has a distinctly characteristic constitution of his/her own (as also of each drug dynamis). Various distinct types of constitution have been given distinct names since the earliest history of systemic medicine both in the East as well as the West. And since the advent of homeopathy in the last century it has been authentically noticed that every individual drug has a special relative affinity for particular types of constitution. This fact was clearly noticed by Hahnemann himself while conducting his human pharmacological experiments (provings) as well as in his critical and meticulous therapeutic experience. This line of observation, work and practical application in approaching the Similimum has been further developed by Dr Grauvogl, Woodward, Burnett, Hughes, O. Lesser and others (Kanjilal 1977).

Furthermore, Bhanja in *Constitution: Drug Pictures & Treatment* argues:

To a Homoeopath, the study of constitution of a patient under treatment is undoubtedly, of paramount importance. The task involved is, however, quite fascinating. Here we study the fountain-head of the living organism, which speaks in the language of various idiosyncrasis, susceptibilities, predispositions, temperaments as well as a series of mental and physical expressions got up by nature as it works through diverse channels in the dynamic plane of the constitution (Bhanja 1993).

Example: Causticum

Constitutional taint: It corresponds to all the three miasms- Psora, sycosis, and syphilis. Scrofulous constitution. It has scrofulous inflammation about ears, eyes, and scalp. Scrofulous children.

Chronic diseases in old, broken down constitutions.

Typical subjects: Dark-haired persons with rigid fibres. Lymphatic, torpid temperament. It is often called for in dyspeptics and consumptives in whom there is a chronic tendency to diarrhoea. Persons who suffer from chronic constipation. Patient is chilly. His conditions are aggravated by washing, bathing, open air, after being drenched. Children who are slow in learning to walk. Persons in whom weakness progresses gradually towards paralysis. Women in whom sexual appetite is wanting. Persons in whom itch has been supressed by mercury and sulphur; burning itch.

Notes and features: Paralytic weakness, paralysis, tension and shortening of muscles, burning, soreness and rawness, cracks, fissures, warts.

Disposition: timid, nervous and fearful, esp. at night. Melancholy with weeping mood. Child cries at the least thing. Tendency to make mistakes when speaking. Indisposition to labour. Mistrust of the future.

Appearance: Yellow colour of face. Eruptions of red pimples on face. Tetters on the lower lip. Painful corns in the feet.

Side affinities: affects right side to a remarkable degree.

Desires: Desire for beer, smoked meat, pungent things.

Aversions: Aversion to sweet things and delicacies.

Modalities. Obliquely contributory: chronic hoarseness. Want of secretion of milk. Difficult first menstruation. Obstruction of speech (Bhanja 1993).

Drilling downwards into literature we see that most of the information comes from two sources, Clarke and Lesser. Clarke (1925) started with an introductory paragraph:

Many observers in all schools have noticed certain tendencies to particular disease-manifestations in certain types of individuals, and among those who have succeeded in reducing the different forms to specific types there is a fairly unanimous selection of the number Three (Clarke 1925).

It is in the writings of Clarke that we see for the first time the merging of the ideas of constitution and miasm.

> After years of patient observation Hahnemann saw that a superficial symptom-resemblance between drug-symptoms and disease-symptoms was sometimes insufficient to show the true specific correspondence. Eventually he tracked down the underlying constitutional dyscrasiae to the three "miasms", and he named them, Syphilis, Sycosis and Psora. The first of these was due to the initial sore of the chancre, the second to the constitutional effects of gonorrhoea and the third to the chronic effects of itch poisoning. The three typical remedies indicated in the three dyscrasiae were (1) Mercury, (2) Thuja, (3) Sulphur. These were the typical remedies of each of the three classes (Clarke 1925).

Clarke was alluding to the clear observation that Hahnemann identified three chronic miasms, and to his mind it was no surprise that these correlated in some ways to the observations of Paracelsus and to Rademacher.

> Rademacher again, also found a three-fold division. His division was an aetiological or causative one, and varied as the peculiar cause at work. In some epidemics one type would rule and the remedy for that type would be Copper. At another season a somewhat different type would prevail and for that Iron would be needed; for a third again Cubic Nitre or Natrum Nitricum would be the remedy. And each of these remedies had allied remedies of its own type (Clarke 1925).

Clarke then introduces the work of von Grauvogl who wrote about three identifiable constitutional types. Edward von Grauvogl (1811-1877) proposed the classification of body types into hydrogenoid, carbo-nitrogenoid, and oxygenoid.

Eduard von Grauvogl's Part 1 & 2 is one of the rarest *homeopathy* books in existence. First published in 1870 no subsequent editions were published due to the printing plates being burned in the Chicago fire of 1871. He discusses three primary constitutions: oxygenoid, hydrogenoid and carbo-nitrogenoid and how they relate to *homeopathic* practice.

1. The Hydrogenoid Constitution is characterised by an excess of Hydrogen and consequently of water in the blood and tissues. 2. The Oxygenoid is characterised by an excess of Oxygen, or, at least, by an exaggerated influence of Oxygen on the organism. 3. The Carbo-nitrogenoid Constitution is characterised by an excess of Carbon and Nitrogen.'

'The Hydrogenoid Constitution corresponds closely with Hahnemann's Sycosis but it covers a much wider area and, is not by any means confined to the acquired or inherited results of gonorrhoeal infection. Intermittent-fevers and periodicity come within its sphere. At the present time Vaccinosis, or the constitutional sufferings from cow-pox infection, should certainly be included under this heading. The antidotal relation to it of Thuja, which is one of Grauvogl's principal remedies for Hydrogenoids is a clear indication that this is so. Moreover, Burnett told me that he regarded Gout as belonging to the Sycotic diseases. The Oxygenoid Constitution is Hahnemann's Syphilis but we have no examples of its treatment as we have of the other two. The Carbo-nitrogenoid Constitution is Hahnemann's Psora'.

Von Grauvogl wrote (Clarke 1925),

If the patient states, that he feels worse in cold, or damp weather, and in the rain, then I know that I have to choose among the remedies which are similar to his disease, such only as contain a greater percentage of a combination of O with C and

H, consequently produce more heat and diminish the influence of the water. Hence the symptoms of a disease in this constitution of the body are aggravated by everything which in any way increases the atoms of water in the organism, by baths, for example, and that all the same whether they are mineral baths or simple water baths; or whatever increases the attractions of the organic molecules for water, as, for example, the eating of animals which have lived in the water, as fishes, etc. All diseases in such constitutions are increased by cold, also by cold and cooling food and drinks, for example, sour milk, hard eggs, cucumbers and mushrooms, but chiefly by living near water, and especially standing water.

Hydrogenoid Constitution

This was characterised by slow nutrition. Retains excessive water in a passive manner. Patient is like a sponge. Oedema of the extremities. Sensitive to the humidity and the seaside. Slow, fatigued, without life, apathetic, heavy and indolent. Poor renal function. Asthmatics, rheumatics, obesity. Round, short limbed, obese. Cold clammy hands. Medicines: Nat Sulph, Nat Carb, Calc Carb, Mag Carb, Phos, Siliea, Iodine, Bromine, Muriaticum, Borax, Thuja, Carbo Veg, Pulsatilla, Conium, Apis, Spigelia, Amm Muriaticum. Corresponds closely with Hahnemann's Sycosis.

From von Grauvogl's practice

Case I:

Catalepsy, etc. Nux and Ipec. in alternation; later Aranea diadema. A woman, 29, of healthy parents still living (the father 89, mother 75), has suffered from her youth according to her statement, on the slightest bodily exertion or mental emotion from palpitation of the heart. The only cause she could think of was that in her youth she was very timid and easily frightened, which she ascribed to hearing children's tales. Physical examination revealed neither valvular nor other defects except rapid action even during complete bodily rest; the pulse was 80. Of children's diseases she had had whooping-cough and nothing else. The colour of her skin is brilliant white, the skin clear, having never presented any eruptions, hair dark-brown, eyes blue, figure slender, form symmetrical. She had already given birth to three children without difficulty, but has suffered with an incessant headache since her last confinement, which was quite normal, and after which she nursed her child for two months, when she weaned it for lack of milk. All this happened six years before she came to see me; The headache occupied no definite place but extended from the forehead over to the occiput, only sometimes it was most severe on the vertex. This headache did not permit her to visit or receive visits from her most intimate friends even, because it was so greatly agg. by talking or hearing others talk that vomiting ensued; and to make the pain at all endurable she had to take to her bed, where she remained three or four days motionless and lying on her back; Not unfrequently pain in the stomach set in which ceased of itself after the discharge of sour water rising in the throat with nausea, and also the eructations of tasteless gas, which was more frequently induced by the ingestion of vegetable acids or vegetables. Her appetite was good but not ravenous; she refused to eat meat, even the smell of it was repugnant to her. The menses, as indeed was indicated by the pain in the vertex, were irregular, scanty and pale, and were generally six to eight days too early. In the interval there was more or less leucorrhoea which was debilitating, and the accession of the menses was announced by a violent colic. The respiration was unrestrained, but in the apex of the right lung there was a dull respiratory murmur, in a small portion without any change of sound on percussion. She never had any cough and the digestion was regular. To the above symptoms were added, since her last confinement also, cataleptic attacks, almost every morning, after waking from an uninterrupted, good, but not refreshing sleep. Thus, if her husband did not notice in the morning that she closed her eyes again shortly after waking, and at the same time sighed once deeply, and at this very moment did not at once shake her shoulders with both hands and call to her aloud, then nothing would arouse her from the motionless insensible condition lasting from one to two hours, in which one could raise her arms and legs in any direction without them returning to their former position. These attacks had come and still came and went without any known cause, but they left behind them no further ailment. As regards the concomitant circumstances of these pains, I learned that they were much more violent in damp weather than in dry and, in fact, her general condition was agg. at such times, so that this woman, who was previously lively and joyful became more and more melancholic. The many physicians who had been consulted, the many cures which had been tried for her, and especially all use of baths, increased her sufferings. I further learned that her headache especially, even aside from considering the influence of the weather, was most violent in the afternoon and evening; that consequently it increased in severity irregularly though periodically, which also pointed to an affection of the nervous system; that she constantly suffered from chilliness, hence the whole winter through was obliged to keep her room very warm, and even in summer she had cold hands and feet, notwithstanding all her clothing and other means for keeping warm...In brief, among all the remedies which might be indicated according to the law of similarity for the case, which certainly was not easily to be cured, there were mainly two of which I knew at once from many years' practice, that they not only produce a more active interchange of substance, and hence would occasion more warmth in the body, and would not only restore the lost power of resistance against the influences of cold and moisture, but would also have an enlivening effect on the nervous system. These two are Nux vomica and Ipecac. I have also observed that each of these remedies had far less effect in these directions when given by itself, alone, than when they were permitted to operate on the organism in succession. I therefore ordered Nux 3 to be taken at 7 or 8 a.m. , and 6 p.m. , and three or four drops of Ipec. 3, every two hours during the day, although it was the fervent desire of this patient to be delivered as soon as possible, first of all and at any price, from the headache which tormented her without ceasing, for this was the most annoying of all her sufferings and hindered her in most of her duties. Had I sought to conform to this wish I should surely have had to select quite other remedies, and probably a long series of them in succession, and most probably too with no favourable result - or no result at all. Hence I told the patient that I could not meet her wishes at once but on the other hand promised her with all assurance the complete restoration of her health and, within the space of a year at furthest, a deliverance from all her sufferings; adding that before her headache could be relieved she would first have to notice a greater sensation of warmth in her body. Besides, I forbade her to take any baths for more than five minutes, and for the time being her accustomed washing in cold water; and also her remaining near water, especially standing water. I forbade her also coffee and, of course, vinegar, fruit and fish. This was on the 1st of May. I visited the patient every eight days, having told her to take the remedies as directed for eight days, and then to set them aside for eight days, and so on. On the 4th of June she stated that she really thought she was not so cold as she had been for many years, for she could now even sit in the shade in the garden, a thing which had hitherto been impossible to her. At the same time the cataleptic attacks had so diminished in intensity that she had often only a mere intimation of them. But headache and palpitation of the heart still unfitted her for all occupation. The cataleptic attacks now happily had returned but seldom for several weeks (except the merest indication of them), and even the headaches were no longer aggravated in the evening, when, at the end of July, her children got measles one after the other. She would not entrust the care of them to anybody but was unspeakably happy that she could sustain the bodily exertions and mental excitements thereupon attendant, which a month before would have been utterly impracticable. During the whole course of the children's sickness I naturally intermittent the use of the Ipecac. and Nux, and only gave her Aconite occasionally, as she was very much alarmed at the condition of one of the children whose disease had become very severe. After this had all passed off without injury for the children as well as for the mother, the whole family went for eight days into the mountains of Bavaria. This agreed very well with all except the mother; for she took a sail upon a lake, which I had expressly forbidden, and after this day felt chilly and cold again, the headache also being notably aggravated. As I had found in my practice that Aranea diadema even more than Nux. and Ipec. diminishes the influence of hydrogen upon the system, and since it was also indicated according to the law of similars, I directed her to take four or five drops every two hours. The warmth of the body soon returned, and for the first time the menses waited for the full four weeks, but was more abundant and of a red colour. It is a pity that in other cases, the Aranea diadema produces very violent haemorrhage, especially from the lungs, which fact calls for caution in the use of this great remedy. After two weeks the patient noticed a marked relief of the headaches which had returned; and after eight days this headache entirely ceased for some days. The cataleptic attacks had already entirely disappeared for about a fortnight and have not returned since. But it was not till the 13th of September that the patient finally assured me that, in the most striking manner, just as if she had been delivered from a bad habit, she had not had the slightest sensation of a headache for four days. Nor has it ever returned again after the lapse of six years. After another fortnight, during which time the patient had personally superintended the removal from her summer residence to the city, a thing which before was not to be thought of, she called my attention to the fact that after having been in the city three days she had experienced increased palpitation of the heart again, as had been the case every year after this change. Now I gave her Puls. 30, since the constitutional conditions for the previous ailments were all removed. As the favourable effects of the 30th began to wear off in a few days I gave Puls 3. This had the desired effect within six days and the heart's action became regular and remained so. I now gave her finally Magnes. sulph. 6, after which even her leucorrhoea diminished, and now disappeared entirely, not to return. Thus, at the end of November of this year this woman was perfectly free from all her sufferings of years' standing. She went into society again and renewed her youth. From the above rule and a large experience I know that neither Puls. nor Magnes. sulph. would have afforded relief so readily had not the constitutional treatment preceded.

Case II:

Hydrogenoid Intermittent. Aranea diadema. A pupil of the Academy of Arts, 23, sent for me because he could no longer pursue his art with love and pleasure; he felt himself so constantly oppressed in the chest that a walk across the room even put him out of breath; He attributed his trouble to an intermittent fever acquired in a university city some months before, which was removed by very large doses of Quinine, of which he often had to take 20 grains at once. Since that time an enlargement of the spleen had remained which reached to the space between third and fourth ribs. At that place a dark mark made on the skin with Nitrate of Silver by the professor of the City Hospital to mark the outlines of the enormous swelling of the spleen was still visible. Below the first line there were other reddish marks, the traces of similar outlines which had indicated the gradual swelling and ascent of the spleen. The heart was pushed to the right and beat feebly, 98 to the minute. The respiration was very short, raised the right side of the thorax only, 30 times to the minute, and audible only at the very apex of the right lung. The appearance of this young man of course indicated disease of the spleen. The upper edge was found again between the third and fourth ribs, though in consequence of earlier improvement, it must previously have stood lower. As soon as I entered the house where he resided and which stood close to the water, I observed that all the walls were very damp. I was now convinced that I should find a disease-form arising from a hydrogenoid constitution, for such a house, especially when it is but little or not at all exposed to the sun, is very sure to harbour disease-forms of the most varied kinds, but which ought not to be treated according to their names as they are set down in the text-books of special Pathology and Therapeutics in which their treatment is struck off after one and the same model. Here, however, the disease was a relapse induced by the damp dwelling. On being questioned the patient said that he was chilly day and night, although it was midsummer, and as often as it rained he has always felt worse. He also acknowledged that especially during the past four weeks, during which time he had lived in this room, he had felt worse than ever. On constitutional grounds, as well as on the strength of the indication of the law of similars, there was no doubt that the remedy indicated was Aranea diadema. He was ordered it in the 2x, four or five drops in a spoonful of water every two hours. After eight days the upper border of the spleen was behind the fifth rib and fell within six weeks to the seventh. The heart returned to its place; and in the part of the lung which had been compressed the respiratory murmur was again distinctly heard, and the patient felt himself well again. Nevertheless I advised him to continue the remedy some time longer...

Case V:

Uterine Fibroma in a Hydrogenoid. Nux and Ipec. A married woman, 28, who gave birth to her last child some years ago without difficulty, and who appeared to have no predisposition to any disease, complained that for six months her abdomen had been greatly enlarging to such an extent that everyone had been congratulating her on a new pregnancy, which, however, could not be the case, as she had none of the usual indications. Her periods were regular, every four weeks as usual and only for a few weeks she had had a constant leucorrhoea. The abdomen was round and everywhere uniformly hard all round in a circumference of about six inches diameter above the symphysis pubis, but it was entirely free from pain even on pressure. An examination showed a condition of the os uteri as in the fourth month of pregnancy. The os was high and directed backwards. Around it, in the bottom of the vagina, the same cartilaginous resistance was felt as externally on the abdomen, and this resistance formed the immediate prolongation of the cervix and thus belonged to the womb ... Thus it could only be considered a fibrous polypus, or, more probably, a round fibroid within the uterus. Owing to the size of the growth an operation was not to be thought of, though to the physiological school any other resource is unknown...This woman did not look at all ill, had a good appetite and slept well, only she became sooner more wearied by her domestic duties than was previously the case, in the discharge of which duties she was very much incommoded by this tumour in her abdomen. This was on April 4th. The remedies which I administered internally so long as I had my eye on the object of the disease alone were attended with no success, and from month to month the abdomen increased in size until - unhappily it was not till September 6th - I enquired about the concomitant circumstances. She acknowledged that she felt chilly every evening, and was worse, that is, there was more rapid enlargement of the abdomen, during moist weather. On this account I prescribed Nux 3 and Ipec. 3 in alternation every two hours, and with such effect that as early as September 26th the tumour had decreased in size to a diameter of three inches, though it could still be distinctly felt above the pubic bone. The cervix had also assumed a convex position and by the 30th of October had become quite perpendicular again; the lips were somewhat swollen, but the leucorrhoea had disappeared. The improvement continued without interruption, during frequent suspension of the remedies, and four years have passed without any complaint from the woman, so that her complete cure was certainly accomplished.

Oxygenoid

In addition to the Hydrogenoid, he introduced the idea of the Oxygenoid constitution. Clarke (1925) wrote,

> It will thus be seen that Grauvogl included under the term "Oxygenoid" much more than is included in Hahnemann's and Bazin's "Syphilis", just as "Hydrogenoids" included more than the results of Gonorrhoea. ... Speaking generally on the remedies for the Oxygenoid constitution, Grauvogl says, that on account of too active an influence of Oxygen on the body this seeks its remedies mainly in the Carbon and Nitrogen series which prevent the oxidation of tissues. "Rademacher places Iron in the first rank, but I put first Hydriodate of Potash - Kali iodatum - because it absorbs all the ozone. Here the carbon and alkalis rich in carbon have a different effect, as Graphites, Petroleum, Kreosote, Benzoic acid, Citric acid, Hydrocyanic acid, Laurocerasus, and, chiefly for inductive reasons, Antozone water, corresponding indeed to iodosmone water. Furthermore, Nitric acid; also many so-called narcotics, especially Aconite. Moreover, China, Quinine and Arsenic (given alone and not in alternation with Nux); and also the metals which are capable of suspending the process of decomposition, hence Chromium and Kali bichromicum". Other symptoms constantly found in oxygenoids are : Excessive elimination of urea and phosphates; Plethora - great quantity of blood; Much oxygen fixed on the haemoglobin; Excessive thinness. Animal heat, strong after meals and feeble in the intervals. Vigorous appetite which persists astonishingly

during illnesses. Abstinence, on the contrary, is badly tolerated. Amel. by Rest and Food. Agg. by Cold, Sea-air, Low altitudes. Oxygenoids are what are commonly called nervous individuals characterised by great physical and mental activity.

Oxygenoid:

Hypersensitive to exaggerated acceleration of chemical reactions and changes. Lower resistence to toxins and poisons → hperthermy. Patient burns up too much energy and does not assimilate well → demineralisation. Over active patient. Pre tubercular. Long limbed, lean. Hyperthyroidism. White spots on the nails. Medicines: Mercury, Kali Iod, Ferrum met, Graphites, Petroleum, Kreosote, Aconite, China, Arsenicum album, Chromium, Kali bichromium, most acid medicines. Closely corresponds with Hahnemann's Syphilis.

Carbo-nitrogenoid Constitution

This constitution is characterised by insufficient oxygenation and the diseases it produces are called diseases of retarded nutrition... General symptoms are great frequency of respirations with shallowness; short breath, frequent pulse, blood charged with melanotic cellules. Constipation or diarrhoea, flatulence, urinary troubles, gouty pains in the head, gouty swellings, vertigo, ataxia, dullness of the head, somnolence, yawning, hypochondriasis, irritability, and extraordinary impatience. Copious uric acid and oxalates in urine. - Epistaxis and haemorrhoids. - Pruritus. - Precocious baldness with perspiration of the head. - Cerebral fatigue. - Unhealthy skin, fetid and acid perspiration, boils, eczema, urticaria. Remedies included Cupr., Phos., Sulph., Camph., Hepar sulph., Aco., Merc., Aur., Argent., Plumb., Plat.,

Ol. tereb., Rhus., Dulc., Cham., Lyc., Bov., Bel., Nux. 30 (alone - not alternated as for Hydrogenoids), Digit., Hyos., Apis., Lob. infl.

Carbo Nitrogenoid:

Slow oxygenation → auto intoxication. Dimilution of oxygen by tissues. Periodic fits of elimination. Psoriasis, eczema, arthritis. Hands dry, lean, like parchment. Fingers crooked. medicines: Cuprum, Phosphorus, Sulphur, Camphor, Hepar Sulp, Mercury, Aurum, Arg Nit, Plumbum, Platina, Rhus Tox, Dulcamarra, Chamomilla, Lycopodium, Belladonna, Nux Vomica, Hyoscyamus, Apis, Lobellia. Corresponds closely with Hahnemann's Psora.

From von Grauvogl's Practice

Case II:

Headache, Vertigo, Dyspnoea, Palpitation, etc. - Arg. nit. A blooming girl of 19, menstruating regularly, suffered for five years without interruption from pressing pains over the whole head, sometimes only on the vertex, sometimes on the left frontal bone, which were agg. by firm pressure on the painful parts, and were ascribed to immoderate dancing in the evening, while the many physicians whose advice was sought had been able to give no relief whatever. On being questioned the patient further states that she suffers from vertigo and is easily tired, whilst at the same time she is losing her memory. On going upstairs her breathing is hurried and she has palpitation of the heart. The tongue is coated white. Appetite and sleep are very good, but she is too sleepy during the day; pains in the stomach here and there, frequently for weeks at a time, with nausea and vomiting even. On feeling the pulse I noticed a trembling of the hands; pulse 98; a burning feeling in the region of the heart; she can breathe pretty deeply without pain, but cannot hold her breath long, and on breathing only vesicular respiration can be heard, yet there is no cough. The urine is pale and poor in solid constituents. Nothing more was to be learned. After the fourth dose of Argent. nit., 2, the girl was relieved of all her headaches and she could afterwards breathe much more easily. Her palpitation was relieved also, and her memory returned in full force, for which an interval of five days only was necessary.

Case III:

Calculous Pyelitis - Arg. nit. A woman, 37, of lively temperament and healthy appearance, who was married and had given birth to one child, and had recovered well from her confinement, had suffered during the last three years, without any known cause, from attacks of so-called nephritic colic recurring periodically every three months. Attempts were made to relieve the excessive pains by the applications of leeches to the region of the kidneys on both sides, and by the use of purgatives, and it was only after the patient was reduced to the last degree by this treatment that the pains gradually remitted. On account of her change of residence I was called in to see her in her last attack and found her in most acute pains in the regions of both kidneys, the pains extending down the ureters to the bladder. She was lying motionless on her back, since every motion of her body caused her inexpressible pain, and touching the region of the kidneys increased these pains in the highest degree. She was perspiring freely; pulse 130; she sought by frequent and short breaths to avoid deep inspiration, for this increased her pains insufferably. The urine contained blood, was scanty, passed often, but only a little at a time and by drops. It contained a visible sediment of crystallised uric acid and pus, with amorphous gravely concretions, some as large as half a lentil. The clear urine above the sediment was acid and gave a deposit when heated with nitric acid. Thus it was clear that I had a case of calculous pyelitis to deal with. She begged to have leeches applied, as she had some already and previously she had always experienced relief from them. But nevertheless, she was afraid to incur the pain of turning on her face, which the application would have necessitated, and so was dissuaded from their use on the promise of receiving relief in some other manner. This I could promise when I prescribed Arg. nit. 2, four or five drops every hour. When I saw her again after six hours she was very grateful to me for such prompt relief and so easily accomplished; for a quarter of an hour after she had taken the first drops she felt greater relief from her pains than was previously the case under the use of leeches. She was able to urinate at once without hindrance, and more copiously, and she was already lying without pain, yet motionless, because the least motion renewed her pains again. On this account she restrained the urine as long as possible; this has been impossible before, but could now be accomplished with ease. Next morning the pulse was 80 again, and she breathed as when in health. After eight days no more uric acid crystals were passed, but only small concretions. She showed me one of the size of a lentil, which she had passed without pain, and that was the last sign of her disease, which had lasted three years. For curiosity I had taken some of the urine on the first day for further examination. Besides what has been already mentioned, it contained no trace of triple phosphates, but the well-known epithelia of the mucous membrane of the pelvis of the kidney. Hence the pus could not have come from the bladder. Three years have now passed without a relapse (Clarke 1925).

Lesser and Nebel

Otto Lesser was against the division of constitutions into causative or biochemical types as done by Hahnemann with his miasms (Psora, Syphilis, Sycosis), Rademacher (Iron, Copper, Natrum nitricum), Grauvogl (Hydrogenoid, Oxygenoid, Carbonitrogenoid) and Schussler (12 tissue remedies). He preferred a more phenomenological approach in drug proving, and in his clinic used the concept of constitution for treating the patient. He argued that by matching the totality of symptoms of disease to the totality of drug symptoms, homeopaths automatically cover the constitution without making any biochemical or causative theory. Each homeopathic medicine has its own constitution developed during proving. Also all human beings have their own peculiar constitutions that can be taken care of by corresponding drug pictures evolved during proving. This is the inductive logic, the phenomenological approach which is the foundation of homeopathic thinking (Lesser 1934). He was no friend of von Grauvogl's ideas.

> Our present attitude toward the question of constitution should approximate reality as far as possible. But actually there are no types but persons. Therefore, we should give to each person his own constitution. We need speak of constitutions only in order to comprehend peculiarities of individuals in certain respects and to describe them with type conceptions. To determine this property as a deviation from an imaginary norm is as foreign to reality as it is useless. It is only by the special relations of a living organism to its environment that we can determine its properties. But it is not the characterization of a man in all respects that interests us, when as physicians we speak of constitution, but chiefly in his tendency to become sick. It is necessary to appreciate this

intimate actual state before one can begin a study of its basis. A division according to inherited and acquired properties does not help us here. For the recognition and utilization the tendencies can be observed in their transient connections; likewise a rigid separation of constitutional anomalies and transitions to disease is not justified in actuality. Our most important task must be the recognition of susceptibility. The more the disposition reveals itself in the total person and not merely in the single organ, the sooner the conception of constitution can be applied. Eventually, we can depart from the conception. It would be better to speak of the anlage, the disposition of the total person. On the one side one can seek to recognize the present individual-historic developmental relations from the inherited and acquired, on the other side the organic configuration of the total disposition from the disposition of the parts. But a worthwhile synthesis is obtained first through the recognition of direction. As through the function of the organic structure the arrangement and meaning of a part becomes comprehensible to practical understanding so also the recognition of "for what purpose" in the anlage first yields a worthwhile unit. All these attempts to fix these indefinitely determined clinically derived dispositions into universal tissue systems, systems of chemical or nervous regulation, must be further supplemented. The division of Grauvogl is nothing more than a further attempt at division which goes back to three types of metabolic utilization; and indeed it is the most radical because it even goes back to the chemical elements of metabolic utilization' (Lesser 1934).

Nor did he have much time for the biochemical opinions of Schüssler.

This is the place to glance at the so-called "biochemistry" (commonly called biochemic therapy) of Schüssler. For the originally homeopathic physician, W. Schüssler, the decisive impression was that the mineral substances natural to the body must have an especially unique position. With grotesque onesidedness he limited his entire therapy to twelve so-called cell or tissue salts: ferr. phosphor., magnes. phosphor., calc. phosphor., kali phosphor., kal. chlorat., kal. sulfur., natrum muriat., natr. phosphor., natr. sulfur., calc. fluorat., silica, calc. Sulfur' (Lesser 1934).

Antoine Nebel, a homeopath in Lausanne, Switzerland formulated his own slant on constitutional typology, as well as developed his own potency machine that prepared Korsakovian dilutions of homeopathic medicines. His categories include: Carbonic, Phosphoric and Fluoric.

Carbonic

Short, fat, overweight or obese
Face generally round or square, and symmetrical
Hands are short and square with short fingers, square on the tips
Rigidity of ligaments
Reactions, and diseases are slow, progressive, chronic and insidious
Obesity, gout, gall stones and kidney stones, chronic eczema, hypertension
Retain water and fat
Sensitive to cold, but do not like direct sun
Prefer peace, order and method
At best a methodical worker, at worst lazy and indifferent
Prone to Psoric and Sycotic disease

Medicines include: the Carbonates of Calcium, Baryta, Kali and Magnesium, Graphites, Carbo Veg, Lycopodium, Sulphur.

Phosphoric

Tall, thin, limbs are very straight when extended Above average height
Face is triangular with a large forehead down to a narrow chin Hands and fingers are long and slender Limbs are very straight
Dentition can be poor
Reactions are quick, but brief due to their weakness Easily tired Prone to loss of weight and de-mineralisation, hyperthyroidism, juvenile acne
Cold sensitive, but need fresh air
Excitable and hypersensitive, with little patience
Often work in fits and starts Suits artistic types
Prone to tubercular diseases

Medicines include: Calc Phos, Phosphorus, Hepar Sulph, Nat mur, Ferrum, Arsenicum Album, Stannum.

Flouric

Variable height, usually rather small and thin Asymmetry of the face and body and often quite flexible
Can be double jointed Teeth are small and irregular with poor enamel that decays easily
Tendency to vascular problems, lumbago, varicose inflammations and ulcerations
Emotionally they are unstable, indecisive, disordered and agitated, can be violent
At best they are bright and intuitive At worst they can be depraved and perverted, vicious and unscrupulous
Prone to the Syphilitic diseases

Medicines include: Fluorine, Calc Fluor, Mercury, Kali Bichromium, Nitric Acid, and the heavy metals.

Vannier's Constitution and Types

Leon Vannier is another who created a threefold classification (Vannier 1998), and he argued that the typological observation of the individual, the morphology, physiognomy, general appearance and demeanour, the handwriting, all contribute to enable us to determine the 'constitution' and the temperament. He went further and argued that the type of human being is defined by the knowledge of constitution and temperament.

> The constitution of the subject is determined by observation of the skeleton, study of form, particularly by examination of the relationship between the different parts. These relationships vary according to the constitution under observation but they never undergo a fundamental change in the course of life. As they were at birth, so they will remain. No treatment can modify them. The constitution is what actually exists while the temperament is what will develop in time. The temperament is a dynamic state depending on the Constitution of the subject which is a static state. The temperament is represented by the sum-total of physical, physiological, biological, psychological and dynamic possibilities of the subject. These possibilities are latent in him at birth. To define the constitution of an individual is to place him in the genus to which it belongs. To determine his temperament is to define the species to which he belongs, characterised by a sum-total of possibilities always remaining the same for a certain group. Constitution is the living material upon which the individual depends for his development. This development may take place according to three different plans and which characterise three types of constitution, designated as: Carbonic, Phosphoric and Fluoric. While studying these constitutions and observing the sensory and functional phenomena which appeared to be matched by certain objective signs, a surprising discovery was made showing their frequent correlation with the signs of our three great homoeopathic remedies: Calcarea carbonica, Calcarea phosphorica and Calcarea fluorica.

Carbonic:

May be described as a rigid individual, holding himself erect, with a stiff gait, slow or quick, but always well controlled, together with a restrained manner. Patient and obstinate, he never gives way; clear and precise, he is well disciplined. Anxious to achieve success he does not shrink responsibilities and is not averse to imposing his authority on others. All the parts are perfectly balanced, thorax and trunk, upper and lower limbs. Body is well built and the dimensions of the various parts are equally well proportionate. The upper and lower dental arches are in a normal relationship. The forearm is always thrust forward in the standing position, not quite straight with the arm in the full extension of the upper limb. The thigh and the leg do not form a perfectly straight line but there is no angular abnormality. The carbonic is steady and reliable, with marked powers of resistance. Controlled and disciplined.

Phosphoric:

Thin and frail individual, tall and slim, with an easy and graceful gait, and pleasant manners. An exalted individual who feels and suffers acutely, a sensitive and delicate nature, prone to spontaneous enthusiasm or sudden despair, whose charming personality is distinctly attractive. Face is usually elongated but always attractive with fine and mobile features. Palate has a tendency towards Gothic arch formation. The arm and forearm in hyperextension are always in a perfect straight line. Lower limbs are without angular formation. The dominant motive in the life of the Phosphoric is the pursuit of perfection.

Fluoric:

Unstable individual, with an awkward gait and an extravagant demeanour. No more capable of controlling his static state than of co-ordinating his own thoughts. They do not hold him well. The dental arches are not in close contact throughout their extent, the protrusion of some of the upper teeth. The arm and forearm form an obtuse angle opening on the posterior aspect and increasing with hyperextension of the upper limb. The thigh and leg show an angular deformation in the form of an obtuse angle opening forward. While instability is the main characteristic of the static state, exaggeration and awkwardness are the dominant characteristics of his movements. Gestures are not in harmony with the feeling expressed. They are exaggerated and often seem useless and awkward. Handwriting: A stroke underlining the signature. They dislike solitude. Must have an opportunity of talking and exchanging ideas in an atmosphere of turmoil in which he seems to revel.

The Carbonic Constitution represents the original constitution (free from all toxic taint) on which the other two Phosphoric and Fluoric engrafterd' (Vannier 1998).

Vannier describes eight basic prototypes, named for Greek and Roman divinities with definite individualizing traits. These are Mars, Saturn, Apollo, Venus, Jupiter, Mercury, Luna, and Terra. Each type is described in terms of dominant characteristics, morphology, mind, character, diseases to which they are prone, and changes that commonly occur with age and in specific circumstances (Vannier 1992)

Constitutional Prescribing in Light of a True Understanding of Constitution

From this wealth of opinion, observation, and clinical

experience, it is clear that generations of homeopaths have attempted to identify the constitution of the patient sitting in front of them, and use that as the basis for a homeopathic prescription. Some of those observations have been grounded in biochemistry, some based on straight observation, some have been made based upon chemical imbalance, and some based on temperament. When I go and visit my family, we all notice the same thing. My father and I cough in exactly the same way. The noise is the same. You sit in a café and observe. There are characteristics of the people you notice - eye colour, body types. Mac users and PC users. Homeopaths have made observations over the years and noticed that some remedies are useful for these types.

David Little is the most contemporary homeopath who has tackled this issue and nailed it in his chapter on *Constitution and Predisposition*. Hahnemann never prescribed 'constitutionally' as we think we know it today, but he did speak a lot about 'constitution'. In the words of Little (2011),

> Hahnemann paid close attention to the constitution in both acute and chronic diseases. Vide Sycosis, The Chronic Diseases, the footnote on page 150. "The miasm of the other common gonorrhoea seem not to penetrate the whole organism, but only to locally stimulate the urinary organs. They yield either to a dose of one drop of fresh parsley juice, when this is indicated by a frequent urgency to urinate, or a small dose of Cannabis, of Cantharides, or of the Copaiva balm, according to their different constitutions and other ailments attending it.' In this example Hahnemann suggests using the constitutional concomitant symptoms to help in the selection of a remedy. He expects homoeopaths to understand that the term "constitution"

simply means the whole living organism. All chronic remedies are "constitutional" in this sense as they reflect the essential nature of the totality of the symptoms. I think we have proved beyond a doubt that Hahnemann had a deep understanding of classical constitution, temperament, inheritance, susceptibility, diathesis and miasms. He also introduced temperamental pictures that included both the natural traits of the individual when healthy compared with the negative changes brought on by illness. Hahnemann's writing and the Paris casebooks include Hippocratic terms like the choleric, phlegmatic, sanguine and nervous temperaments. Each of these temperaments is associated with positive and negative qualities and predispositions toward certain disease states, signs, befallments and symptoms. They are also prone to particular diathetic states such as the venous, lymphatic and leuco-phlegmatic constitutions. If one studies material of the first generation of homoeopaths they will find such references with their concomitant signs and symptoms.

Hahnemann's writings demonstrate the important relationships between the congenital constitution, inheritance, predisposition and diathesis. The individual constitution and temperament is the most important feature in individualizing the symptoms of the chronic miasms. In the Chronic Diseases Hahnemann pointed out that the physical constitution, the mental temperament, hereditary dispositions, habits, lifestyle as well as environmental factors like diet are the most important conditioning factors in the symptoms of the miasms. This careful assessment of inheritance (nature) and environmental factors (nurture) is found in no other system of healing. Vide page 102 of the *Chronic Diseases*.

"The awakening of the internal Psora which has hitherto

slumbered and been latent, and, as it were kept bound by a good bodily constitution and favorable external circumstances, as well as its breaking out into more serious ailments and maladies, is announced by the increase of the symptoms given above as indicating the slumbering Psora, and also by a numberless multitude of various other signs and complaints. These are varied according to the difference in the bodily constitution of a man, his hereditary disposition, the various errors in his education and habits, his manner of living and diet, his employment, his turn of mind, his morality, etc.

Hahnemann wrote that the same disease state (such as psoric miasm) is varied according to the differences in "bodily constitution" and "hereditary disposition" as well as the patient's turn of mind, morals, diet, etc. This is because the human constitution and temperament (Nature) are the most important influences in the development of disease signs and symptoms. The next most important factors are environment, climate, diet and stress (nurture). For these reasons, a homoeopathic remedy should be similar to the negative changes found in the constitution and temperament as presented by the signs, befallments and symptoms. Hahnemann repeats a similar refrain in aphorism 81 of the Organon where he discusses the influence of the congenital bodily constitutions (angebornen Koerper-Constitutionen). The diversity of human constitutions and the environments in which human beings live are a major contributing factor in the development of the manifold symptoms of psora and the miasms. As the infectious agents of the miasms have been passed through millions of human beings over the course of hundreds of generations its symptoms have greatly mutated. For hundreds of thousands of years the infectious miasms have been present either in endemic pockets or as universal epidemics. The effects of the miasms have been found in the remains of the most ancient human beings and are found on every continent in every culture. It is no wonder that the symptoms produced by the universal miasms have been mistaken for manifold different diseases.

To untangle these issues, Little looks at the difference between Diathesis, Inherited and Acquired Constitutions:

> The idea of a diathesis is very closely linked with the inherited constitutional predispositions to particular symptoms. What does Diathesis mean? The Greek term, diathesis, is very closely linked with the inherited and acquired miasms and constitutional predispositions to particular symptom syndromes.
> 1. A diathesis is an inherited or acquired condition of the organism which makes it susceptible to peculiar disease states; a constitutional predisposition toward certain disorders. From the Greek, diathesis, dia-asunder and tithenai-to place.
> 2. A constitutional state which mistunes the body, and/or mind.
> 3. Diathetic constitutions are a category of constitutional predisposition or susceptibility to certain disorders, i.e., lymphatic, venous, leuco-phlegmatic, scrofulous, psoric, sycotic, etc. A diathesis is a permanent (hereditary or acquired) condition of the body that renders it liable to certain special diseases or affections; a constitutional predisposition or tendency. This word comes from the Greek for disposition or state. Thus a diathesis is a constitutional state that can be physical and psychological as well as inherited or acquired. The concept of diathesis is closely linked to both predisposition and the inherited miasms in Homoeopathy.

This material is very cryptic to most modern homoeopaths yet those who have put this system to work find it practical and indispensable to daily practice (Little 2011).

Ingredients Needed for a Constitutional Prescription

As a consequence, the homeopath looking constitutionally and with the broadest possible perspective during the homeopathic case taking is observing as much as possible. The significant factors of the entire medical history (the disease timeline), acute and chronic causations (the aetiological constellation), the chronic miasms, and the seven attendant circumstances form the basis of proper case taking (Aphorism 5). On this solid foundation the objective signs, coincidental befallments and subjective symptoms of the body and soul are recorded in detail (Aphorism 6). Little (*Hahnemann on Constitution and Temperament 2011*) goes into some further detail, and in a contemporary context highlights these seven attendant circumstances:

1. **The discernible body constitution** (especially in chronic cases). This category of symptoms includes a comparison of the physical constitution during a time of relative health with the negative changes brought on by diseases. It also includes Hippocratic diathetic constitution (the scrofulous, lymphatic, venous, nervous, rheumatic constitutions, etc.), a description of the physique (tall or thin, short or fat, loose or tight tissue types, etc) and the state of the vitality (weak, strong, unstable, etc). Rubrics of this nature are found in *Hering's Guiding Symptoms* and *Knerr's Repertory* as well as throughout many repertories.

2. **The mental and emotional character.** This refers to the character of the Geist (intellect) & Gemuet (emotional disposition). In this statement Hahnemann uses the term "charakter", which means personality rather than just transient mental conditions. This implies more than merely recording unrelated mental symptoms. One must understand "who" they are treating by constructing a complete psychological profile. This includes all the qualities related to emotional disposition, rational spirit and intellect as well as the soul. Rubrics related to these states are found through the mental sections of most homoeopathic repertories. Rubrics related to Hippocratic temperaments (choleric, phlegmatic, sanguine, melancholic) are found in *Hering's Guiding Symptoms* and *Knerr's Repertory*. Strictly speaking, these temperamental rubrics relate to the complete mind/body complex.

3. **The occupation.** The occupation that a person chooses is often characteristic of the individual's innate talents and desires. It also is an area that reveals many occupational hazards that may produce diseases as well as maintaining causes that obstruct the cure. These areas can reveal important symptoms as well as being relevant to the case management procedures.

4. **Lifestyle and habits.** These are cardinal general symptoms. How a person chooses to live and what they like to do are very characteristic symptoms. These symptoms offer great insights into the personality of the patient and their negative mental states. Investigating how a person lives often reveals indiscretions in diet, rest, and exercise as well as substance abuse and other areas that produce unneeded stress and strain.

5. **Civic and domestic relationships.** These rubrics include family dynamics as well as social relationships. How a person relates to their mate, family relations, children, friends, co-workers and society offers many signs and symptoms. These situational rubrics are a very important source of significant symptoms. Dysfunctional relationships produce illness as well as forming maintaining causes that keep up the disease state.

6. **Age.** Stages of life are a very important part of time and progression in Homoeopathy. The critical times are conception, birth, childhood, puberty, adolescence, middle age, and old age. Some remedies work particularly well on babies while other are more suited to the elderly. Some work well at both extremes of life. Hering recorded this in the section of the *Guiding Symptoms* called States of Life and Constitution.

7. **Sex and sexuality.** Some remedies are relatively more characteristic of females while some are more reflective of males. Some cover problems unique to the female and others male. The sexuality of a human being is closely connected to their physical and emotional health. The frustration of the orgasm reflex and the human need for intimacy leads to physical and psychosexual disorders. A person's sexual ethics, sexual fantasies, sexual performance, and their sense of sexual satisfaction are a rich source of symptoms.'

The time and progression, causation, the physical constitution, mental temperament and the 7 attendant circumstances are the foundation of homoeopathic case taking. Without these internal and situational rubrics the totality of the symptoms is incomplete. Who are they? What do they look like?

What is the mental and emotional character like? What kind of lifestyle do they have? What are their habits? How do they relate to other people? What are their family relationships like? How are they aging? What is their sexuality like? These areas of study include personal and group factors. This is very important if the homoeopath is to understand the layers by which complex chronic diseases have formed and recognize the reversal of the symptoms during cure.

On the basis of the study of the timeline, constitution, temperament, causation, miasms and the 7 attendant circumstances the detailed study of the disease symptoms is continued (Little 2011).

Mappa Mundi and Temperaments

Many homeopaths, but in particular Norland (2003), Reves (1993), de Rosa (2011), Fraser (2004) and Sherr, have taken time to write about and teach a system of identifying patient traits and symptoms, and then also materia medica profiles through using another system of identifying temperaments. Students of those teachers are encouraged to map the symptoms of the patient on a medicine wheel and familiarise themselves with those same characteristics in medicine profiles. David Little has also written on the subject. These essentially come from Galen with various additions from medieval medicine, alchemy, and Jungian psychology.

The use of Hippocratic temperaments (choleric, phlegmatic, sanguine and melancholic) expands the study of constitution in homoeopathy because it includes physiognomy and the natural groupings of human beings into four major and twelve minor mind-body types. This 2500 year old system is the oldest living tradition in western medicine. These classical methods offer much insight into the nature of the innate constitution and temperament as well as potential diathesis toward particular signs, befallments and symptoms. Physiognomy is defined as: "Physiognomy, the art of judging character from the appearance, esp., from the face; general appearance of anything; character, aspect-Greek- physiognomy, a shortened form of physiognomoni-physis, nature, gnomon-onos, an interpreter." A homoeopathic physiognomist is an interpreter of natural temperament, heredity, predisposition, miasms and constitutional diathesis, as well as the present state of the spirit, mind and body. Let us look at the definition of the key terms, temperament, and constitution. What does temperament mean? The word temperament has different levels of meaning depending on usage. Temperament from Latin, temperare; to temper, restrain, compound, moderate (Little 2011).

1. Choleric – yellow bile

Characteristic medicines: Sulphur, Nux vomica

The Emotions of the Choleric	
Born leader	Bossy
Dynamic and active	Impatient
Compulsive need for change	Quick-tempered
Must correct wrongs	Can't Relax
Strong-willed and decisive	Too impetuous
Unemotional	Enjoys controversy and arguments
Not easily discouraged	Won't give up when losing
Independent and self sufficient	Comes on too strong
Exudes confidence	Inflexible
Can run anything	Is not complimentary
Is unsympathetic	Dislikes tears and emotions

2. Melancholic – black bile

Characteristic medicines: Arsenicum album, Alumina

The Emotions of the Melancholy	
Deep and thoughtful	Remembers the negatives
Analytical	Moody and depressed
Serious and purposeful	Enjoys being hurt
Genius prone	Has false humility
Talented and creative	Off in another world
Artistic or musical	Low self-image
Philosophical and poetic	Has selective hearing
Appreciative of beauty	Self-centred
Sensitive to others	Too introspective
Self-sacrificing	Guilt feelings
Conscientious	Persecution complex
Idealistic	Tends to hypochondria

3. Sanguine - blood

Characteristic medicines: Calc carb

The Emotions of the Sanguine's	
Appealing personality	Compulsive talker
Talkative, Storyteller	Exaggerates and elaborates
Life of the Party	Dwells on trivia
Good sense of humour	Can't remember names
Memory for colour	Scares others off
Physically holds on to listener	Too happy for some
Emotional and demonstrative	Has restless energy
Enthusiastic and expressive	Egotistical
Cheerful and bubbling over	Blusters and complains
Curious	Naive, gets taken in
Good on stage	Has loud voice and laugh
Wide-eyed and innocent	Controlled by circumstances
Lives in the present	Gets angry easily
Changeable disposition	Seems phony to some
Sincere at heart	Never grows up, stays a child

4. Phlegmatic – phlegm

Characteristic medicines: Pulsatilla

The Phlegmatic's Emotions	The Phlegmatic's Emotions
Low-key personality	Unenthusiastic
Easygoing and relaxed	Fearful and worried
Calm, cool and collected	Indecisive
Well balanced	Avoids responsibility
Consistent life	Quiet will of iron
Quiet but witty	Selfish
Sympathetic and kind	Shy and reticent
Keeps emotions hidden	Too compromising
Happily reconciled to life	Self-righteous
All-purpose person	

In summary, there is a lot that is attractive about this theory. Beautiful student assignments and fantastic artistic lectures have been based around the analysis of a remedy or patients and their classification using the mappa mundi. This elemental theory in good hands can be very elegant. But again, it becomes less convincing (just like miasmatic theory), when you realise that different authors classify remedies differently. I was taught that *Calc Carb* was a phlegmatic remedy, and that *Lycopodium* was more melancholic in contrast to the previous table. But in good hands, most patients can be classified as choleric, melancholic, sanguine or phlegmatic. Moreover, remedy profiles can be viewed from the perspective of the tension of opposites that exist within their defined symptom pictures, and proving symptoms mapped on the mappa mundi.

The four major constitutions are called the choleric, phlegmatic, sanguine and melancholic or nervous temperaments. The twelve minor types are mixtures of the major type. They are the cholero-phlegmatic, the sangino-phlegmatic, the nervo-phlegmatic, the phlegmo-choleric, the sanguino- choleric, nervocholeric, the cholero-sanguine, the phlegmo-sanguine, and the nervo-sanguine, the cholero-nervous, phlegmo-nervous and sanguino-nervous. Each of these temperaments represents a natural grouping of constitutional types that have similar mental and physical qualities (Little 2011).

To take it further and drill deeper:

Little on the Phlegmatic Temperament

What did Hahnemann mean by the "phlegmatic temperament"? To understand this one must study the teaching of Hippocrates and Hahnemann very closely. The data on the Hippocratic temperaments represent 2,500 years of continuous clinical observation. The homoeopaths of the 19th century were very familiar with the Hippocratic canon and most knew the constitutional temperaments. The archetypal images of the four temperaments and humours are still in use even in the modern English language. For instance, the word "temperamental" still means to be very sensitive or overly emotional. At the same time to be in "good" or "bad humor" denotes a happy or distressed state of mind. A person may also be "full of humor" or "humorless" depending on the nature of their personality or mood.

Somebody may be referred to as being in a "dark mood" or to be "melancholic" when he or she is depressed. The word, melancholic, is derived from the word "black" (melan) and the term "bile" which denotes a dark humour or inwardly sullen state of mind. We also say that some people have a "bitter temperament' or while others have a "sour disposition". To be bitter is defined as a state of intense antagonism or hostility whereas to be sour is defined as being austere, morose, or peevish. These states are associated with the choleric and melancholic humour. Terms like these have their roots in the tastes of the four humours i.e., bitter (bile), sweet (blood), salty (phlegm), and sour (atrabile). To be "jaundiced" not only means to turn yellow because of excess bile but also to be prejudiced, envious and resentful. To "turn white" is a common expression associated with a state of fear. To "see red" means to be violently enraged which is related to the term "sanguinary" which means to be ready to shed blood. To feel "blue" is defined as being depressed in spirits, dejected or melancholic. These terms are closely related to the colors of the four humours, yellow (bile), white (phlegm), red (blood), and atrabile (blue-black).

All of these terms are based on the doctrines of the ancient Greeks and the nature of instinctive, innate body language. The Hippocratic theory of temperaments is closely related to the psychological and the physiological functions of the psycho-neuro-endocrine system (PNE) and morphological structures. The intrinsic connection between constitutional development and the neuro-endocrine secretions are well known in modern medicine. Nevertheless, the 2500-year-old Hippocratic system is still much more advanced in its observations of human temperament. The following rubrics are part of a collection taken from traditional sources and a clinical study spanning more than a decade.

The Temperament of the Phlegmatic

The water element is related to the emotional sensitivity and gives a person an ability to have deep feeling tones. This is why the phlegmatic temperament is psychic, sympathetic, mediumistic, and empathetic. When they are in "pleasant humour" they are imaginative, sensitive, artistic, romantic, sentimental and sympathetic. They are gentle, sweet, mild, and timid and have a receptive, yielding disposition with a tendency to try to please everyone. They like comfortable, safe situations and when they are with friends they come out and can be quite playful, frivolous, and jovial and like to tease.

Their strengths are that they are very sensitive, imaginative, sympathetic, adaptable, peaceful, tolerant, gentle, placid, soft, receptive, considerate and calm. Their weaknesses are that they become easily attached and are prone to be sad, tearful, indecisive, vulnerable, unsure, fearful, timid, envious, hesitant, changeable, submissive, indifferent, silent, reticent, unforgiving, mournful, pitiable and stubborn.

Under stress phlegmatic types easily become tearful, fearful, sentimental and very moody. The phlegmatic type experiences changeable moods that come in waves and tides like an emotional ocean where one moment they seem happy and the next sad. Their emotional state changes like the phases of the moon. When their mental skies are cloudy they rain down a shower of tears that gives them a sense of relief and allows them to return to bright sunny clarity. They may cry for happy or sad reasons, and sometimes, for no reason at all! If they are under prolonged stress they become sad and withdrawn as if a dark cloud has settled over them and they become shy, inward and dreamy.

Phlegmatics make very strong emotional connections with their loved ones and sexual partners, and suffer greatly from loss if these relationships do not work out. They suffer deeply from a sense of abandonment if they feel they are not appreciated and are easily hurt. They are worse when exposed to too much excitement, over stimulating environments, and when forced to do things in a hurry. In their own private way they can be stubborn, irritable, and they easily suffer from inward grief with silent peevishness. They are prone to passive aggression. As the individual breaks down under stress the phlegmatic temperament becomes more insecure, indecisive, cold, careless, listless, apathetic and suffers from nervous exhaustion. They may even become completely dull, blank, slow and stupid and appear like an idiot.

Phlegmatic Bodily Constitution (Generals)

In the Hippocratic tradition the seat of a phlegmatic's inner energy is in the cool moist fluids of the brain and pituitary gland and its influence spreads through the lymphatic channels and the veins and has its outer lower seat in the lower abdomen. The negative pole of the "natural forces" that governs the anabolic processes of nutritional transformations and the generative seed rules the phlegmatic constitution. They rule the lymphatic system level of the five-fold defense mechanism and often suffer from autointoxication due to imbalances of the toxin-antitoxin axis.

The body of the phlegmatic temperament is large boned, well rounded, and has soft tissue with flaccid muscles that tire easily. They easily suffer from water retention that makes them look and feel heavy, fleshy and fat. They easily put on weight on the hips, sacrum and thighs. The phlegmatic temperament moves with leisurely graceful motions and has difficulty doing things quickly because rapid motion makes them feel confused. Under continual stress the phlegmatic constitution suffers alternating emotional states, and becomes tired, weak, slow, chilly, and prone to edema.

The phlegmatic constitution has a round face, soft features, and deep watery eyes that swim with emotion. The sclera and the iris of their eyes often have grayish white spots and the iris may show a white ring around its outer edge. This ring like effect is called a lymphatic rosary in iridology. The face of a phlegmatic is round with soft, oval features and is often slightly bloated. Their skin is commonly cold, moist, whitish, pale, pasty and translucent with blue and green veins showing through.

They are worse from cold food and drinks. The phlegmatic type may like open air because it stimulates them but they do not like cold wind. They have a tendency to cold clammy perspiration that may be < aggravated by emotions. All complaints are < worse by cold, cloudy weather, winter and dampness, and are better > in warmer, dry climates and warm influences. They also can be worse < cold and heat as their temperature control is extremely unstable. They suffer from skin diseases that are accompanied by swelling and clear discharges that may change from bland to more irritating clear or white secretions. They also have a tendency to form lesions with white scales. A phlegmatic type usually feels cold easily and is < worse by cold, damp environments and cold food and drink. Correspondingly, phlegmatic types are > better warm drier environments and warm food and drinks.

The tongue of a phlegmatic is pale, swollen and may be watery or coated with a white coating. The phlegmatic pulse is usually slow, soft, wide and slippery. It is strong in the first phases of an illness but it becomes weak and stagnates as a disease becomes chronic. The hands of the phlegmatic temperament are cold, thick, soft, humid, swollen, and plump and their skin is white, pale and puffy. Their fingers are often short with thick tips and the joints are reasonably lax. The nails of the phlegmatic are often wide, white, pale, and soft and the moons are not very predominant.

When they shake hands their palm feels soft, wet, and cold, and their grip is weak. Phlegmatic women tend to hug softly and often do not offer a kiss as a greeting. If they do kiss, it is usually on the cheek, which causes them to blush and look sideways. Von Grauvogl called them the hydrogenoid type because of their tendency to hold water weight and to be < worse by damp cold atmospheres, watery foods, or living near bodies of water.

Physiognomists of the past have called the phlegmatic constitution such names as the venous, lymphatic, abdominal and thymus types. Morphologically speaking, Sheldon considered these constitutions to be pure endomorphs because of their large organs and lack of somatic structures. For this reason he called them the viscerotonic persons. In Danielopolu's system the phlegmatics are called vagotonic persons because they have overactive parasympathetic nervous systems that suppress the function of the sympathetic nervous system. This is related to many of their predispositions to hypofunction, coldness, slow metabolism, water retention, weight gain, etc.

Phlegmatic Predispositions (Diathesis and Miasms)

The phlegmatic temperament is prone to water retention, cold stomachs, insufficient secretion of digestive juices (such as hydrochloric acid), poor assimilation, anemia, and flatulence. The phlegmatic temperament is prone to poor circulation, lymphatic stagnation, non-inflammatory swollen glands, watery swelling, autointoxication, glandular swellings, increased mucus and serous secretions and watery discharges of clear or whitish color. They have a tendency toward hypo-pituitary, hypothyroid, low blood pressure, slow metabolism, low temperature, and lack of energy. The phlegmatic has a tendency to disorders of the genito-urinary system and their urine is frequent, pale and in larger quantities. Their arthritic problems manifest with cold white swellings that are < cold and damp and often better > warm applications and dry weather.

They are prone to taking cold with watery discharges and chilliness and flushes of heat. They easily accumulate water in the lungs and have much phlegm and mucus that produces complications. Tendency toward urinary infections (acute miasms), NSU, frequent urination and yeast infections with watery milky discharges. The sycotic miasm tends to produce an abundance of phlegmatic humours and the phlegmatic temperament.

Now we can see that the phlegmatic temperament represents a portrait of a group of individuals who share similar natural traits and reactions to environment as well as predispositions toward certain signs and symptoms. This system includes mentals and generals, thermals, desires, aversions, sensations, modalities and pathological generals as well as particular symptoms of the regions of the body. It also assesses the vitality of the life force as well as the inherited and acquired miasms, predispositions and diathesis. One can see that this system of constitution and temperament is much more advanced than any modern constitutional concepts (glandular and morphological types which have few symptoms) as it employs similar data to Hahnemannian Homoeopathy. Thus the ancient wisdom of Pythagoras and Hippocrates has found its home in the medicine of the future, Homoeopathy.

Phlegmatic Remedies

The phlegmatic, leuco-phlegmatic temperament as well as the lymphatic and hydrogenoid constitution is ruled by the same element (water). These constitutions are reflected in a group of well-proven remedies. It is easy to see the similarities between this phlegmatic constitution and Pulsatilla. It is also similar to well known remedies such as Agnus cast., Aloe, Asterias rubens, Ammonium carb., Calc carb., Capsicum, Carbo veg., Cyclamen, Dulcamara, Graphites, Hepar sulph, Mercurius, Natrum carb, Natrum chlor, Natrum sulph., Sepia, Thuja., etc..

The carbon group of mineral remedies are very similar to the phlegmatic temperament, leuco-phlegmatic and lymphatic constitutions. Such remedies include Am-carb., Calc-carb., Carbo-v., Graphites, Kali carb., Natrum carb, etc.. The Natrums also have a tendency to phlegmatic states Nat-c., Nat-chlr, Nat-m., Nat-s. The Ammoniums, and Antimoniums also are similar as demonstrated by Am-c., Am-m., and Ant-c., Ant-t., Animal remedies include Asterias Rubens, Calcarea, Sepia (water creatures) and Apis. Many anti-sycotic remedies also are similar as there is a connection between phlegmatic states and sycosis. Here you find Agnus Cast., Thuja, Asterias rubens, Natrum sulph., Calc carb., etc.. Plant remedies include Aloe, Dulcamara, Pulsatilla, Cyclamen, Thuja, etc. Here is a repertory rubric with sources for the phlegmatic temperament and lymphatic constitutions (Little 2011).

For significant work on the other temperaments, see Norland (2003) and Fraser (2002, 2004, 2008).

Conclusions

It is clear that Hahnemann did make reference to temperamental portraits. As Little (2011) points out:

> The employment of this, as of all other medicines, is most suitable when not only the corporeal affections of the medicine correspond in similarity to the corporal symptoms of the disease, but also when the mental and emotional alterations peculiar to the drug encounter similar states in the disease states to be cured, or at least in the temperament of the subject of treatment. Hence the medicinal employment of Pulsatilla will be all the more efficacious when, in affections for which this plant is suitable in respect to the corporeal symptoms, there is at the same time in the patient a timid lachrymose disposition, with a tendency to inward grief and silent peevishness, or at all events a mild and yielding disposition, especially when the patient in his normal state of health was good tempered and mild (or even frivolous and good humouredly waggish) It is therefore especially adapted for slow phlegmatic temperaments; on the other hand it is but little suitable for persons who form their resolutions with rapidity, and are quick in their movements, even though they may appear to be good tempered."

In the words of Little (2011), 'the above quote is a constitutional portrait. Hahnemann's picture includes attributes of the natural constitution (timid lachrymose disposition, slow phlegmatic temperament), positive natural traits during a time of health and happiness (good tempered, mild, good humouredly waggish) and negative emotions brought on by disease (inward grief, silent peevishness). This portrait includes natural, positive and negative qualities. As one can see from the above quotes this information was included within the totality of the symptoms.

Pulsatilla is "adapted for slow phlegmatic temperaments", while on the other hand it is less suitable for those who "form resolutions with rapidity' and are "quick in their movements". Such data establishes constitutional portraits as well as the use of temperamental counter indications as elimination rubrics. Pulsatilla is rarely indicated in those constitutions that make quick resolutions or move rapidly because this remedy does not normally suit that type of patient. This temperamental picture demonstrates several of the essential elements of the Pulsatilla proving. This demonstrates that Hahnemann was the first to open the field of investigation into constitution and temperament in Homoeopathy. Hahnemann's Paris casebooks show that the Founder used Hippocratic terminology. Rima Handley noted in her Later Hahnemann that the Founder wrote in his casebooks that Mme del a Nois was "sanguine" and Eugene Perry was "choleric" Hahnemann also occasionally used the diathetic terms. For example, he wrote that Claire Christallo (DF-5) was "disposed to scrofula" and called another patient "lymphatic". Ms. Handley wrote that Hahnemann did not seem to use constitution, temperament or diathesis in his prescribing. While it is true that Hahnemann did not give remedies because a person was "sanguine", this is not the complete picture. Negative changes in a formerly healthy constitution and temperament are part of the totality of the symptoms. Handley also wrote that Hahnemann had no idea of the modern usage of constitution or essence. This is most certainly true in the sense of "essence constitutional prescribing" advocated by a few Neo-Kentian practitioners in the 1970s. Although Hahnemann did not use their method of so-called "essence prescribing", he most certainly did introduce the idea of the Wesen (essence, nature and genius) in The Organon. Hahnemann's essence is the Gestalt of a disease as expressed by the characteristic symptoms of the mistuning of the vital force. This Essence contains the essential nature of the totality of the characteristic symptoms that leads to the most suitable homoeopathic remedy. This is the true Esse (Little 2011).

But how practical is temperament really? How many cases that do well in a homeopaths clinic are helped with constitutional prescribing? We need research. Will a patient show up in the clinic with an uncomplicated list of phlegmatic symptoms and nothing else? In reality, this theory like so many theories in homeopathic medicine creates the opportunity for more interpretation and speculation. Without doubt, some cases do get better, but is that a significant number?

Of Practical Use

1. *Rubrics related to constitutional diathesis include; Hysterical, constitutions; Hemorrhagic, constitutions; Lymphatic, constitutions; Venous, constitutions; Plethoric, constitutions; Rheumatic, constitutions; Scrofulous, constitution; Paralytic, constitutions; Gouty, constitutions; Tubercular, constitutions; Asthmatic constitutions; and their similar remedies. "Lymphatic, constitutions -am-c., Apis, arn, ars, aster, aur-m., bapt, BAR-C., Bar-m, BELL., CALC., calc-ar., Cann-i., Carb-v., Chin., dulc., FERR., GRAPH., Hep., kalm., Lyc., MERC., murx., Nat-m., nit-ac., Petr., phos., Puls., Rhus-t., Sep., Sil., Sulph., thuj."*

2. *Rubrics related to the bodily constitution include; Lean, thin people; Large fat, people, bloated; Emaciated constitutions; Fibre, lax, constitutions; Fibre rigid, constitutions; Tall lean, constitutions; Dwarfish, constitutions; and their similar remedies. "Fibre, lax., constitutions-agar., bar-c., bor.,*

CALC., calc-p., Caps., cinnam., hep., KALI-C., MAG-C., MERC., OP., PHOS., SABAD., Sil., spong."

3. Rubrics related to the Hippocratic temperaments and humours include; Bilious, constitutions; Choleric, constitutions; Phlegmatic, constitutions; Sanguine constitutions; Melancholic, constitutions; Nervous, constitutions and their remedies. "Bilious, constitutions; acon., Aesc., ail., ambr., ant-c., ant-t., ars., Bell., berb., BRY., cann-i., CARD-M., Cham., CHEL., CHIN., chion., chol., Cocc., Ip., iris., Lach., lept., mag-m., Merc., nat-s., NUX V., Phos., plat., ptel., PSOS., Puls., sang., sep., Sulph."

4. Rubrics related to the miasms include; Psoric, constitutions; Sycotic constitutions; Tubercular, constitutions; Syphilitic, constitutions; Cancerous constitutions (mixed miasms). "SYPHILITIC, constitutions-Ars., aec-t., AUR., Benz-ac., Clem., Cor-r., Crot-h., cund., euph., ferr-i., Fl-ac., Guai., Kali-b., KALI-I., MERC., Merc-c., Merc-d., Merc-i-f., Mez., NIT-AC., Petr., Phos., Ph-ac., Phyt., Sars., Sil., Still., sulph., SYPH., Thuj.

Constitutional prescribing is not the same as chronic prescribing, since the patient does not have to exhibit any sign of chronic disease pathology to require a constitutional medicine. Constitutional prescribing does not simply address the present disturbance, but also the past and future. It is treating the patient's susceptibility, the propensity to repeated acutes, and any existing chronic disease that this style of prescribing supports.

True constitutional prescribing is the choice of a medicine based on the characteristics of a person based on observation or biotype. This is distinct from Kentian prescribing. It is valuable for the percentage of patients that have clearly identifiable characteristics as agreed upon and learned in materia medica profiles, and for healthy people.

Further Reading

- Watson — *Guide to the Methodologies of Homeopathy*
- Clarke — *Constitutional Medicine With Especial Reference to the Three Constitutions of Von Grauvogl*
- Vannier — *Typology in Homoeopathy*
- Mathur — *Principles of Prescribing*
- Lesser — *Text book of Homoeopathic Materia Medica*
- Little — *Hahnemann on Constitution and Temperament*
- Fraser — *Using Mappa Mundi in Homoeopathy*
- Norland — *The Four Elements in Homeopathy- Mappa Mundi of elements and associated temperaments.*
- Eizayaga — *Genotype Constitution/Phenotype Constitution, Prevention through Constitutional Medicine.*
- de Rosa — *Mappa Mundi method and its application to homeopathy*

Chapter 5

Vital Sensation
Shilpa Bhouraskar

It is difficult to know where to begin when talking about Sensation Method in modern and contemporary homeopathy. Whole books need to be devoted to it and much discussion had. Over the years, literally thousands of homeopaths around the world have attended Rajan Sankaran's seminars and been taught by the man, or his followers and advocates of the method. My first introduction to his work face-to-face was in 1994 in London. It was an experience for sure. His ideas have clearly changed over the years and the early work from The Spirit of Homeopathy, The Substance of Homeopathy, The System of Homeopathy and even the early work on the plants have been superseded as he has himself grown and taken a generation of homeopaths with him.

When interviewing Sankaran for the Case Taking book that precedes this one, what was most striking was that in his hands, with his grounding in the study and practice of medicine, in the principles of homeopathic medicine there is no disconnection between what is being suggested with his Sensation Method and, let's call it traditional homeopathic medicine as we know from Hahnemann, Kent and the other icons of homeopathy. But this is not the case worldwide, and as was articulated in that interview, by many other homeopaths in print, in articles, and to him directly the unfortunate consequences of Sensation Method is that poorly trained homeopaths have been taking poorly understood concepts and articulating them to a bewildered public who are genuinely concerned and homeopathy has been ridiculed as a consequence.

This is not to dispute the method in any way. New ideas need to be added. But new ideas also have to have critical-thinking, reflection and evaluation applied to them and in any mature profession debate about their value is a necessary part of evolution of an idea.

For the contribution of this chapter I turned to the Sydney-based homeopath Shilpa Bhouraskar. When she arrived in Sydney in 2004 it was immediately clear that this was a voice, grounded in orthodox homeopathic thinking and method, but who had the flexibility in practice to apply different methods when appropriate. Even more astounding was that in her teaching work she was able to articulate clearly to students the value of this new idea and keep it in context. In doing so she was able to translate that this was an idea that deserved passionate enthusiasm but also critical thinking. Even better was that she was able to demonstrate when it was appropriate and when not in her clinical training work. Many patients and now hundreds of students have been able to see this method in skilled hands and applied with discrimination and appropriateness.

She is the developer of the HomeoQuest homeopathic software, and with a background from India and with her skilled teaching she is in a great place to contribute a chapter on this important method of homeopathy. In 2010 she wrote a powerful e-book on methodology and homeopathy. It was on the back of that than I asked Shilpa to write a chapter, not only explaining Sensation Method but also placing it in its true context alongside the other interpretations of homeopathic method. Shilpa has been in practice since 1994.

AG

Contents

- Introduction
- The Evolution of Homeopathy in Stages
- Stage 1
- Stage 2
- Stage 3
- Stage 4
- Comparison of Stages, Disease and Medicine Understanding
- Application of the Stages in Practice
- Confirm Your Prescription Through All the Four Stages
- A Case Example Incorporating All Stages
- Which Approach to Use and When
- Circumstances When Stage 1 and 2 Are Best Suited
- Disease Circumstances
- Homeopath's Circumstances
- Patient Circumstances
- Circumstances When Stage 3 or 4 Are Best Suited
- Disease Circumstances
- Homeopath's Circumstances
- Patient Circumstances
- The Sensation Method Compared With the Earlier Methods
- Conclusion
- Further Reading

In this chapter you will:

1. Learn the historical and theoretical development of the Sensation Method
2. Understand the components of the method
3. Explore the issues behind when to apply it
4. Grasp its depth through case study

Chapter 5

Vital Sensation
Shilpa Bhouraskar

Introduction

My experiences and journey using the Sensation Method would be incomplete without sharing my previous journey as a homeopathic medical student, and later as a practitioner in the last 14 years of my practice.

The best time during my homeopathic training was our hospital clinical sessions. It was when we actually observed the homeopathic theory being applied in practice. Our homeopathic hospital in Mumbai, India had a blend of practitioners who worked using different methods in homeopathy. The practitioners ranged from those who used combinations of different tissue salts for medical conditions to pure Hahnemannian homeopaths with decades of experience in eliciting the exact keynotes even in comatose patients. Further, there were those who had mastered the art of eliciting elaborate remedy pictures based on not just the totality, but also on observing the way a patient entered the clinic and shook their hands. And finally, we had Sankaran who did not just stop at the peculiar keynotes. He elicited the depths of someone's mental state and dreams to understand and match the delusion.

Looking back, I think it was a wonderful way to expose us to different methods of prescribing. It helped us identify an approach that appealed to our logic and comfort level, and go into the details so we could incorporate this method in future practice.

Let me share some observations I made during that period. I realised that different successful practitioners would find totally different remedies for the same patient (based on their approach). Although every well-chosen remedy gave results in some form, it was clear that some approaches yielded remedies that produced more consistent and deeper cures than the other. The interesting fact was that not every approach was suited to every patient, and not every approach appealed to every homeopath. Further certain types of patients chose certain practitioners, and this choice was not necessarily based on the practitioner who was able to produce the best results, but it was something to do with their individuality and the approach they chose to use, and the outcome the patient expected from homeopathy.

I remember a patient who always demanded immediate relief for his severe acute headaches, which did not respond to the strongest painkillers. He was always in a hurry, never had more than five minutes to spare, and was never interested in any thing other than pain relief. But every time he had an episode, his extremely confident homeopath provided that relief for him. Within minutes he chose a remedy for him on just a few of his keynote symptoms. We were in complete awe of this homeopath that asked the least questions and chose the best objective keynotes. For this patient, this homeopathic approach was simply magical.

However, I could see how he was just unsuited to the homeopath next door. His case taking involved precision and art to understand the innermost disturbance in a patient. He had the patience to wait and understand his patient without being too fussed about the time or remedy. He preferred minimal repetition even during acutes. But in the follow ups, we were amazed at deeper changes produced not just in the patient's overall health but life in general. Needless to say, he has his own large following of patients who seek more than just symptom relief.

Eventually at the end of my internship, I reached some conclusions. Firstly, I found certain homeopathic approaches produced better results than others, and as a clinician I realised that an approach was not independent of a patient. So as everything in homeopathy, it was all about individualisation of an approach. Secondly, I needed to gain enough experience on applying these different approaches for individual patients. The idea was to work at places where hundreds of patients visit regularly, and experience first hand which approaches work and which don't under some supervision. I worked voluntarily for various charitable institutes around Mumbai, and at homeopathic camps in rural centres in my state that offered free homeopathy services. I also assisted busy practitioners who had no time to spend an hour with every patient. I shared their case load for free and practised meticulous case taking. Everything that I learned from the hospital Out Patient Department at various seminars and workshops was directly being applied on the patients. Soon it gave me enough experience to formulate my own practice as a homeopath.

The Evolution of Homeopathy in Stages

Today after 14 years of private practice, I have realised there is a fascinating connection between the different homeopathic approaches since the discovery of homeopathy.

Using this knowledge I determine the most suitable approach for a patient based on the patient's exact needs. This is very helpful in clinical practice because it creates an immediate positive patient -practitioner relationship.

Further, I build upon this initial relationship, and offer to work with them through the different stages, depending on how far they want to go in the treatment process. This way, I use the best of homeopathy based on a patient's needs, and ultimately provide greater patient satisfaction.

To explain this process, let me start by sharing the fascinating connection between the different approaches in homeopathy. I have divided them into four stages as they evolved during the homeopathic time line.

Stage 1

This was initially how Hahnemann discovered homeopathy. He had learned first hand that Cinchona had been used to treat intermittent fevers. He then observed that Cinchona bark produced fever with chills. This was similar to the symptom of intermittent fevers. This was the Law of Similars at work. This model is similar to the allopathic way of using homeopathic remedies where medicines are chosen on the basis of the name of a disease or a disease diagnosis. Homeopathic combination remedies available in pharmacies for various diseases work at this stage.

Stage 2

Very soon, Hahnemann realised the name isn't important, and any fever with symptoms similar to those produced by Cinchona, irrespective of the diagnosis, can be treated with Cinchona bark. Understanding the specific Cinchona fever led to this breakthrough. And this is where the evolution began.

This model is similar to using homeopathic remedies for local, particular symptoms, which is very closely related to pathophysiology. The therapeutic medicines based on common and peculiar disease symptoms work at this stage.

Stage 3

Eventually, practitioners realised that differentiating the different types of fevers in patients was necessary to determine which fevers would benefit from Cinchona. It was then seen that differentiation of two similar diseases in different people was possible based on symptoms that belonged to the person and not disease.

This was the dawn of person-specific treatment, the striking advantage of homeopathy over conventional medicine. Then, the model of using physical and mental generals, and peculiar, queer, rare, striking (PQRS) symptoms related to an individual, not just a disease developed. This model has been, and continues to be, the most popular and widely used in homeopathy.

Even though Hahnemann was the first homeopath to discover this stage in homeopathy, the two major influences that revolutionised this stage were Bönninghausen and Kent. Both of them spoke about the same fundamental concept - the individual comes before the disease - but expressed that in a variety of different ways. It is largely a matter of understanding the symptoms of an individual (physical, mental, general and constitutional symptoms) beyond just disease symptoms that helps to individualise two individuals suffering from a similar disease.

Bönninghausen identified the concomitants as an expression of individuality in a case, while Kent proposed a pyramid or hierarchy of symptoms with mental symptoms being the most important at the apex, and the physical symptoms at the bottom. Patients were being perceived as personalities with different constitutional traits, which gave rise to understanding of remedies as drug pictures and essences. Now it was not enough to know the local symptoms of Cinchona, an understanding of the individual personality and constitution of Cinchona was required.

It was Kentian homeopathy that remained popular throughout history, and strongly influenced the way homeopathy is practised, even today in most parts of the world. It is also known as classical homeopathy or constitutional homeopathy.

Stage 4

Stage 4 is where the latest developments of homeopathy have evolved today, beyond the so-called Hahnemannian homeopathy methods.

The underlying philosophy of homeopathy perceives disease as a disturbance in the vital force, and this disturbance is initially expressed as constitutional traits, and then disease signs and symptoms. Stage 4 is trying to find the core disturbance of vital force before it is expressed as symptoms. This case taking process has been revolutionised by Rajan Sankaran, and he calls it the understanding of the Vital Sensation.

These are not mind or body symptoms but sensations equally expressed at both levels – somewhere where the body and mind meet. It is trying to get at the root of the patient's vitality and existence. He describes it as the closest expression of the disturbed vital force or the energy. This is disease expression never assessed before, a level beyond the individual and the individual's constitution.

So it is about understanding the vital sensation of *China* in a patient, a sensation is an experience beyond the mental and physical symptoms of *China*. Sankaran stumbled across this method while tying to find the common themes of plant remedies in the same family.

The kingdom analysis is not new, it is one of the newer ways of understanding the common themes of particular kingdoms and their sub-kingdoms, and then understanding and prescribing remedies based on that developed by homeopaths, such as Jan Scholten, Massimo Mangialavori and Sankaran.

However it was Sankaran who actually took the understanding of kingdom analysis further to reach a deeper level of eliciting the sensations beyond symptoms.

Another homeopath, Irene Schlingensiepen – Brysch in her book *The Source of Homeopathy* further fine tunes this stage. She goes beyond the understanding of the sensation during the case taking process until she dives into the very source structure of an individual. It is an attempt to understand the very source of 'China the substance' within a patient.

Thus Stage 4 homeopathy is this fascinating process of eliciting and connecting the source within an individual to the source of the remedy itself.

Through homeopathic evolution at every stage, you are one step closer to understanding the entire disease in its totality, the disease in an individual as well as the individual in disease. It is taking a journey towards someone's inner core and finding where that person's vitality is disturbed.

For me, this represents a useful classification of various approaches and methods of prescribing in homeopathy. It bridges the old and new approaches, as well as reduces the confusion in understanding the wide spectrum of homeopathic practice. It helped me classify the case taking, case analysis, miasmatic approach, remedy understanding, potency selection, and every other part of case management no matter which approach I chose.

As a teacher it helped me explain to my students the connection between the differences in each approach, such as the differences between the classical and non-classical methods, or the differences between the traditional Kentian and non-traditional Sensation Method, as well as the subtle differences between the delusion and Sensation Method proposed by Sankaran.

Comparison of Stages, Disease and Medicine Understanding

Here is one example of how the deepening of patient understanding in stages relates to the depth in medicine understanding. I have used the remedy China Officinalis as an example in the following table to explain this concept:

Disease in Individual		Individual in Disease	
Stage 1	Stage 2	Stage 3	Stage 4
Disease diagnosis	Disease particular symptoms (common and PQRS)	General symptoms and constitutional traits (common and PQRS)	Vital sensation, source and energy
Malaria fever	China fever	China constitution	China Sensation
Malaria is characterised clinically by fever (usually periodic), varying degrees of anaemia and splenic enlargement, and a range of syndromes resulting from the physiological and pathological involvement of certain organs, including the brain, liver and kidneys.	Symptoms include periodic fever well marked paroxysms, shuddering chills from every drink, cold hands and feet, hot face, profuse sweat, etc.	People who were once stout, healthy, remarkably active and industrious become broken down by exhausting discharges and suffer pale face, sunken eyes, over sensitivity to touch, pain, draft of air. Sufferers show great physical prostration and become mentally apathetic, dull, indifferent, etc.	Over stimulation which aggravates mentally and physically, for example desires stimulants, ideas, plans, etc. but is stuck in a position where none of these desires can be fulfilled, and faces attacks from time to time.

Application of the Stages in Practice
Confirm Your Prescription Through All the Four Stages

Research and my personal experience both show the accuracy of prescription increases as you reach the higher stages. However, the most amazing cures result when you match the case through its evolution to the remedy understanding and its corresponding evolution. Most successful homeopaths acknowledge this fact from experience.

Kent mentions this in his articles on treating pathological diseases with homeopathy, and discusses how the constitutional remedy (Stage 3) needs to cover the pathology (Stage 1). Eizayaga talks about this in explaining his triangle, and incorporating the lesional layer (Stage 1 and 2), fundamental layer (Stage 3) and constitutional layer (Stage 3) when prescribing the simillimum. Sankaran, in the newest and most successful Sensation Method, talks about the knowledge of levels and disease understanding, which closely relates to the stages in homeopathy. He explains how he has had the most success when he enters a case from chief complaint (Stage 1) to reach the levels of sensation, energy and beyond (Stage 4).

This is critical because when he worked using the delusional method, his case taking had a greater emphasis on the mental state and the delusion, whereas the need for the remedy covering the physical particulars and pathology was secondary and sometimes ignored. However, with the Sensation Method, there is a balance in the whole case-taking process that has improved the success rate considerably.

Thus incorporating all four stages in your understanding helps multiple confirmations of your remedy, and cures are more consistent, rather than sporadic miracle cures.

A Case Example Incorporating All Stages

Case Taking

Female 62 years. Came to the student clinic.

Information Collected by the Student

This intake basically provided information at Stage 1 and 2, with some Stage 3 information as well. The patient presented with psoriasis she had for the last six years on the left side of her scalp, spreading to forehead and left arm. She experienced extreme itching and tightness, constant shedding of dandruff-like particles. Her symptoms were aggravated by stress, and were worse during winter and very hot summer days. She avoids dark clothes.

Past History

- Consistently painful menses since puberty
- Endometriosis and backache
- PMS - Irritable but didn't express it, contained it within
- Extremely anaemic in pre-teen and early teen years
- Fungal infection of toes in her 30s
- At 40, hormonal treatment for endometriosis
- Sinusitis
- Psoriasis of scalp, treated with tar shampoo. But took *Pulsatilla*, which cleared it, as well as the sinusitis.
- Since menopause – hypertension and hyperlipedemia for which she sought allopathic treatment

Current Situation

- Extremely responsible at work
- Duty conscious, moral and very particular about being tidy
- Dreams of being persecuted, which she related to her strict

Catholic upbringing.

She was prescribed a few remedies including *Kali brom* 200 and then *Carcinosinum* 200, which didn't do much, and the psoriasis continued to spread.

Information from the Questionnaire

This completed the information at Stage 3.

Physical Generals

- Flatulence when I eat a lot of yogurt
- Craving salt, cheese, yogurt
- Aversion – fatty rich food, sweets
- Aversion to drafts
- Loves open air
- Perspiration – feet, stains clothing
- Menses heavy painful, with bloating and headache

Upsetting Moments/Situations in the Patient's Own Words

I had a good relationship with my sister, especially long distance, she lives on her own and can't tolerate people around her for a long period of time. When she comes to Sydney, she likes to go off on her own, but loves to be part of us as well. Sometimes she goes ballistic and you just want to run away. It doesn't happen often anymore, as she lives in Europe.

Shocked when my sister in law said she did not to want to see me, as she didn't like family. I felt hurt at the time, but since then have become very indifferent. I still do the right thing by her, but if I don't see her ever again, that's fine by me. She lives in Sydney and since her husband died, she does want to see us.

I was shocked, numbed with disbelief of the way my daughter treated me as past my use by date seven years ago; I cried often when at home, but just kept quiet within myself, I did talk to my husband a lot, he tried to help, but though he had a good relationship with our daughter, he had not connected with her like I did. I was depressed, but did not take medication.

Nine years ago I worked for a boss that didn't like me. I sometimes felt she would like to stick a knife in me and I did try to get another job at the time, but without success. It was stressful and I talked a lot about my woes at home. I changed and kept telling myself I really liked her and she was a great person. When I finally left this employer for a part-time job, we parted as friends.

As a migrant, I have always had to rely on myself, having no relatives as a support, this has been stressful in the past when decisions had to be made, hoping that the right one were taken. All my family lives overseas.

Dreams

As a child/teenager, I used to dream I was persecuted, which was very frightening, they did subside when I married and became a quieter sleeper, my sleepwalking disappeared as well, thanks to my husband. I still remember having to run and keep running from I still do not know whom, till I woke up.

I dream of work and wake up in panic about things or jobs I had forgotten to do at work. In reality I am extremely diligent. The fear is very real, like if I get caught, my life will be over! It has had no association with my real life.

Fantasies

> I wish I had plenty of money to travel first class or business class to Europe and USA so I can visit my family regularly, I miss them a lot.

Although I could have prescribed based on this information, I asked her if she wanted to go a bit further to confirm the prescription, and increase the accuracy of understanding her case. She agreed, and I took the interview to Stage 4 - the Sensation Method.

Interview at Stage 4

The sensation homeopathy is the process of eliciting and understanding the sensation in a patient, and matching it with the most appropriate remedy. In the analysis, the Kingdom, miasm and the source of the remedy are also confirmed to greatly increase the accuracy of your prescription. I highly encourage any interested reader to refer to the various books and cases written on the Sensation Method by Dr Rajan Sankaran to get an in-depth understanding of the method. This case is just a glimpse into the process, and although the process is very systematic, it is flexible enough for all practitioners to find their own way of reaching the sensation. I have provided the case in a question and answer format in the patient's own words. My comments and thought process are in italics at every juncture.

How are you doing?

> I have decided to stop paid work because it's too much. I dream a lot about work, keep everything going. The sessions in the clinic have made me focus on myself, I have never allowed myself to

focus on myself. Always been hurried through life. It's a crazy life I am leading. Lots of dreams of work. I wake up in the middle of night and I dreamt of things that did not happen at work.

In what way?

Panic and chaotic. No assistance to help me. Mind was spinning. I was doing things I normally don't have to do as a part of my work. They are giving me more and more responsibilities thinking she is easy and can do it. They make you run.

She is talking at the emotional level. Her state is quite compensated. This suggests what potency I have to give her, i.e. 200. To enter her case, I decide to start with the chief complaint, which is Level 1.

When did the psoriasis flare up?

It was six years back when daughter packed and left for US. I don't have support network.

I said don't marry, you will be stuck but she married within two months.

What did you feel? (emotional level)

I felt betrayed. We were good friends. We had a harmonious family. Husband is more easy going, I may be more radical. He evens and balances out. We said all right it's her life. Then she asked me to arrange her wedding in Sydney for her friends. I did organise it, but she totally ignored me. Used us as her parents. We didn't leave on a very nice footing. It felt as if punched in the stomach by someone I loved and cherished. The gloom lasted for two and a half years. I cried a lot. I am not the one who normally cries. I don't have family around.

Talk about that?

When children grow up, they need guidance from someone who has been through that, its easier to make a decision, easier if you share responsibility in decision making, e.g. if your kids are sick, they might say its ok its just chicken pox. Or in my case my son is hyperactive. I would want to discuss with people who have that experience. It's a big responsibility to bring up that child, educate and help him live in this world.

He is now a very responsible and balanced person. He is the one who is easy and daughter was difficult.

Responsibility is important and instilled in me since childhood. Must do this must do that. So now even though I wanted to continue working till end of the year, I let go. I am happy I made that decision.

Even with daughter I wanted people to help me find a path.

You do bring up kids to eventually lose them, but I was opposed to the way we were in no uncertain terms. As if we were past due date. No longer necessary, unimportant, don't exist for her. Don't need you. No communication possible.

As we moved a lot after my birth in South America to Holland, South Africa, I became quite self reliant.

You don't whinge and get things moving, Sort everything yourself. Become independent personally and financially.

We see that family is important and that she needs people around. If she loses them, it upsets her, but she has compensated by becoming self-reliant and independent. This is still her emotional level. However she mentions responsibility often and I need to understand what it means to her.

Talk about responsibility?

I have dreams of responsibility. Panic fear as if not done my duty, ashamed. I was responsible for running the place (*at her work place*). People expect me to do it. Always been like that. They control, and I try to give my best and give 100% because I think I can but at my health's detriment. I could not get out because I had to get that centre going. It's not my home. I tried to do it at home.

When I was caring for people, realised life is valuable and you do the best for them. Heightened my responsibility towards work. They shouldn't die during what you administer them so I changed my job from that situation. It would be terrible if they die. You have to do the right thing.

This connects with the dreams she had as a child. Catholic upbringing of doing the right thing.

I have been given a set of rules or life planned for me, and you try and do the best of your abilities. Doing everything correctly and not making mistakes.

Thus responsibility is needing to care for people at home or work or else she feels extremely guilty as if she has done wrong. This is again the emotional level. So now I use another point of entry to get to a deeper level.

What are your hobbies and interests?

I love perfumes. I did aromatherapy and Swedish massage at college.

In hobbies I like embroidery, creating something from nothing, e.g. needle work, something really nice.

I love gardening, plants, herbs. I cook with fresh herbs.

I love to see things grow.

Plant and nurture them. Fertilize them right, mulching.

I may have been a farmer in former life. I love to work with nature. So healing to work with nature, smells, colours.

Because animals and plants are unconditional. They give back so much.

You don't have to give something to receive something.

With people I find you need to give more. They expect a lot out of you.

I listen to people complain, and if you want to complain they don't listen. And the ones that are true friends always seem to be leaving. It's disappointing but I pack and leave so often you get used to saying goodbye.

This was the turning point of the case for me; it was a deeper connection between all situations in her life - the daughter's incident and moving and leaving family as a child, work, etc. all together from a completely unrelated situation and this is the connection of the case. When you reach this point, everything just flows beautifully and you don't need to ask a lot of questions.

I love to cook and go out of my way when I have friends coming over.

But I would love to be able to do it with my family, mum and dad.

I should have been brought up in an Italian family. The unit of an extended family.

Togetherness and exuberance.

It gives me great pleasure, nice food, happy company, which I have to create with strangers. I had a huge extended family. I talk to my sister, what do you think, take other's point of view.

I want to create that family with my grandchildren and its just not there.

I don't hate her but I am removed. 'I don't care attitude' in order to not get hurt anymore.

She is talking about her daughter.

She is not going to affect me anymore. You don't get involved because you don't want to go through that feeling of darkness. No emotion is there. Initially anger, now I don't care.

This denotes the miasm – because it is the reaction to a situation – i.e. acceptance and avoidance - could be sycosis.

Once with my son's condition during one of the bleak times, there was an aura of vibration all around me. Enveloped me in love. I felt he will be alright and nothing will happen to him anymore.

I tried to get it back through Reiki and meditation, but it never came back.

This is the energy of her case.

Talk about that?

Exceptional love.

Change in my life.

I don't become frightened of death anymore because there is something wonderful outside this world. Extremely happy. As if all the care in the world taken away It was just letting everything go, about my son. (He was 20 then.) Letting go of the responsibility.

I was in a cocoon. The experience left very slowly. It was caring warmth floating light like an angel that can help.

What is the opposite feeling?
This will explain the polarity of the sensation.

Aloneness. Responsibility you have to shoulder alone. Thinking of answers to a problem all on your own, duties to make him a well-balanced individual. In a greater extended family you can rely on others; family takes part in your growing up.

Thanks to homeopathy I have been able to make a clear decision. We were away from all that.

Case Analysis
At Stage 4 - Sankaran's Sensation Method

Sensation
The problem has to do with structure. She needs relationships, a unit of friends, family. Any stress is related to losing this structure. This is the Mineral kingdom.

What relationships provide her is love, care, nourishment and a sense of identity.

These are themes of Row 3 in the periodic table.

Other themes in Row 3 are a strong sense of right and wrong, morality, issues of trust, being conscious of appearance and extreme sense of being forsaken, etc.

What is the other part of the sensation? There is a sense of being let down or betrayed, and having no relationship or structure whatsoever.

These are Column 1 and 17 themes within Row 3 using the periodic table.

So the remedy is *Natrum Mur*.

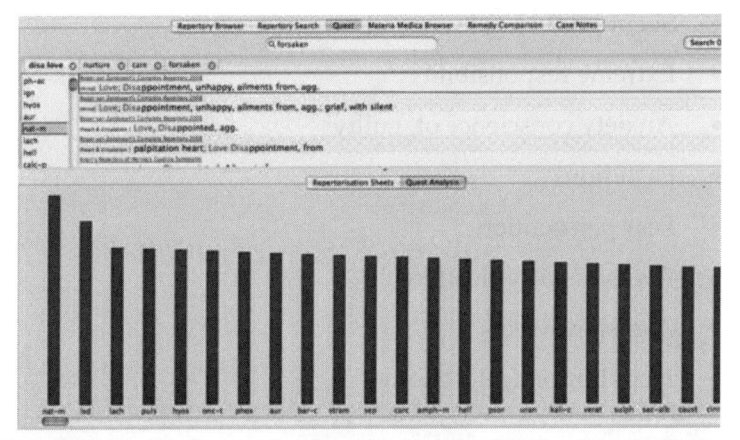

Illustration 1: Sankaran Analysis using the HomeoQuest Software

The *Natrum Mur* Sensation

Disappointed by relations, friends, family whom they trust, love and depend on. Completely no one to care for and love unconditionally. Sankaran's miasmatic analysis

This is a situation where she is acutely disappointed and betrayed periodically, but she has just accepted it with an 'I don't care' attitude

Malarial miasm – between Sycosis and Acute

Being stuck in a situation of dependence and suffering acute periodic attacks (disappointments, recurrences, etc)

At Stage 3 - Kentian analysis
Totality of her case

- Disappointment and unhappy love
- Silent grief
- Extreme responsibility
- Anxiety conscience of, guilty
- Fastidious
- Fear persecution
- Aversion fatty rich food
- Aversion sweets
- Perspiration feet, staining

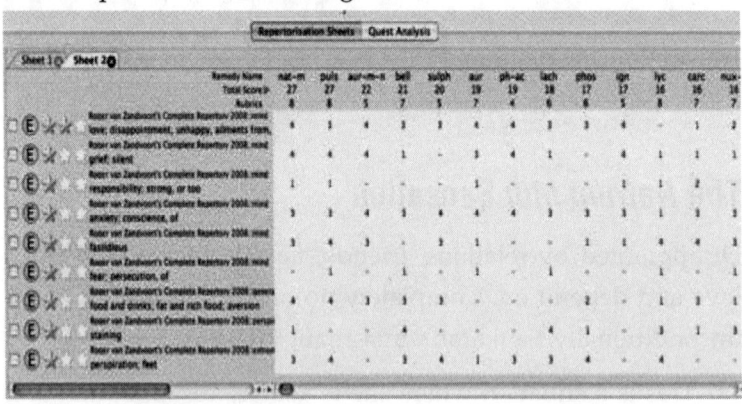

Illustration 2: Kentian Analysis using the HomeoQuest Software

The first two remedies were *Natrum Muriaticum* and *Pulsatilla*. If I had not taken the case at Stage 4, I would have referred to Materia Medica to confirm my prescription.

Interestingly, *Pulsatilla* had helped her quite well during the last episode of psoriasis.

However having taken the case at the Sensation level, I am certain it's a Mineral because it's a problem related to structure and everything falls in place.

Kentian Miasmatic analysis

- Miasm in Constitutional Traits – Sycosis
- Disappointment
- Silent grief
- Responsibility
- Fastidious
- Moral
- Guilt
- Fear persecution
- Fear failure

Miasm in Physical Symptoms – Sycosis

Chief complaint

Psoriasis – chronic, recurring itchy, excessive flaking, accumulation, raised patches, etc- sycosis.

Other Past Complaints

All of the following complaints are rooted in the sycotic miasm:

- PMS
- Endometriosis
- Hyperlipidemia

- Fungal infection
- Sinusitis

So the miasm of the case is Sycosis, which is covered by *Natrum muriaticum*. It is a multi-miasmatic remedy with a predominance of Psora and Sycosis according to Kentian analysis. Now let's confirm the remedy at Stage 1 and 2 for the disease psoriasis.

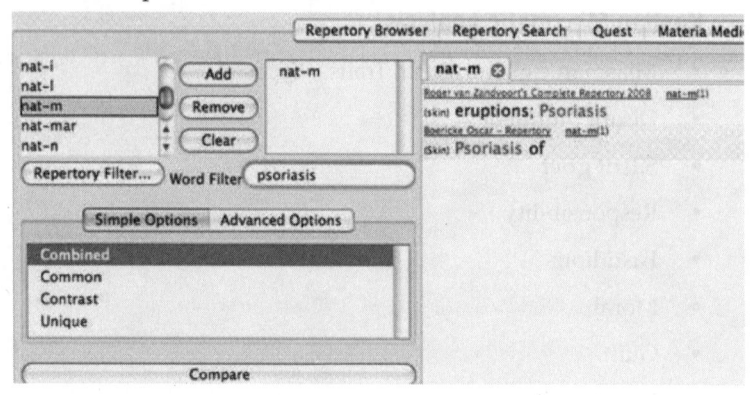

Illustration 3: Clinical Rubrics

Prescription

Natrum Muriaticum 200

Follow Up

Three months later

I have been remarkably well after the remedy you gave. Not painful, itchiness or thick scales. It feels only like dandruff.

Dreams - All my dreams have been about work and failure, but now I have been able to let go. I don't wake up in panic. It wasn't vivid either. I am taking care of myself now. I am still a person who likes to hold people, but I have put my boundaries out.

My whole life had been one big race against time and now I can take my time. A real wonderful feeling.

Two weeks ago I sneezed a lot, but that went away in a day. No discharge or anything.

All I can say that the psoriasis doesn't rule my life anymore.

Six months later

Things are improving. Hair growing on a bald spot on my head!! I had that spot for eight years. Psoriasis not getting worse.

I am sleeping really well. No more dreams about work. Pleasant ones taking my dog for a walk.

It used to be very red inflamed now it's pink. It's not as aggressive anymore or as unpleasant. No new spots or lesions. Its not as thick anymore, everything would build up before.

There is an improvement.

I have been really good emotionally. I have started to relax. I don't think of work anymore. I am cleaning up cupboards, but doing it in my own time.

We were apprehensive going to New York, but it was good. I am happy with my life, come to terms with my life and situation.

Being away from work helps as well

Previously I had to clean windows. Now there is less pressure on me.

I sleep really well.

I sleep non stop from 8-5am.

Very much more relaxed about life in general.

New hair growing on my bald patches. That's good.

Nine months later

After *Nat Mur* 1M - 1 dose.

Daughter was stand offish. I took the dose on a Saturday and on Sunday, I send her an email saying that if you don't want to keep this relationship, then so be it, and she has been much obliging and I am surprised, that I have been always someone always pleasing people and now I take a strong stand and say that's it. I don't bother too much about me. It's been a relief to me. It's like a burden has come off me. If you are pleasing somebody all the time because you are worried you will not have a lasting relation. Now I have evolved and grown and the people that really appreciate me will stay anyway. And the people that won't are not real friends anyway.

I am not really scared anymore in relationship area. I know who I am and take it or leave it.

People around also involve my husband, and like my daughter even he said it's time to take stance with my daughter. So I wrote we love her and if she can't be bother communicating parent to child neither do we. And she said no I do want to keep in touch and she phoned the next day.

I have decided to take matters in my hand and not leave it to others to take things in their hands. It is now what my husband and I want. This is something which is growing. It's reached its peak after the last dose.

It's no use getting upset abut things. If people don't make you happy, so be it. It was never really good anyway.

Ten months later

I am really good. It's not a big patch any more. Just three small patches.

My blood pressure is really low. (She was on anti-hypertensives. This was a possibility of the remedy having a favourable effect on her blood pressure so I advised her to look into adjusting the dose with her GP).

It's not as itchy.

Husband very surprised. It's not like it used to be. It was one big white mess."

Dreams – "A happy one. I am with a group of people. I have never met them in real life but they are friends in my dream.

I slept like a baby. I totally slept through the last night's thunderstorm.

So I might need to monitor it more.

Two years later

She continues to remain well and hadn't required any more medicines. Thus this case could have been solved using any method or strategy. *Nat Mur* was strongly indicated at Stage 3 analysis, even before we took the interview using the Sensation Method at Stage 4. However I used the Sensation Method eventually as a confirmation when I realised she was ready for it and an ideal patient for the same.

We have all these tools today that were never available

before. This is just one way of using the best homeopathy has to offer today.

Which Approach to Use and When

Most homeopaths choose to restrict themselves to working at just one particular stage and do so quite successfully. Throughout history, there have been successful homeopaths pioneering every stage in homeopathy.

My experience as a homeopath is that there are practical difficulties in applying just one particular stage in real life homeopathy in all cases.

Here you need to be flexible enough to adapt your case taking to fit the circumstances and get the best results possible. Thus having the knowledge, skills and understanding of working at every stage can tremendously benefit our practice and expand our scope as homeopaths. This process is about finding solutions to problems and helping patients in the quickest and most practical way rather than struggling to work with a so-called ideal method.

Although some of my most amazing cures have occurred by confirming the prescription right up to the fourth stage using the Sensation Method, it is not an approach that suits all patients, especially in their first interview. There are cases where you simply have to limit yourself to understanding approaches at one of the lower stages.

Let's look at various circumstances where working with approaches at certain specific stages are the most appropriate:

Circumstances When Stage 1 and 2 Are Best Suited

Disease Circumstances

- Patients with gross pathological diseases where good individualising symptoms are lacking due to progression of the disease itself
- Patients in a hospital setting who want complementary homeopathy
- Comatose patients
- New-born infants or children
- Animals
- Patients who cannot communicate well due to mental or physical disabilities
- One-sided diseases

Homeopath's Circumstances

- Focussed solely on the main disease and its removal
- Looking for a direct, practical approach

Patient Circumstances

- Not every patient is comfortable going through the detailed life history, or even experiencing the deepest sensations in a clinical situation, especially if they are new to homeopathy and coming from an allopathic view of looking at disease separately from the person.

Circumstances When Stage 3 or 4 Are Best Suited

Disease Circumstances

- Most diseases where there is a definite mind body co-relation
- Diseases that are more general and have a well-defined plethora of PQRS symptoms

Homeopath's Circumstances

- Ready to look beyond the disease and into the person
- Ready to dive into the hidden, unknown interior of the person to look for a cause beyond the material level

At Stage 4, Sankaran says it is the world of the non-sense. You might never understand what they say but everything they say connects beautifully to the story of the source. This is a skill that comes with practice. The homeopath has to be willing to provide that space for the patient to express this sensation in an unprejudiced manner.

Patient Circumstances

- Looking for options and answers beyond the medical explanation of disease and health
- Knowing that there is a mind body co-relation in sickness and experiences it everyday in life
- Willing to journey with you to find that innermost state of disturbance in sensation and energy

Having said that, the experience of colleagues and students in countries where homeopathy is not well known, or when people are still unsure of the therapy and the therapist, most patients do not wish to go further than their symptom picture in the first interview. Stage 3 involves talking about their mental and physical general state in great detail, and at Stage 4 some questions that lead them to the sensation can be frustrating or uncomfortable for someone who did not expect this level of depth during the consult.

However, during the follow-ups they are generally more receptive. Trust, practice and education are the keys when you need to take them to the deeper stages. Until that happens, provide relief for symptoms using other methods at an earlier stage where the patient is comfortable. Letting patients set the pace in their own healing journeys makes a huge difference.

Having said that, any case can be taken at any stage, and homeopaths that are skilled enough at a particular stage can treat every case using their own method of choice quite successfully.

For me, it is about working with patients rather than forcing them to work along with me. It's just my experience that working at their pace and meeting their needs and expectations provides a much more satisfying outcome in the long run. It's a slower but a more enjoyable process of moving toward the same goal.

The Sensation Method Compared With the Earlier Methods

Let us now focus on Stage 4 – the Sensation Method specifically and look at the advantages and disadvantages of using it as compared to the traditional approaches at Stage 3.

Advantages		Disadvantages	
Stages 3 Traditional homeopathy	Stage 4 Sensation homeopathy	Stages 3 Traditional homeopathy	Stage 4 Sensation homeopathy
For the Homeopath			
They are working in their comfort zone and using tried and tested methods and medications.	When you have determined the correct sensation, there is little doubt about the prescription as the remedy covers all stages when you have travelled through the levels. Follow ups are short and highly satisfying and cure process is much more efficient with lesser efforts. You are no longer restricted to provings and repertorial data. The whole universe is your materia medica.	Every follow up is a time-consuming process unless you accidently hit upon a remedy matching all stages. In complex cases, you need a good grasp of Hahnemannian and Post-Hahnemannian miasms, with experience working in layers to produce a cure.	Developing additional skill set for case taking and understanding remedies and their sensations. Comparatively lesser clinical confirmation for your prescription. The time and commitment required for the initial consult is more. Lastly if the sensation is not understood clearly at the end, you have to retake the case and still give the patient a remedy. This can be time consuming and frustrating for the patient.

For the Patient			
Depending on the approach and accuracy of the remedy, they can expect some form of improvement right from the first follow up. The remedy given is more or less proven and hence they have good clinical confirmation to back their case.	The initial consult itself creates a level of awareness and initiates the healing process. They will need just one remedy through out the cure process in minimal doses. Once the sensation and remedy are confirmed it makes it all worthwhile. Follow ups are a breeze and the cure process is much deeper, and makes profound positive impacts on their lives.	The cure process can be time consuming. The follow ups can be extensive and frequent. Changes in medicine and dosages can occur depending on the stage before they are cured.	Unless the exact sensation is found, there is no prescription unless the homeopath uses another approach. There could be one or multiple retakes before the homeopath understands the exact sensation. If they need a completely new remedy, there is a waiting period before the remedy is available from pharmacies and might even include making a new remedy from scratch. During the case taking, they enter into a world of nonsense, which can create a sense of unease and discomfort at times for the patient.

Conclusion

The Sensation Method has unleashed the homeopathic potential as never before. For me, it represents a critical stage in the advancement of homeopathy which had been stagnant for a longer part of the last century at Stage 3.

Contemporary homeopathic practice today is developing a broad spectrum competency of approaches at every stage in homeopathy, and the purpose of this chapter is to introduce the Sensation Method as a part of this broad spectrum that encompasses homeopathy.

Thanks to this method, it is wonderful to have the choice and the means today to be able to understand the disease and the healing process one step further. And for the right patient, at the right time, and at the right pace, it is a journey worth undertaking.

Further Reading

- Bhouraskar — *The Quest for the Simillimum*
- Sankaran — *The Spirit of Homeopathy*
- Sankaran — *The Substance of Homeopathy*
- Sankaran — *The Soul of Remedies*
- Sankaran — *The System of Homeopathy*
- Sankaran — *The Sensation in Homeopathy*
- Sankaran — *Sensation Refined*
- Sankaran — *Structure*
- Sankaran — *The Other Song*

Chapter 6

Miasmatic Prescribing
Jennifer Osborne

Watson (1991) provides a great chapter on practical simple prescribing based on miasmatic indications. He described two main variations of the technique:

1. The use of nosodes
2. The use of anti-miasmatic remedies

1 The Use of Nosodes

While nosodes have a limited presence in the repertory there is no shortage of clarity on their indications based on the remedy profiles that we find in contemporary materia medicas and journals. He argued there were two times to give nosodes,

- when they are indicated
- when indicated remedies fail

Overwhelmingly, the best results using these remedies come when they are prescribed as the best pattern match to the symptoms in the case. When there are Medorrhinum symptoms then give Medorrhinum. Tuberculinum symptoms? Give Tuberculinum. Simple. But in addition, the appropriate nosode is often necessary when 'indicated remedies fail'. This quote is repeated over and over in the homeopathic literature. Of course it assumes that the remedy given was a close similar and not, as could be the case, an entirely inappropriate remedy. But of course we can never tell and we can never know. Watson (1991) argues that when a well selected remedy for some reason doesn't act, it may well indicate the presence of an active miasm that requires treatment with the appropriate nosode.

There are other reasons as well for giving a nosode. When the patient constantly relapses, or where some acute condition fails to resolve homeopaths over the years have had success by prescribing a nosode. Similarly he argues that often a miasm obscures the symptom picture and one way of gaining some clarity when nothing else seems accurate is to give the indicated nosode. Watson gives some excellent examples. A six year old boy with porphyria, pink teeth, intolerance to light and who looked 'goblin like' was given a dose of Syphillinum after a number of prescriptions.

2 The use of anti-miasmatic remedies

To the consternation of many students of homeopathy, there is no real agreement on the classification of most remedies into their miasmatic pigeonhole. One author says this, another author says that. Agrawal has these remedies, Choudhury that, Sankaran another. What is known is that all the deeper acting remedies have been credited with anti-mismatic properties, ever since the relationship between psora and sulphur was understood. It is therefore considered possible to treat by employing remedies that are similar to the indicated misam in the case. Just for starters, there are rubrics in the repertory for Syphilis, Psora, Sycosis etc.

But it is the job of the homeopath to determine the dominant miasm in the case. It is often easier said than done, and there can be *considerable overlaps, with features of more than one miasm being identifiable. Watson (1991) argues that there are several factors to be taken into account when determining the dominant miasm. Firstly, family history gives some indication, especially where there are prevalences of certain diseases in the recent past or even the distant past of the patient. In addition, there is their personal medical history where patterns of illnesses can be traced throughout the patient's life, including presenting symptoms that can be matched to an indicated miasmatic disposition. Some remedies will previously have acted well and this often indicates a miasmatic tendency. Watson (1991) gives the example of where Thuja, Staphisagria and Natrum Sulph may well have been used in the past with some success. Clearly the miasmatic disposition is sycotic and the nosode will be Medorrhinum.*

There is no doubt that the lists of remedies associated with different miasms are useful at times. These clusters of remedies can be employed immediately and usefully to eliminate a significant number of possibilities. We know that our Indian colleagues teach homeopathy from this miasmatic perspective, and every Indian student knows the miasmatic classification of each remedy. To their eyes, this makes homeopathy much easier to practice because all that is required is taking the symptoms of the case and making sure that the remedy chosen comes from that miasmatic classification. Simple.

Of course there is a serious precedent here because this is exactly how Hahnemann seemed to be practicing towards the end of his life. We know from this case books and the work of Rima Handley (1997) that virtually every patient received the remedy Sulphur. This has been interpreted by some as the prescribing of a senile old man enamoured of his new dashing wife. The evidence for this was that he prescribes Sulphur even in cases where the remedy was not indicated at all by the presenting symptoms. Others have seen it as simply prescribing the best anti-miasmatic remedy for the indicated miasm, psora. Handley's (1997) work on Hahnemann's casebooks from his Paris years identified that his preferred method was to give Sulphur usually at the outset diluted in water and alcohol and repeated at regular intervals, daily or every other day, the optimum dose. Hahnemann continued with this until such time as new symptoms emerged or previous symptoms intensified and the new symptom profile indicating the next remedy developed. He would then either stop the Sulphur, or in some few cases, would continue to give it while treating the new aspect of the disorder with a different remedy in a centesimal potency.

Hahnemann's theory of chronic disease is not without its problems. Over the years I have heard it described as:

1. *Too simplistic.*
2. *Ignoring other infectious diseases.*
3. *An interesting historical sideshow.*

Many homeopaths have speculated that Hahnemann's three miasms may well have been useful in the early 1800s, but subsequent developments in health of large populations meant that other new miasms such as cancer and tuberculosis also became as relevant. Some homeopaths stopped there. But many others have gone further and argued that these two additions to Hahnemann's classification are also of that time and that we have since moved on. Towards the end of the 20th century, we have identified AIDS, HIV, SARS, swine flu etc, and some such as Watson (1991), have speculated that even radiation, heavy metal, petrochemicals and electro-magnetic frequencies (EMF's) etc are equally strong miasmatic influences on health.

There are some such as Dimitriadis (2005) who have rightly lambasted educators of homeopathy for its poor and overly liberal interpretations of the clear theory of Hahnemann to the ultimate detriment of the profession through poor prescribing. To untangle the issues and provide some clarity, I asked an Australian homeopath Jennifer Osborne to contribute. Jennifer is a homeopathic phenomenon. When I first met her in 2008 she was surrounded by a bunch of her committed, dedicated and vociferous students at a conference in Sydney. Her enthusiasm and passion for homeopathy was infectious. Soon after I came to know and appreciate more of her skills when we worked together in the department of Homeopathy at Endeavour College of Natural Health. In practice for 12 years, she has inspired a generation of students in Brisbane and Melbourne in Australia with her knowledge and wisdom. She holds special energy for this area, miasmatic disease. Her medical knowledge from an incarnation as a registered nurse makes her a force to be reckoned with in a debate about the value and contemporary use of Hahnemann's Theory of Chronic Disease. Her brief was not to explore the theory as such (this will be left for another publication) but to describe 'miasmatic prescribing'.

AG

Contents

- What Is Miasmatic Prescribing?
- Nosodes as the Simillimum and Intercurrents
- Other Application of Intercurrents
- Other Benefits of a Knowledge and Understanding of Miasms

In this chapter you will:

1. Explore the use of nosodes
2. Understand the application of anti-miasmatic remedies
3. Consider the relevance and application of inter-current remedies
4. Learn the importance of searching for the dominant miasm in a case

Chapter 6

Miasmatic Prescribing
Jennifer Osborne

Faithfulness in Tracing the Picture of the Disease

fidê'lity *n. 1. Faithfulness, loyalty, (to); strict conformity to truth of fact; exact correspondence to the original; precision of reproduction (HIGH fidê'lity)*

In Aphorism 83, Hahnemann urges us to exercise 'fidelity' in tracing the picture of disease. From the above definition in the Oxford dictionary, fidelity means faithfulness, loyalty and perhaps Hahnemann is urging us to strictly and precisely reproduce the facts. But what exactly does this mean? Many homeopaths have many views of this one aphorism, and even more regarding his theory of chronic disease.

Hahnemann proposes that disease progresses in a measurable and consistent way that can be applied to both physical pathology, and according to some modern homeopaths, mental and emotional symptomatology. These modern homeopaths assert that spiritual, psychosocial and cultural aspects are also considered to be an important aspect of these disease states that have all influenced human evolution from biblical times through to modern day.

His chronic diseases consisted of the Psoric, Sycotic, and Syphilitic miasms. Modern homeopaths have expanded upon this to include the additional chronic diseases of the Tubercular and Cancer miasms. They originate from the diseases of Scabies, Gonorrhea, Syphilis, Tuberculosis and Cancer.

So let us start by defining 'miasm'. The Oxford only contains the word 'miasma' as an infectious or noxious emanation or defilement. If we turn to others for its definition, such as Murphy (2007), we find a much more useful idea that as homeopaths we can utilise; 'a *pre-disposition to certain groups of chronic symptoms of disease.*'

Kurz, 2005 notes that as homeopathic students;

> ...we are all taught about chronic diseases & how they relate to the miasms, we read in all the classic texts about the importance of miasmatic prescribing in the treatment of chronic diseases, yet they grew virtually absent in the everyday practice of homoeopaths. Reading through the published accounts of cured cases, we seem to be doing quite well without them...... who introduced it...why it took him so long...& how they helped homoeopathy become more effective, and why they have fallen out of use are some of the questions that come to mind.

He further goes on to say that:

> ...thoughts like these are likely the reason that we study Hahnemann's theory on chronic diseases but do not practice it – nor do not know how to practice it.

So what do we know about them currently? We know that they originated from the Greek word for 'taint' or 'stain.' The concept was first introduced by Hippocrates around 400BC and it was used to refer to the disease-baring agent that was carried within dirty water or bad air. In Hahnemann's era, this belief was still quite popular and believed to be responsible for the spread of epidemics.

Hahnemann himself did not include miasms in his initial framework, and between 1796 and 1828, miasms had not even entered into Homeopathic teaching. In his *Chronic Diseases,* he speaks of his increasing frustration at not being able to cure deep-seated chronic diseases.

In his preface he writes:

> ...when such a relapse would take place the homoeopathic physician would give the remedy most fitting among the medicines then known as if directed against a new disease, and this would be attended by pretty good success, which for the time would again bring the patient to a better state ... In the former case, however in which merely troubles which seemed to be removed were renewed, the remedy which had been serviceable the first time would prove less useful and when repeated again it would help still less. ...these new symptoms were at times not at all improved, especially when the obstacles (mode of living) hindered the recovery....

He stated that although Homeopathy was very successful in the treatment of acute disease, it did not seem to be able to assist within the realm of the slow onset, progressive chronic diseases. The stage had been set for the emergence of miasmatic theory. It has been interpreted that Hahnemann thought that a miasm demonstrated a constitutional weakness that was hereditary and based upon a parasitic infection that could be passed down from generation to generation.

This is exceptionally intriguing if one considers the current understanding of genetic inheritance, which is accepted today as scientific fact. The point of difference being that from a 'miasmatic' perspective, this then creates a condition of 'fertile soil' for the incoming disease-bearing agent when conditions are ripe to affect a change within the vital organism. The weakness already exists. It is not the result of an external agent.

Hahnemann traced constitutional weaknesses back to three initial parasitic diseases; scabies, gonorrhoea and syphilis respectively. According to Hahnemann, these three diseases are the root of all disease. He introduced the corresponding miasms: psora, sycosis and syphilis.

For a more modern perspective, we can turn to the interpretation of Little (1998) who agrees that:

>...in Hahnemannian Homoeopathy the word "miasm" means the effects of microorganisms on the vital force including the symptoms that are transmitted to the following generations. These chronic miasms are capable of producing degenerative illnesses, auto-immune diseases and lead the organism toward immuno-deficiency disorders.

Morell (1996) states that:

>...the theory suggests that if 100% of all disease is miasmatic, then 85% is due to the primary and atavistic miasm Hahnemann called Psora. The remaining 15% of all disease he held to be either syphilitic or sycotic, being derived from suppressed Syphilis or suppressed Gonorrhoea. Hahnemann unlike Kent later attached no moral dimension whatsoever to the sexual nature of the two latter miasms. Kent of course, emphasised this a great deal....

Clarke (1985) agrees.

The large majority of chronic diseases Hahnemann traced to the chronic miasm he termed "psora," and he maintained on the skin of the miasm was an eruption of itching vesicles, of which the itch vesicle was a type. It has of which the itch vesicle was a type.

Hahnemann himself ascribed the itch to 'the production of nine-tenths of chronic diseases.' Clarke (1985) maintains in his *Homeopathy Explained*, which, in spite of the presence of the insect Hahnemann emphasised that,

> ...this was not the whole of the disease - just as the tubercle bacillus is not the whole of pulmonary consumption. If it were, no doctors would escape consumption, since they inhale the bacillus constantly from their patients. 'The itch,' Hahnemann maintained, 'is chiefly an internal disease'. 'Psora is an internal disease – a sort of internal itch – and may exist with or without an eruption upon the skin.' 'Psora forms the basis of the itch.' To the reckless suppression of the chief external symptoms of psora Hahnemann ascribed the prevalence of chronic disorders.

Today homeopaths are still divided in acceptance of the theory which was originally greeted with a combination of disbelief and derision by many but the most devoted of his followers. The importance of chronic disease theory in clinical practice today continues to have many advocates and opponents. If we are to accept the premise that this miasmatic predisposition exists, then what exactly are the implications for current clinical practice? How do we apply this knowledge to our case work and final prescription?

Rather than revisiting this theory in detail, the purpose of this particular chapter is to outline how to apply miasmatic theory to current clinical practice in a practical way.

What Is Miasmatic Prescribing?

So what exactly is miasmatic prescribing? Most of us consider the use of nosodes when asking this question. Hahnemann himself opposed the use of Isopathy and medicines made from disease products initially. Why would we require nosodes when heavy doses of *Sulphur* were applied externally in the treatment of scabies just as the application of mercury was utilised to treat syphilis? The same would also apply in the use of *Thuja* with its capability to produce the characteristic discharges similar to that of gonorrhoea. If we consider this, do we need nosodes at all?

Had it not been for Hering and his significant contributions to proving these substances, Hahnemann may not have then been able to accept the eventual use of *Psorinum*. These days, nosodes are selected just like any other homeopathic medicine. They are chosen according to the Law of Similars, and form a valuable addition to our materia medica. Some homeopaths, in consideration of miasmatic theory, routinely prescribe a nosode followed by the simillimum, depending on what they perceive as the primary presenting miasm. In doing so, the underlying belief is that they are assisting in the removal of these 'hereditary' weaknesses. Other practitioners consider the presenting miasm, and then prescribe what they consider to be constitutionally using the miasm as a guiding tool for medicinal selection.

Nosodes as the Simillimum and Intercurrents

Let's examine how we could apply the use of miasmatic theory into our practice. Many homeopaths today describe their prescription as being 'Constitutional.' The simillimum is determined after what is considered to be a detailed consultation encompassing the 'totality' of the symptoms, which includes the mental, emotional and physical aspects of the person's case including past and family history. The simillimum is therefore determined as the closest match between the medicinal picture and the patient picture. Finding the simillimum is the ultimate aim of the homeopathic practitioner.

However, we may consider that there is also a 'miasmatic simillimum' that is based on the patients presenting or fundamental miasm, and determined by taking an accurate family and past history of the patient.

This is generally considered to be a miasmatic nosode, often referred to as an 'intercurrent' or complimentary medicine. Intercurrent prescribing is referred to by Owen (2007) as, 'a prescription between an effective constitutional medicine.' Therefore the goal or intention behind an intercurrent medicine or prescription is to open up the case. According to Owen, he states the following about intercurrents:

> ...patient will only need or receive one homeopathic remedy that covers all their symptoms, in practice, especially in more complex cases, patients seek out different inter-current treatment for particular symptoms. This type of prescription could be due to a particular symptom needing treatment, or an overlying acute picture etc.

The use of nosodes is considered the most common aspect of intercurrent prescribing. In this case, the practitioner uses the specific nosode that corresponds to the presenting miasm. The main nosodes are:

- Psorinum for Psora

- Medorrhinum for Sycosis
- Syphilinum for Syphilis

In this style of case management, the homeopathic practitioner uses the nosode as the 'intercurrent' between the constitutional prescription in order to attain cure. An example of this would be the use of the nosode *Syphilinum* in a case of *Mercurius*. The practitioner determines the constitutional simillimum to be *Mercurius* and prescribes *Merc Sol* 30c, which works well until the potency is exhausted. Symptoms may return and the practitioner increases the potency to *Merc Sol* 200c and then *Merc Sol* 1M. After moving to the 1M potency, no change has resulted but the simillimum is unquestioned. The practitioner determines that an 'obstacle to cure' exists and the intercurrent or nosode of *Syphilinum* 200c is given. In this example, the potency is selected as the last potency that was effective, in this case the *Mercurius* 200c. At this point, if there is no noted response to the nosode, another dose of an increased potency may be given before returning to the original simillimum of *Mercurius* once again at the last effective potency of 200c.

This process results in the original simillimum continuing to be effective in its movement towards cure. *Syphilinum* was selected as the miasmatic intercurrent because the case was determined to be syphilitic in nature, and is further supported by the prescription of *Mercurius* within the case. This example demonstrates the need for an understanding of the miasms and the symptoms belonging to a particular miasm. This understanding can assist in differential diagnosis when consulting the materia medica, and ultimately the final selection of medicine.

In intercurrent prescribing, the nosode is only used when an obstacle to cure is perceived, and the constitutional medicine is no longer effective. In all other instances, the nosode is only indicated when it is considered to be the simillimum.

Hahnemann himself worked his way towards cure by using complimentary or 'intercurrent' medicines that were similar in action to the simillimum. If there was no evidence of miasm or acute disease present, he used intercurrent prescribing. An example of this is *Pulsatilla* 30c, *Pulsatilla* 200c, *Pulsatilla* 1M, with no response, and then Silica 200c before returning to *Pulsatilla* 200c. This approach is often referred to as 'zigzagging' towards cure. In zigzagging towards cure, Hahnemann discovered the well-known Psoric triad of *Sulphur, Psorinum* and *Arsenicum*, which is useful in cases that include eczema, itching and asthma.

It is important to note that anything that impacts upon the vital force, such as an acute disease, could activate or worsen one of the inherited chronic miasms, and therefore is to be treated as separate. The nosode of the acute disease may also be useful during the acute phase of illness, such as the Herpes nosode in a case of chickenpox. Many homeopaths still prefer to prescribe homeopathically using a 'similar' medicine such as *Rhus Tox* to treat this condition. This point of contention is often where the debate over homeopathic philosophy comes into play, and has been hotly contested regarding homeopathy verses isopathy and 'similars' verses 'same.' Personal practitioner preference and training contribute significantly to the stance one takes.

The astute practitioner needs to be able to differentiate between an acute disease and an acute exacerbation of a chronic disease, as outlined by Hahnemann in aphorism 73 regarding latent Psora when considering the use of nosodes.

The recognition of the disease, the ability to predict its progression, and the subsequent awareness of deterioration within a case, all serve to alert the practitioner to the need for an immediate case review (Aphorism 167), as well as support the understanding of the theory of chronic disease and the ability to trace the picture of disease. The question that we ask at this point is do we prescribe an acute medicine for the acute picture, or do we prescribe for the chronic/constitutional state?

If we are considering the treatment of an active, acute, miasmatic state, we are advised not to give the nosode if the state is not exposed. The use of the nosode is only indicated when it is the simillimum to the case. If the miasm is not active, it is not available for treatment. In this case, we would prescribe the simillimum for the case, and only use the miasmatic nosode if it ceased to work as illustrated in the intercurrent examples previously stated.

Other Application of Intercurrents

Another treatment protocol that might be considered at this stage is one commonly discussed within homeopathic education and supported by many practitioners. Always start with the simillimum to the case, and proceed with a nosode only when there is an obstacle or blockage to cure that prevents the vital force from fully expressing itself. A blockage is removed when the vital force is stronger and the simillimum starts to or continues to work as it did previously. During this period, clarity of the symptom picture emerges for the practitioner, including improved vitality for the patient.

It is worth mentioning that there are two other accepted forms of intercurrent prescribing apart from the use of nosodes and zigzagging towards cure. These accepted forms of prescribing include isopathy and the use of sarcodes, and aetiological medicines based upon causation. An 'aetiological simillimum' is selected (also referred to as 'never well since...'), for example the use of *Natrum Sulphuricum* in the case of a longstanding head injury that is still impacting the case and creating an obstacle to cure.

In applying the use of nosodes from a chronic disease perspective, it is important to note that the same rules apply. A curative response is one whereby the case progresses according to well-defined principles, such as those outlined within the *Organon* and Hering's observations on cure. An improvement in the vital force often expressed as increased vitality and the disappearance of key mental symptoms within the case.

An intercurrent prescription can result in a number of outcomes. If there is no reaction to the intercurrent medicine after one dose, return to the simillimum after a week in the last effective dose and potency. At this point the original medicine continues to move towards cure. This is considered a successful prescription. If after a single dose of the nosode there is a significant improvement and movement towards cure, then the intercurrent medicine is now deemed the curative one and is continued until its effects cease to continue, and the original simillimum is then once again returned to at the last effective potency. Alternatively, some homeopaths advocate returning to the original simillimum after one week if the response is only moderate, which can still result in a successful prescription.

It is also possible that the intercurrent medicine acts

curatively and no further prescription is required. This is one whereby the intercurrent medicine has been deemed as the acute medicine for the case and is often demonstrated in clinical practice.

Lastly, the intercurrent medicine or nosode may be given, but upon return to the simillimum, the case does not continue towards cure. This is considered to be the wrong intercurrent and the prescription must be considered again.

Other Benefits of a Knowledge and Understanding of Miasms

The use of nosodes provides the homeopathic practitioner with a valuable tool in the treatment of chronic disease. It is commonly said that if students are to understand the miasm, they need to be familiar with the materia medica pictures of the corresponding nosode.

What other benefits can a knowledge and understanding of the miasms provide? How does the miasm go together with selecting it for the totality of symptoms? Kurz, 2005, notes the following: 'If we consider the totality and prescribe for it, why do we need to take the miasm into account in addition?' This is an important question. Surely if we prescribe according to the Law of Similars, then an understanding of miasms is irrelevant?

Roberts (1936) in his *Principles and Art of Cure by Homœopathy* provides us with an insight into their importance in the following passage:

> In treating patients suffering from these stigmata (miasms), this classification is of inestimable value, for it immediately

throws the simillimum into a class of remedies corresponding with the accentuation of the stigma (miasm) that is outstanding in the case, and this should be considered in the totality; it will often throw light upon the choice of a simillimum that is applicable to the individual case and stage of development.

If we accept that the presence of Psora weakens the constitution, and this is recognisable in a predictable and definable expression of specific symptoms, this provides us with valuable insight into the understanding of suppression and the treatment of such. These symptoms are viewed as pertaining to the Psoric miasm. For treatment of this particular chronic disease, you need to recognise the miasmatic presentation of the patient, and select the corresponding antipsoric medicine with this miasmatic presentation in mind. This is Hahnemann's concept of how to treat chronic disease.

The application of this concept to clinical practice is staggering. Along with providing the homeopathic practitioner with valuable insight into the materia medica of our medicines (another example of this may be Galen's temperaments) and allowing us to differentiate on its basis, the concept of miasms more importantly provides us with knowledge into the progression of disease. Understanding the suppression of symptoms behind the presenting case provides the homeopath with a tangible plan for case management – a firm anchor upon which to navigate through the rough waters in the journey of a case.

An understanding of the progression of disease is an essential element in determining how we understand the progression of a case, and how we need to continue within the case. Often the homeopathic student can get lost in the middle of a case, and it is at this point that our homeopathic philosophy and understanding of the concept of miasms can assist us greatly in moving towards a successful prescription. We need to be able to understand the totality of the case as the patient sits before us within one micro consultation, as well as the larger macro view of the case history in its entirety, including those aspects of the case that have preceded the individual that may have significantly contributed to current susceptibility and weakness of constitution.

Even before Hahnemann died, Hering had contributed the idea of two further miasms by identifying the infection tuberculosis and its resultant two venereal miasms, sycosis and syphilis, and two non-venereal, psora and pseudo-psora. Today Sankaran suggests many more miasms for our consideration. Whilst many homeopaths may express concern over this ever-growing abundance of what they consider to be an alarming amount of miasms, the underlying principle is the same. Any acute infection that is suppressed can become a longstanding chronic disease, and weaken the overall constitution that prevents an individual from achieving optimal health.

This concept is straightforward and has been overcomplicated by many. To illustrate simply, Herpes Zoster once suppressed by allopathic medications could internalise and present later as a much more chronic disease if the life conditions of an individual or following generations are conducive. Another example of this may be Multiple Sclerosis. The understanding of suppression and the disease being driven inwardly into a more chronic expression, in this case from acute affection of the nerve ganglia to a chronic affection of the nerve system, is a logical leap to make. This is an example of tracing the picture of disease, and has implications for our selection of medicines. If we reflect upon the origin and progression of the disease within a case, we can then apply the medicines that are 'similar' in action in a curative way. This can only significantly contribute to our materia medica knowledge and our understanding of which medicines would be useful to us in this example.

In years of studying and teaching miasmatic theory, one idea has been uppermost in the thoughts of many homeopaths. Hahnemann was in fact a doctor of the medical art, and to him medical science and disease knowledge contributed to his understanding and subsequent development of homeopathy. They were inextricably intertwined and one informed the other, hence the emergence of his chronic disease theory.

In any application of the Law of Similars, the question has to be asked if this knowledge is necessary. If we match the patient picture to the medicinal picture, and discover the curative medicine, why do we need to understand and be able to trace the picture of disease?

We need to do so for one important reason. It is not for the successful cases whereby the simillimum is found that we need to understand chronic disease. It is for the unsuccessful cases where we do not know how to proceed, and could through our lack of understanding, do more harm than good.

Understanding the progression of disease in our patient's lives can become a valuable tool and provide the framework for the aspiring practitioner, which can inform both our preventative practice and our initial and ongoing case management strategies.

Perhaps the final word should come from the founder himself in his introduction to *Chronic Diseases:*

> Since the years 1816 and 1817 I have been occupied day and night in efforts to discover the reason why the known Homeopathic remedies did not affect a true cure of the above mentioned chronic diseases; and sought to secure a more accurate, and, if possible, a correct insight into the true nature of these thousands of chronic diseases, which remained uncured despite the incontrovertible truth of the Homeopathic doctrine.
>
> When behold! The Giver of all good permitted me, after unceasing meditation, indefatigable research, careful observation and the most accurate experiments to solve this sublime problem for the benefit of mankind (Hahnemann, *The Chronic Diseases* 1835).

References

Agrawal, Y.R. (1995) *A Comparative Study of Chronic Miasms*, Vijay, New Delhi, India.

Allen, H.C. (1910) *Allen's Keynotes and Characteristics with Comparisons with Bowel Nosodes*, B. Jain Publishers, New Delhi, India.

Allen, J.H. (1994) *The Chronic Miasms: Psora and Pseudo-Psora*, B. Jain Publishers, New Delhi, India.

Allen, J.H. (1994) *The Chronic Miasms: Sycosis*, B. Jain Publishers, New Delhi, India.

Bailey, P. (1998) *Carcinosinium: A Clinical Materia Medica*, Palmyra, Western Australia.

Banerjea, S. (1991) *Miasmatic Diagnosis: Practical Tips with Clinical Comparisons*, B. Jain Publishers, New Delhi, India.

Bentley, G. (2003) *Appearance and Circumstance*, Pennon Publishing, Melbourne, Australia.

Bentley, G. (2006) *Homeopathic Facial Analysis*, Pennon Publishing, Australia.

Bentley, G. (2008) *Soul and Survival: The common human experience*, Pennon Publishing, Australia.

Boerike, W. (1996) *Pocket Manual of Homoeopathic Materia Medica*, Motilal Banarsidass, India.

Choudhury, H. (2001) *Indication of Miasm*, B. Jain Publishers, New Delhi, India.

Clarke, J. (1985) *Homoeopathy Explained*, B. Jain Publishers, New Delhi, India.

Foubister, D. (1993) *The Carcinosin Drug Picture*, Indian Books and Periodicals Syndicate, New Delhi, India.

Fraser, P. (2002) *The AIDS Miasm Contemporary Disease and the New Remedies*, Winter Press, United Kingdom.

Fraser, P. (2008) *Using Miasms in Homoeopathy*, Winter Press, West Wickham.

Gupta, A. (1989) *Organon of Medicine: At a glance*, B. Jain Publishers, New Delhi, India.

Hahnemann, S. (1994) *Organon of Medicine, 5th and 6th editions combined, trans. Dudgeon 5th edn & trans. Boericke 6th edn, Medi-T*, available at www.homeoint.org/books/hahorgan/index.htm

Hahnemann, S. (1978) *Organon of Medicine, 6th edn, trans W. Boericke*, B. Jain Publishers, New Delhi, India.

Hahnemann, S. (2005) *The Chronic Diseases: Their Peculiar Nature & Their Homoeopathic Cure, vol 1 & 2*, B. Jain Publishers, New Delhi.

Hahnemann, S. *Organon*, Brewster-O'Rielly, W. (1996) *Organon of the Medical Art*, Birdcage Books, Redmond, Wash.

Hering, C. (1997) *The Guiding Symptoms of Our Materia Medica*, B. Jain Publishing, New Delhi, India.

Heudens-Mast, H. (2005) *The Foundation of the Chronic Miasms in the Practice of Homeopathy*, Lutea Press, Florida.

Julian, O. (1997) *Julian's Materia Medica of Nosodes*, B. Jain Publishers, New Delhi, India.

Klein, L. (2009) *Miasms and Nosodes*, Narayana Publishers, Germany.

Kurz, C. (2005) *Imagine Homeopathy: A book of Experiments, Images & Metaphors*. Thieme, New York.

Little, D. (1998) *What are miasms?* http://www.wholehealthnow.com/homeopathy_pro/dl-miasms-03.html

Morell, P. (1996) *Hahnemann's Miasm theory and Miasm remedies* http://www.homeoint.org/morrell/articles/index.htm

Morrison, R. (1993) *Desktop Guide to Keynote & Confirmatory Symptoms*, Hahnemann Clinic Publishing, California.

Murphy, R. (2007) *Case Analysis & Prescribing Techniques*, B. Jain Publishers, New Delhi.

Norland, M. (2003) *Signatures Miasms Aids - Spiritual Aspects of Homeopathy*, B. Jain Publishers, New Delhi, India.

Ortega, P. (1980) *Notes on the Miasms*, National Homoeopathic Pharmacy of Homeopatia de Mexico A.C.

Owen, D. (2007) *Principles & Practice of Homeopathy: The Therapeutic & Healing Process*, Churchill Livingstone Elsevier.

Rehman, A. (1997) *Encyclopedia of Remedy Relationships*, Thieme, Heidelberg.

Roberts, H.A. (1990) *The Principles and Art of Cure of Homeopathy*, B. Jain Publishers, New Delhi, India.

Sankaran, P. (1978) *Some Notes on the Nosodes*, Homeopathic Medical Publishers, Bombay, India.

Sankaran, R. (1999) *The Substance of Homoeopathy*, Homoeopathic Medical Publishers, Bombay, India.

Sankaran, R. (1994) *The Substance of Homoeopathy*, Homoeopathic Medical Publishers, Mumbai, Mumbai, India.

Sankaran, R. (1999) *The Spirit of Homoeopathy*, Homoeopathic Medical Publishers, Mumbai, India.

Saxton, J. (2006) *Miasms as Practical Tools*, Beaconsfield Publishers, Beaconsfield.

Speight, P. (1961) *A Comparison of the Chronic Miasms*, Health Science Press, Rustington.

Zee, H. (2000) *Miasms in Labour*, Stichting Alonnissos, The Netherlands.

Further Reading

- Choudhury — *Indication of Miasm*
- Coulter — *AIDS and Syphilis - a hidden link*
- Dimitriadis — *The Theory of Chronic Diseases According to Hahnemann*
- Dimitriadis — *Homeopathic Diagnosis Hahnemann through Bönninghausen*

Chapter 7

Jan Scholten's Group Analysis
Greg Cope

I remember first seeing Jan Scholten in 1993. I had been studying for a number of years but this was the first conference I'd ever been to and I was bewildered. It was one of those English conferences in the 1990s with hundreds of people. Scholten made a stir with his presentation. His book Homeopathy and the Minerals, known to students worldwide as 'the green one,' was still literally warm off the press. And with the first few sentences of the seminar presentation, some got up and walked out because what was being suggested was clearly not homeopathy. The idea of group thinking, and the concept of prescribing a homeopathic remedy on the basis other than from a proving, was too painful to hear for some. Yet others sat up in their seats because what was being said and articulated was quite stunning and in fact revolutionary. Within a year or so, his Homeopathy and the Elements was published (the blue book) and the initial idea of putting together known indications from different minerals gave way to a style of prescribing using the most fundamental map of nature, the periodic table.

To my mind, Scholten's work represents a completely different direction in homeopathic medicine, as important as the shift from Hahnemannian homeopathy to Kentian homeopathy under the influence of Swedenborg in the 1870s and 80s. It is an utterly new direction. For this chapter I've turned to an advocate of the method and someone who is using it with considerable success over and over in practice. Greg Cope began practising homeopathy in 2003. Known throughout Australia for his considerable technological skill and support of the Archibel software packages, Radar, Encyclopaedia Homoeopathica and now Opus, Greg has been a really calming influence on many homeopaths that have chosen the electronic pathway. But it is since he has been teaching and lecturing in homeopathic medicine at Endeavour College of Natural Health that he has really made a mark. Now a full-time senior lecturer on campus in Brisbane, he continues to both practice and inspire a new generation of students.

AG

Contents

- Jan Scholten
- Group Analysis
- Reverse Law of Similars
- Homeopathy and the Minerals
- Homeopathy and the Elements
- The Plant Kingdom
- Prescribing Techniques
- References and Further Reading

In this chapter you will:

1. Learn the historical and theoretical development of Scholten's work
2. Understand how it has evolved over time
3. Familiarise yourselves with the basics of the method
4. Observe the method demonstrated through case studies

Chapter 7
Jan Scholten's Group Analysis
Greg Cope

Jan Scholten

Although now well known within our profession, Jan's journey to become a homeopath was not a direct one. After graduating from high school, Jan began his tertiary studies in the field of biochemistry. Finding this field too materialistic, he turned his attention to the study of philosophy in an effort to discover the nature of life. Disappointed again by what seemed to him an intellectual exercise rather than a practical tool to discover the true meaning of things, Jan then turned his attention to the study of medicine in the hopes that the study of human health would reveal what had eluded him in his study of philosophy. It was during his internships that Jan was confronted with the awareness that medical treatment was not helping patients as he had expected, and in fact there were many that were made worse by it.

Like Hahnemann before him, when confronted with the outcome of allopathic treatment, Jan abandoned medicine but unlike Hahnemann, opened a gallery of modern art. Although running a gallery was something that he loved as a hobby, this venture proved financially unviable and so Jan returned his attention to general practice and sought ways to be a GP without the negative consequences for patients he had seen during his study of medicine. This led him to the study of acupuncture and homeopathy, eventually choosing homeopathy as his preferred profession. He chose homeopathy due to the astonishing results seen even in cases in which his allopathic studies had classified as incurable, and because of his desire to become a master in one field rather than a dabbler in many. Though a long and circuitous path to becoming a homeopath, the influences of biochemistry, philosophy, medicine, Chinese medicine and even art form a foundational part of Jan's practice of homeopathy, together with many other influences. Perhaps it is a sign of universal irony that Jan abandoned practice as an acupuncturist in order to focus pointedly on the profession that would require him to synthesise the knowledge of all the previous professions he had studied before.

Like many before him, Jan struggled with the application of homeopathy in clinical practice. So many cases saw staggering results that were beyond his expectations, but others were failures. By focussing on the cases where no result was achieved, Jan began to challenge the way he perceived disease and its cure. It was during this time that he studied under teachers Alphons Geukens, Jost Kunzli, Roger Morrison, Bill Gray, and especially he gives credit to George Vithoulkas and Rajan Sankaran who altered the way Jan understood homeopathy. It was particularly the work of Clarke, Morrison and Vithoulkas in the area of Group Analysis that inspired Jan to start working in a new way.

Group Analysis

The idea of studying homeopathic medicines in groups based on chemical or natural similarity is far from new. Although aware of this possibility, Hahnemann rejected it, fearful that the practice of baseless speculation prevalent in allopathic practice in his time would also take over homeopathy. It was perhaps Ernest A. Farrington who was the first to bring such ideas back into broad appeal having arranged medicines by their kingdom and chemical relationships in an attempt to assist his students to 'bring some system out of this chaos of materia medica'. Published posthumously as *Clinical Materia Medica* in 1887, this series of lectures by Farrington became the foundation of a new approach to group analysis in homeopathy. Farrington's focus was on the study of existing materia medica, and improving its understanding and utilisation by students of homeopathy. It was later with the work of Kent that Group Analysis was first applied significantly to the mineral kingdom to generate new materia medica of unproven or little known medicines.

Like Farrington before him, James Tyler Kent sought a method to teach materia medica to students of homeopathy that would enliven the medicine pictures and promote better retention of the mass of symptoms found in our provings and materia medica. Though he acknowledged that this method was far from perfect, Kent began publishing his lectures on materia medica, which became the beginning of the concept of essence prescribing in homeopathy.

Perhaps more than other homeopaths before him, Kent expanded the definition of totality of symptoms as discussed by Hahnemann to include a substantial focus on the symptoms of the mind and the symptoms of the person as a whole, rather than symptoms of their diseased parts. Influenced by the ideas of Christian philosopher Emanuel Swedenborg, Kent assigned greater importance to the mental and general symptoms, identifying them as belonging to a higher plane than purely local affections. He subsequently began the development of 'essences' or narrative stories involving common presentations of the medicine pictures. Excited by this new way of studying medicines, the homeopathic profession requested more and more work from Kent, leading him to make a commitment to publish a new medicine each month. Many consider that this relentless demand for new medicines to be published led Kent to author experimental work from his practice based on the use of unproven or little known mineral salts with symptoms derived from group analysis.

Perhaps out of fidelity to the principles of Hahnemann who rejected such work, Kent doesn't provide us with clear details of how he came to develop his materia medica for these new mineral salts, and even suggests that for at least some of these medicines, provings existed. These provings are unpublished or unknown if this is the case. Observers have speculated that it was one of Kent's other substantial contributions to the profession, his repertory, which was the tool use to generate these new medicine symptoms. It has been speculated that Kent focussed on the rubrics in his repertory, and where he found a rubric containing two separate elements as proven medicines, he also considered that their combined salt may have the same symptom. So he experimented in his practice with this information in an attempt to confirm his ideas and expand the number and understanding of medicines. Kent acknowledged the experimental nature of this information and recommended further research by proving to confirm or negate his ideas. Nonetheless, he fell under heavy criticism for deviating from the strict methodology of Hahnemann, particularly by Henry Clay Allen who railed against his publication of unproven medicines at the Homeopathic Congress of 1908. Kent subsequently retracted these synthetic medicines from the second edition of his *Lectures on Materia Medica* and never again published this work. It was returned to the profession after his death by his students in *New Remedies, Clinical Cases, Lesser Writings* and has since been reincorporated into his *Lectures on Materia Medica* by modern publishers.

Reverse Law of Similars

Inspired by the work of Vithoulkas, Sankaran, Geukens and others, Jan began to search for the essence of his patients during case taking, and to perceive a more detailed and deeper totality than he had previously. The problem remained that cases would present where Jan was able to understand the case very well through the process of case taking, but found difficulty in matching the patient's essence to that of a suitable similar medicine. Out of this struggle was born the reverse law of similars, in which he recognised that an unknown picture requires an unknown medicine. The challenge became how to find an unknown medicine to prescribe for a patient with an unknown disease picture.

Homeopathy and the Minerals

Jan recognised that there were many remedies in homeopathy, about which a very large amount of information was known;

these remedies were known as the polycrests, but there were many others about which little to nothing was known that we could expect should be equally as important as the best known of our polycrests. Working on the theory that there are no small remedies in homeopathy only little known ones, Jan began to examine how to use these lesser known minerals in his practice. Working as Kent and others before him had done, Jan began to look at the component cations and anions of the mineral salts to try to understand their key themes and symptoms. Why if *Nat-mur*, *Calc-carb* and *Nat-carb* are such important medicines, do we never prescribe *Calc-mur*? Surely it should be considered for many patients he thought. Jan began looking in his practice at cases that had been highly successful with well-known medicines, and further examined his clinical experience to understand the core indications for the medicines elemental components. Finding commonalities in his clinical experience, Jan began to apply these ideas to new or little known medicines, such as *Calc-mur*, in order to generate new materia medica.

Jan's information is drawn from a wide variety of places, some commonly used in homeopathy, others much less so. Of course with the mineral salts it is an area of focus in chemistry, but other information that go into his remedy profiles comes from nutrition, toxicology and any other area of study that examines the interaction between the substance and human economy. Jan also studied the use of the material in industry and the environment and other applications from the perspective of the doctrine of signatures. His writings contain references to numerology derived from the chemical structure of elements, the mythology frequently found related to the name given to an element, provings conducted by Jan and his colleagues, both classical and meditative or abbreviated in form.

Testing this information in the clinic and refining it based on successful application, Jan published his first book *Homeopathy and the Minerals* in 1993 detailing the rewards of his experiments in the clinic, and that of his colleagues at the Homeopatisch Artsencentrum Utrecht. Included was information on the calcareas, magnesiums, kalis, natrums, barytas, acidums, ammoniums, nitricums, fluoratums, cabonicums, muriaticums, sulphuricums, phosphoricums, bromatums, iodatums, as well as some initial ideas on ferrum, vanadium, kali-bich, chromium and manganum. By focusing on the well-known salts in homeopathy, and formulating themes for the best known anions and cations, Jan introduced a significant number of new remedies to homeopathic practice, which have since established themselves as polycrest remedies in many practitioners' practices. *Calc-carb* and *Calc-phos* were joined by *Calc-mur* and *Calc-fluor* as developed medicine pictures, and little known or unheard of remedies like *Calc-nit, Calc-iod, Calc-brom* and more became part of some homeopaths regular practice, even when these combinations had not yet become so common for Jan himself. Like most group analysis, Jan provided primarily mental symptom suggestions, some physical generals and a few indications for physical particular symptoms. *Calcarea* become crystallized into central themes such as 'what others will say about him', 'sensitive to criticism', 'insecurity' 'fears', 'protection and withdrawal' and general characteristics well known in *Calc-carb*. Like the Institute of Clinical Research (ICR) before him, Jan found the carbon salts provided a good description of the metal and could be largely used as a basis for further group analysis.

A new aspect to group analysis work that had not been proposed before, Jan found that very often in his cured cases the anion was found to be consistently relatable to a type of relationship in the patient's life connected to their disease state. Jan had found the Carbons often accompanied father issues, the muriaticums with the mother, sulphur the partner, and the phosphoricums with peer relationships, such as siblings, neighbours and friends. Suddenly if someone was concerned about the opinion of him expressed by his friends, *Calc-phos* could be considered. If sensitive to criticism from the partner *Calc-sulph*, or *Calc-mur* if feeling sensitive to what others think of them as a mother. Although Scholten's themes for the anions are broader and more developed than only a relationship type, this new approach to prescribing allowed many new medicines to be prescribed, and considered with simplicity when a case was understood at a deeper level. Where remedy differentiation may have been very difficult in some cases previously, it became very simple to consider that a tired mother may need *Muriatic* (mother) *Acidum* (exhaustion), and the small medicine picture in existing materia medicas would confirm the prescription. Like Sankaran's situational materia medica approach being developed at the same time, this necessitated a new approach to case taking. Understanding the way a disease fitted into a patient's life and story, and the inter-dependence of each on the other was an essential aspect of prescribing. Scholten found he had to ask his clients more questions to understand them and find the essence of the case, but once the client was understood, analysis often became much easier when related to the themes of an anion and cation in combination. Scholten also started to look at broader relationships, finding some similarities between *Vanadium, Kali-bichromium, Chromium, Manganum* and *Ferrum*, substances, which are closely related in the periodic table. This work in *Homeopathy and the Mineral's* lead the way for what was to follow in Jan's next major contribution *Homeopathy and the Elements*.

Homeopathy and the Elements

In Jan's first book, his focus was on looking at the essences of anions and cations, and examining new combinations and expanding the knowledge of existing combinations. Although many of the salts produced were new to homeopathy, the element components were typically well known in several well utilised polycrests. *Homeopathy and the Elements* significantly changed this, as Jan turned his attention to introducing entirely new elements into the homeopaths medicinal armament. By combining these new elements into salts with other known elements, there was a dramatic explosion of medicines into practice that were formerly unheard of, and in some cases not even possible to potentise and produce medicines from.

Jan started to look at the relationships between elements in the rows and columns of the periodic table. Developed by chemists, there are various versions of the periodic table. Russian chemist Dmitri Mendeleev published the first significant periodic table, containing the 63 known elements at the time. By recognising repeating patterns or 'periods' of similar reactions between different elements, Mendeleev was able to identify elements with chemical similarity before the underlying atomic structures that explained these 'periods' was understood. Many homeopathic medicines that are known to be similar to another from the proving symptoms in homeopathic medicine, are found to occur in the same row or column of the periodic table as their similar medicine. Phosporus, Arsenicum and Nitrogen, all in the 15th column of the periodic table are well known for their similarities. For example, Scholten had already identified similarities between *Ferrum, Chromium, Vanadium* and others from the fourth row of the periodic table; *Platina* and *Palladium* are often recognised as very similar and occur directly above and below each other; and *Platina* occurs beside *Aurum* to which it is also known as being similar. By expanding these known similarities, Scholten began to predict the qualities of entirely unknown medicines from areas of the periodic table that had previously been entirely unexplored.

ELEMENT THEORY TABLE STAGE (COLUMN) KEYWORDS	Period / Series / Row Keywords Click any Series / row for element keynotes	STAGES 1.-9 DETAIL STAGES 10-18 DETAIL
Hydrogen Series	Being, Existence, True, Real, Space, Space-less, Time, Timeless, Smell, Unborn Fetus, Body-less	
Carbon Series	I, Ego, Person, Individual, Self-worth, Value, Meaning, Ethics, Good, Bad, Hero, Borderline, Magic, Myth, Vitality, Lust, Possessions, Naïve, Birth, Touch, Body, Life, Child	
Silicium Series	Other, You, Friend, Relations, Communicate, Love, Hate, Neighborhood, Language, Learn, Play, Presentation, Clothes, Taste, Teenager, Puberty, Family, Home	
Ferrum Series	Worker, Task, Work, Duty, Craft, Ability, Use, Perfectionism, Routine, Order, Rules, Control, Observed, Exam, Criticized, Failure, Guilt, Crime, Orientation, Adult, Village	
Argentum Series	Inventor, Creation, Inspiration, Ideas, Science, Art, Culture, Unique, Admiration, Aesthetics, Beauty, Mysticism, Show, Performance, Queen, Ambition, Hearing, Voice, Middle age, City, Country	
Lanthanide Series	Autonomy, Self, Own, Independence, Free, Space, Self-control, Spiritual, Individuation, Therapy, Reflective, Secret, Alone, Isolated, Deep, Tense, Serving, Power, Vision, Eye, Light, Auto-immune	
Aurum Series	King, Leader, Management, Responsible, Serious, Heavy, Power, Dictator, Dignified, Haughty, Wealth, Alone, Isolation, Failure, Hurt, Religion, Sexuality, Vision, Eye, Ripe age, Country, World	
Uranium Series	Magic, Intuition, Old age, Universe, Genetic	

©Archibel S.A.

Jan identified that each horizontal row of the periodic table related to an area or sphere of life. The first row containing only 2 elements, hydrogen and helium, was found to relate to 'being' itself. Like Hamlet there are only two choices in this row, 'to be or not to be'. Themes of being, or not being, incarnation, and the differentiation between the real and the unreal may indicate one of these medicines. Progressing on developmentally, the second row of the period table title 'Carbon series' is related to the individual's self worth, defining who they are and if they are perceived as a good or a bad person. Followed by the Silica series with its' focus on relationships, the Ferrum series' themes of work, Argentum series' art and creativity, the Lanthanide series' autonomy, the Gold series' leadership and the Uranium series' magic and intuition. Each stage is a development beyond the one before, and mirrors a common progression of life stages as the aging process progresses. Each row can also be related to physical concepts, with more superficial tissue types nearer the top of the periodic table, the deeper and more vital organs towards the bottom where the elements are generally more toxic or even radioactive.

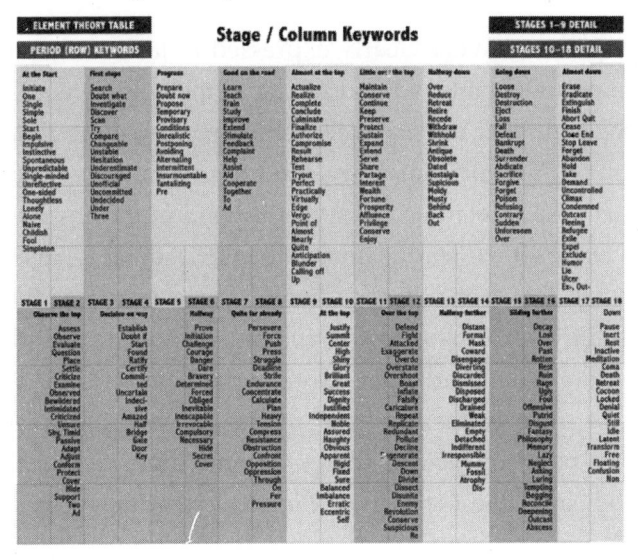

©Archibel S.A.

Having identified the area of life that is a focus for the client or the cause of disease, the practitioner can determine the series or row/s of the periodic table indicated. From here it becomes necessary to choose which element from the row. To assist with this choice, Jan identified a pattern of sequential development that occurs within an individual row. In the same way that the rows display a development from the top to the bottom, the vertical columns display a development starting from the left and progressing to the right-hand side. The concepts of the horizontal row are found to begin in the first column, progressively develop to a mature expression in the tenth column, and from there onwards decline until they fall apart and disintegrate as they move towards the right of the row.

| Cs | Ba | La | Hf | Ta | W | Re | Os | Ir | Pt | Au | Hg | Tl | Pb | Bi | Po | At | Rn |

This pattern is very clearly expressed in Jan's early work with the periodic table, when looking at the gold series. This series has a number of very well-known medicines at various stages along the horizontal row, and are commonly seen to express concepts relating to leadership and authority. *Baryta* in stage two near the start is unable to take leadership, instead they are dependant on others and prefer someone to lead them. Towards the centre of this row *Platina* and *Aurum* are confident in their worth, and in their more postive aspect are well known for their leadership over others. As we progress past the centre point of *Platina*, things become more destructive, with medicines like *Mercury* or *Plumbum* often suggested as potential prescriptions for dictators losing control of their leadership role. By identifying these well-known points along the series and comparing them to other well-known medicines in other rows, it is then possible to speculate on how other well unknown medicines in the row may be similar and be considered as prescriptions in practice.

- Perhaps the leader who is more confident than *Baryta*, but less confident than *Platina* needs an element that occurs somewhere between them.
- If the client is a forceful and pushy leader, who reminds the practitioner of the forceful essence of *Ferrum* (stage 8 in the Ferrum series), then this client may benefit from *Osmium* (stage 8 in the Aurum series) as they are a leader (*Aurum*) rather than a worker (*Ferrum*).
- If a client is concerned about losing a friend, we may identify 'friend' as in indication of the Silica series, and concern about relationships, and 'losing' as an indication that an element from the right-hand side where things fall apart is needed. Hence, we can consider *Phosphorus* who does not want to lose (stage 15) a friend (silicea series), and feel like they are alone on an island as the famous delusion rubric describes them.
- By combining two elements together, someone whose disease is related to the concept or essence of being a forceful leader for their friends, may need the medicine *Osmium-Phosphoricum*.

By utilising this method, Jan introduced hundreds of new medicines as possible prescriptions, and by extending the idea further was able to introduce an entirely new group to the materia medica with the publication of his book *Secret Lanthanides*.

The Plant Kingdom

As Jan's work progressed with using the periodic table to classify the stages of development of the mineral kingdom, he started to see similar classifications in other areas. The 18 stages of the periodic table were seen to express the pace of a person's symptoms, in much the same way as Sankaran's system of 10 miasms does. Scholten has expressed that he finds the 18 stages a more complete model, but that there are parallels and overlaps between the two systems. Jan has begun to apply the 18 stages of the periodic table as a universal classification system and is now utilising it in the homeopathic classification of plants. In much the same way as Jan tried to discover the themes of a series or horizontal row of the periodic table, Jan began to look for themes and concepts in the natural orders of plant families. Having identified themes for a natural order of plants through the study of cured cases, materia medica, conducting provings and source material lore, Jan then started to map the medicines in a natural order to the already known themes of the 18 stages of the periodic table. This mapping allowed a way to access theses medicines in a way similar to the minerals, and also to predict the symptoms that may be found in little known members of the natural order. Further, in the same way that the periodic table showed a vertical line of development from the Hydrogen series at the top, progressing to the Uranium series at the bottom, the plant families demonstrate a growth from the more prehistoric species, to the more recently evolved as identified by genetic mapping of the Angiosperm Phylogeny Group (APG). Often it can be seen that the elemental composition of older plants is more similar to the elements near the top of the periodic table, and the most recent plants to evolve contain the lower elements such as the lanthanides.

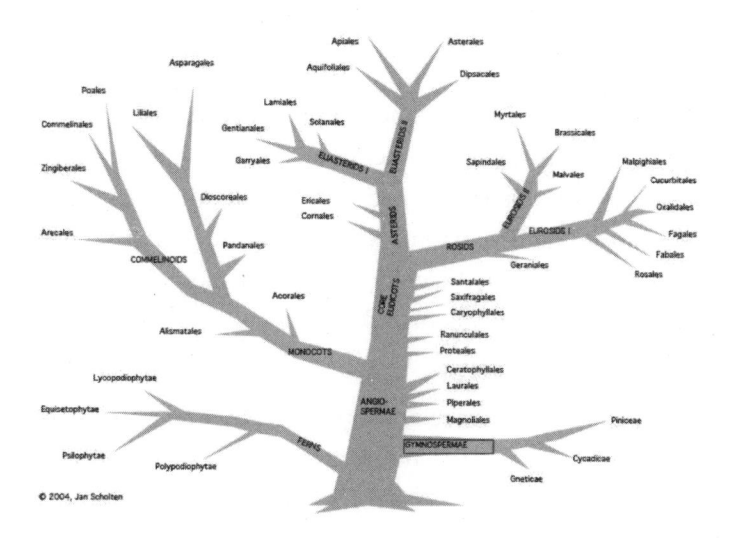

[taxonomy tree diagram]

http://www.janscholten.com/janscholten/Downloads_files/taxonomy%20tree.jpg

Prescribing Techniques

An interesting aspect of Jan's prescribing method is that although he perceives the need for a great variety of medicines in order to match the wide variety of disease presentations that are seen in practice, his approach to potency and posology is quite simple. The majority of remedy pictures described by Jan are accompanied by successful cases from practice, and a common trend is quite clear. Most prescriptions occur in a high potency, typically 1M or the nearest equivalent available from pharmacies, though Jan suggests that potency is of little consequence for most prescriptions so presumably a lower or even higher potency would be equally satisfactory if that was the only potency available. Dry and liquid doses are treated the same, with repetition used as needed. A common prescription seen is 1M, repeated several times over some months.

In contrast with other modern homeopaths using essence style prescribing, Jan will frequently change the medicine when the symptoms of the patient indicate the need. Jan has expressed that he doesn't subscribe to the idea that remedies are patients, or that medicine is the 'constitution'. He describes the medicine as the problem and so when the problem changes so will the medicine.

The highly speculative and predictive nature of Jan's work has often attracted criticism from more classically oriented homeopaths who have more conservative views or who feel we should continue to emulate the approach of Hahnemann. Although some of these homeopaths acknowledge the patterns of concepts growing down and across the periodic table that Jan has highlighted. Luc De Schepper offers a book *Homeopathy and the Periodic Table* which affirms Scholten's observation, but rejects the degree to which remedies can be understood through prediction. Others like Vithoulkas have rejected the work completely, despite the similarity in the origin of the concept, due to the amount of speculation and deviation from classical methodology, which may be more acceptable to our allopathic peers who are looking at the plausibility of homeopathic medicine. Many practitioners however attest that they find significant clinical success with Jan's method, and often are able to solve cases with which they have failed previously. A unique feature of Jan's publications is that he will often show cases where he has prescribed sometimes dozens of classically indicated medicines over many years with little effect, until his understanding of this new method reached a stage of development where he was finally able to find a new medicine that matched the case and healed the client. In my own practice, my greatest successes with the method have been with cases where Jan's method allowed me to consider a medicine I would not have otherwise, and that was confirmed by information found in classical materia medicas. However, there are also many cases where no classical information exists, and the medicine has still proved to be an effective prescription. Medicines like *Baryta-phos, Calc-nit* have become polycrests in my practice, with frequency of prescription in chronic disease far outnumbering prescriptions of even the best known medicines such as the ubiquitous *Sulphur*.

Case example

48 year old Rachael presents with anxiety issues. She has been treated homeopathically for some years by her friend and self-prescribes a lot also. She's had a large number of medicines over many years. She has been using *Arsenicum album* 6c several times a day recently which helps with her anxiety. She tried some *Arsenicum* 30c which aggravated her substantially. Since stopping the *Arsenicum* 30c the aggravation has reduced, but there has been no subsequent improvement so she decided to see a practitioner and see if she can get a better effect.

She has had anxiety symptoms since 6 years ago when her mother died. It was like she lost her joy in life then. She started experiencing blackouts when driving or in a stressful situation. She had her first panic attack while driving. She now can't drive on a motorway, it's too stressful and terrifying, so she can travel only short distances. This is a big problem as she runs a small farm and is the delivery driver for their product. She feels like fear is stalking her all the time. Rachael says she feels unsafe outside of her house, and driving takes her away from where she feels safest. She's always afraid something bad may happen. She anticipates things that might happen when she is away from home, or that she may have a panic attack. Home is the one place where she is happy. On the motorway she feels claustrophobic, like she is trapped on the motorway and can't escape it when she wants to. She feels overwhelmed by her life situation, she cannot cope, worries a lot about her children especially. She used to be social and had a lot of fun, but now she is averse to people coming to visit her and she is too anxious to go out a lot as she is so scared to drive. She gets alarming thoughts, or is easily startled; even answering the phone is very stressful for her.

She worries a lot about her family, her husband is very distant from their children and doesn't show any warm emotions to them. Her son hates his father because of this, and bullies her in order to get attention from his father. If her husband says something negative to one of their children, it causes her to have a panic attack. She feels like a solo mother when she sees her husband emotionally hurting their children with his distant emotions. She was like a mother to her sibling also from a young age, so is used to caring for others. There were lots of problems with her daughter at the time her panic attacks started, problems with her learning at school and being cranky with her mother. Rachael was very worried about her then and her daughter became distant and reclusive. Rachael has a lot of fights with her son, and she feels that coming home is like coming into darkness or a war zone because of that. She can't relax and enjoy her time at home like she used to. He targets her to pick a fight. She would be happier if her son wouldn't be like that, it's because of his father he behaves that way.

She gets palpitations and feels like something heavy on her chest and stomach with the anxiety. It can feel like her heart is on a stalk that sticks out of her chest and it beats very fiercely. She's had chest pain and nausea, EEG reveals nothing abnormal and the symptoms are assumed to be anxiety related. Her friend suggested *Crategus* for the palpitations which helps her a little bit. She's also taken betablockers, aspirin and takes antihistamines for her hay-fever. She has tried many anti-depressants, none worked and the doctors said they can't help her anxiety. She saw a psychologist who didn't help either.

She has been getting hot flushes the last couple of years, peri-menopausal symptoms. She gets really heavy periods that are excruciating painful. She never had premenstrual symptoms until recently. She has a lot of mood swings and irritability now. The anxiety seemed to get worse also after her friend prescribed *Sabina* for some of the menstrual problems. She's also currently using *Sepia* for mood swings. She did try also *Folliculinum* which aggravated her mood swings. Her libido is quite low. She has ovulation pains, that travels up the rectum, vagina, stomach. The pain is so bad she cannot walk. Also before her period she gets more anxiety and palpitations.

Her appetite is poor; she does crave steak and shellfish. She doesn't like sweets very much. She has a high fluid intake, can be up to 3 litres a day in warm weather. She generally prefers cooler weather, and is aggravated by heat. She gets a feeling of heat rushing in her blood during the summer months.

She had a dream that she was shot three times in the chest, the gunman was shooting someone else also and she was trying to see if they were dead too. She had an out of body experience in the dream, could feel the wounds, she was dying on the floor, but the ambulance officers were having a cup of tea before they would leave to come help her. Her sleep is very poor, has been a long time since she had good sleep and is aggravated by the sleeplessness. She takes *Rescue Remedy* which sometimes helps. She is easily woken by noises in the house, especially her son who is up late watching TV and the pets.

She has suffered from reflux and irritable bowel syndrome in the past. Her abdomen feels bloated and tender. The abdominal symptoms seem to happen more around her period or ovulation. It can wake her at night, she takes a variety of medications and antacids to control the symptoms. She's prone to loose bowel motions with the reflux, and sometimes nausea.

I gave Rachael a few medicines while understanding more of her case and finding a medicine that was more fitting and effective. She responded well to the first prescription of *Cocculus* 1M, her period pain reduced though not the bleeding volume, her anxiety reduced a little, and panic attacks became much less frequent. Her old irritable bowel symptoms also returned after *Cocculus*. Subsequent repetitions of *Cocculus* and potency changes had no further effect and she slowly deteriorated to her previous state. Given her general *Calcarea* appearance and anxiety, I then gave several doses of *Calcarea-carbonica* over some weeks in 200c which reduced her anxiety, but aggravated her palpitations immediately after each repetition, as well as her digestive symptoms and hay-fever which didn't then improve. At this point Rachael self-prescribed *Ignatia* which antidoted the positive action that *Calcarea* initially offered and caused a number of new symptoms and also an aggravation of existing symptoms. *Gelsemium* 200c settled the aggravation she experienced following the use of *Ignatia*, but didn't improve her chronic state at all.

At this point I retook her case, and started looking at more options than the common medicines indicated by reportorial analysis. Rachael's symptoms are clearly based around very common concerns, family, work, the structures of daily living. This is an area of life which tends to indicate elements from the upper part of the periodic table. From a repertorial analysis you may consider *Argentum-nitricum* for this case, though there were no apparent indications for the Silver series component, nor anything from the Aurum, Lanthanides, Uranium or Actinides series. *Nitricum* however was strongly indicated. Scholten often comments that the Carbon series to which *Nitricum* belongs can be difficult to spot as the concerns of this series are so common that we may not identify them as symptoms. Carbon relates to the self and it seemed an area of weakness and worthwhile to consider for Rachael. She spoke often of the people in her life, her children and husband in particular, though not in a way that indicated the issue was connected to relationships and hence the Silica series. Instead she spoke about the effect of a situation on her, and her feelings of safety, comfort and ability. Carbon may be related to the development of a strong self of self, and a weakness in this area and the many fears such as Rachael describes may indicate a

Carbon series medicine. *Nitrogen* is strongly indicated in many of her symptoms such as the anxiety, phobias, feelings of claustrophobia, aggravation from heat, violent palpitations, menstrual flooding and hot flushes. Rachael also described her impulsive and alarming thoughts, something often seen in *Argentum-nitricum*. Nitrogen belongs to row 15 of the periodic table which being past the high point of stage 10 relates to loss. In the Carbon series it is particularly the loss of vitality and a loss of sense of self. Scholten describes this as a loss of (or desire for) joy. Rachael in fact used this word often during consultations, describing the death of her mother and her rocky relationship with her son as things that stole her joy from her. She also describes a feeling of threat and danger, which fits with the description of the Nitrates given by Sankaran and others.

Given her general *Calcarea* nature it is easy to consider *Calcarea-nitricum*. Many of the concepts of *Calcarea* can be seen in her case. In particular her response to the *Nitricum* feeling of threat, anxiety and joylessness is to retreat into her place of safety, her home, much like the oyster into its shell. This tendency to retreat strongly indicates stage 2 of the periodic table, with its passivity and contraction. This is the row containing some of our very bashful mineral medicines, such as the *Calcareas, Barytas,* and *Magnesiums. Calcarea* in particular retreats from Ferrum series concepts such as work, task and the surrounding village or community, things which were clearly happening for Rachael and impacting on her ability to run her business.

I prescribed *Calcarea-nitricum* 200c, 3 doses twelve hours apart. Rachael responded well and quickly to the new medicine.

Her next period was very good with much reduced pain and flow, her palpitations decreased, her anxiety was a lot less and she started to enjoy going back out driving again and going to places away from her house. She started to confront the situations with her son and things with him improved because of this. She continued to repeat the medicine periodically for some time, every one to two weeks she took a dose. She returned to the clinic three month later having had her first moment of panic since the medicine change, some palpitations and an increase in premenstrual symptoms. These settled quickly with *Calcarea-nitricum* 1M in a single dose.

References

Scholten, J. (2000) *Homeopathy and the Elements* Stichting Alonnissos, The Netherlands.

Scholten, J. (2005) *Secret Lanthanides* Stichting Alonnissos, The Netherlands.

Scholten, J. (2010) *Schema of the Periodic Table,* Archibel S.A., Belgium.

Suijis, M. (2008) *Actinides the 7th Series of the Periodic Table,* Archibel S.A., Belgium.

Scholten, J. (1993) *Homeopathy and Minerals* Stichting Alonnissos, Utrecht, The Netherlands.

Kent, J.T. (2005) *Lectures on Materia Medica,* B. Jain Publishers, New Delhi, India.

Kent, J.T. (2005) *New Remedies, Clinical Cases, Lesser Writings,* B. Jain Publishers, New Delhi, India.

Bettelheim, M. (1998) *General, Organic & Biochemistry,* Saunders College Publishing, United States of America.

Mastin, J.W. (1905) *The Critique Volume XII,* The Denver Journal Publishing Company, United States of America.

Lesser, O. (1935) *Textbook of Homeopathic Materia Medica,* Archibel S.A., Belgium.

Farrington, E.A. (1908) *Clinical Materia Medica,* Archibel S.A., Belgium.

Dhawale, M.L. (2003) *ICR Hahnemannian Totality Symposium Part II,* Dr. M.L. Dhawale Memorial Trust: Mumbai, India.

Sankaran, R. (2000) *The System of Homoeopathy,* Homoeopathic Medical Publishers, India.

Morrison, R. (2006) *Carbon: Organic & Hydrocarbon Remedies in Homeopathy,* Hahnemann Clinic Publishing, USA.

Schepper, L. (2003), *Homeopathy and the Periodic Table,* Full of Life Publications, Sante Fe.

http://www.homeoint.org/morrell/articles/pm_kentn.htm

http://www.wholehealthnow.com/homeopathy_pro/henry_c_allen.html

http://www.janscholten.com/janscholten/Life.html

Jackson, R. (1998) *American Homeopath,* Archibel, S.A., Belgium.

Further Reading

- Scholten   *Homeopathy and the Elements*
- Scholten   *Secret Lanthanides*
- Scholten   *Schema of the Periodic Table*
- Scholten   *Homeopathy and Minerals*
- Farrington   *Clinical Materia Medica*
- de Schepper   *Homeopathy and the Periodic Table*

Chapter 8

Eizayaga
Ben Gadd

I invited a friend and colleague, Ben Gadd to write a chapter on the work of Dr. Francisco Xavier Eizayaga. Many homeopaths have found themselves moving towards the work of this Argentinian homeopath who created an excellent model and framework for understanding the complexity of homeopathic case analysis and prescribing.

It is an approach to prescribing that is very appropriate in cases with advanced pathology and for when there are degenerative diseases, and also cases where there are complications with drug use. It is well suited to complex cases with multiple causes and where many remedies are indicated. My own experience is that complex and confusing cases are often simplified by applying this model. Where no single remedy emerges from a chronic case taking, it makes perfect sense to separate the lesional, from the fundamental, from the constitutional and from the miasmatic layer.

Of course it is ultimately a map and not the territory and therefore like all theories, there are times that its limitations manifest. It is sometimes not easy to determine exactly if the symptom is lesional or fundamental or constitutional. Often these things are self evident, but in reality, in complex cases where there are skin diseases, or complex pathologies and degenerative conditions, it requires a sharp mind to pigeonhole and separate out all of the symptoms. But a working relationship and a deep understanding of this system is overwhelmingly beneficial. In this chapter, Ben untangles the issues. AG

Contents

- Introduction
- About Eizayaga
- Treating the Patient versus Treating the Disease
- Different Types of Similitude
- Totality of Symptoms
- Classification of Symptoms
- Classification of Diseases
- Layers
- Fundamental Layer
- Constitutional Layer
- Miasmatic Layer
- Prescribing
- Posology
- Repertory
- Criticisms of Eizayaga's Approach
- Case Example
- Analysis
- Conclusion
- References

In this chapter you will:

1. See the value of this synthetic and wholistic approach to working with complex cases
2. Explore the development of the method
3. Understand the disadvantages and criticism of the method
4. Learn its pragmatic value through the study of cases

Chapter 8

Eizayaga
Ben Gadd

Introduction

The ability to utilise different practice methods is essential for the homeopath. If we have a case that suits a certain method - a specific process to find the simillimum - and we choose a different one, we may not achieve the best outcome for our patient. Even if we do, we are likely to have arrived at that outcome by a route that is more complicated than necessary.

In general, while it is likely that practitioners will have a few methods that they are particularly good at, or use most often, it is best for homeopaths to be skilled in all methods. The benefit of Eizayaga's framework is that it provides a structure or roadmap for looking at each case. Even if we are not using the approach as Eizayaga suggests, we can still use his way of classifying symptoms and 'mapping the terrain' of the case to discover the most appropriate method to use. Mapping the terrain can help us to determine where the focus of the case lies. Once we understand this emphasis, selecting the most appropriate method (and medicine) becomes easier.

For example, here is a case of a patient who is nine and a half weeks pregnant and complaining of persistent and disabling morning sickness:

Presenting Complaint
- Constant nausea. Sour feeling in chest
- Retching, gagging < sight or smell or food < meat << any odour
- Constant dizziness < being in a car
- Had nausea for 25 weeks during first pregnancy
- Experiencing a horrible depression. "How am I going to go on? Terrible thoughts of terminating the pregnancy. The emotional part of this is the worst thing. Need to be on my own. Angry. Can't bear to be touched - makes me nauseous."
- Eating >>
- Nausea << before eating < motion
- Thirst ++
- Used to desire pickles (+2) but can't tolerate now. Desires salt (+1) but < nausea

Medical History
- Irritable bowel syndrome
- Anxiety & OCD. Taken antidepressants for past 8 years, with some >
- Gastro-oesophageal reflux disease
- Sinusitis. Hay fever

Generals

- Hot +++, << heat, "makes me cranky"
- meat/chicken, chocolate, sweets, pickles
- Vegemite
- Sleeps well, could sleep & sleep
- Menses regular. Dysmenorrhoea. Dark thick blood, clotting ++

Mentals

Hyper, anxious, fidgety, always touching things. Feeling that if I don't touch a certain object, then something bad will happen to my family. Constant thoughts of "what if", e.g., what if someone puts the cat in the microwave? Might have suicidal thoughts, then five minutes later I'm thinking "am I crazy"?

Analysing this case can be a challenge. Clearly the treatment focus needs to be on the morning sickness, but what symptoms are we to consider to find the medicine? How wide do we need to make the totality of symptoms? Must the medicine contain the mental and emotional elements? Does it matter that she is hot?

An Eizayaga approach first maps the terrain, differentiating symptoms into different layers. Importantly, symptoms from each layer are not mixed together. Such a mixing of symptoms will in all likelihood produce an unreliable prescription. *Sepia* was tried (as a totality prescription) with no effect on the morning sickness. The following is a repertorisation of the lesion layer symptoms from the Boger-Bönninghausen repertory:

stomach, nausea and vomiting, agg, pregnancy during (20)

stomach, nausea and vomiting, retching and gagging (81)

stomach, amel, eating after (52)

stomach, agg, motion (27)

stomach, agg, touch (55)

generalities, agg, odor, strong, (39)

Nux vomica produced an immediate and significant improvement in the morning sickness. It is interesting to note that *Nux-v.* does not correspond with other aspects of this case. For example, it is usually considered a cold medicine and contra-indicated in hot patients (Ghegas, 1996).

Although Nux-v worked well for the morning sickness, it was not indicated at any point in the further treatment of this patient's chronic complaints. Separate lesion layer prescriptions were made for the IBS, hay fever, menstrual symptoms, and anxiety/OCD symptoms, before moving on to the fundamental and miasmatic layers. These layers will be defined later in this chapter.

Before looking at cases through a layered approach, we will briefly introduce Eizayaga, and look at his views on different types of similitude, totality of symptoms, and on the classification of symptoms and diseases.

About Eizayaga

Dr Francisco Xavier Eizayaga (1921-2001) was born in Argentina. He graduated from the University of Buenos Aires, and worked as a urologist, before becoming the Chief of Urology at the Municipal Hospital of Vicente Lopez.

In 1949 and 1950, he studied homeopathy at the Asociación Mèdica Homeopática Argentina, where he became assistant professor in 1954, and a professor of the postgraduate school in 1964. Eight years later, he published his Treatise on Homeopathic Medicine (*Tratado de Medicina Homeopática*). He published many other works, including Kent's Modern Repertory, and was the editor of the journal *Homeopatía*. He gave many seminars in both North and South America, and also lectured in England and Spain (Eizayaga, 2002).

Treating the Patient versus Treating the Disease

Eizayaga became increasingly popular in America and Europe, which Winston (2004) suggests was a reaction to (or perhaps a rebalancing of) teachings that were primarily Kentian, or heavily focused on an essence or centralist understanding of cases and prescribing.

As referred to in Chapter 2 on Hahnemannian prescribing, homeopathy distinguishes between the idea of treating the disease and treating the person. Over time, some homeopaths have moved toward the idea that patients have a constitution, which is unchanging and unaffected by disease (although the constitution determines the susceptibility). Homeopathic treatment using a constitutional medicine will result in a resolution of the disease that the patient is presenting. In the teaching clinic, this is often seen in students who, at the suggestion that the symptoms of the patient correspond with the symptoms of the medicine *Sepia*, say, "But he/she *isn't* a sepia!" They believe that a patient's personality traits and characteristics are the primary indications for the prescription.

As discussed in Chapter two, Hahnemann did not talk about treating constitutions, but rather, about treating disease based on its characteristic symptoms. Arguably, the importance of treating the disease becomes more incidental the further down the Swedenborgian track one progresses. This includes the ideas of treating an essence, a core delusion, a sensation; the thread that runs through the case. If the practitioner understands the centre of the case, as the argument goes, the medicine that represents the centre is given, and everything comes right. This idea sounds beautiful in its simplicity, but is in fact difficult to achieve in practice. If one studies the cases of Hahnemann, Bönninghausen, Kent, Lippe, and other great homeopaths of the past, this is clearly not how homeopathy was practiced. All of these homeopaths treated disease.

An interesting facet of the Eizayaga approach is that we get to examine and utilise both the symptoms of the disease, and the symptoms of the patient. Sometimes these correspond in the same medicine. Often, they do not.

Different Types of Similitude

Eizayaga discusses different types of similitude in his *Treatise on Homeopathic Medicine* (Eizayaga, 1991). This idea is central to any discussion of method; if homeopathy is the application of the law of similars, the question becomes, what has to be similar to what? Arguably, anything can be similar to anything, depending on how far one widens the field of analogy.

In Aphorism 25 of *The Organon*, Hahnemann states that the medicine that has 'demonstrated its power of producing the greatest number of symptoms similar to those observable in the case of disease under treatment' will remove the symptoms of disease. Here, Hahnemann raises the idea of 'quantitative' similitude between the medicine and the natural disease symptoms.

However in Aphorism 153, Hahnemann tells us that the most outstanding, unexpected, rare, peculiar, and characteristic symptoms in the patient are to be chiefly considered in finding the medicine. Here we have the importance of the 'qualitative' similitude.

Hahnemann also differentiated between different types of similitude among various pathogenetic (proving) symptoms. The pathogenesis of a dynamised medicine, which is able to arouse dynamic symptoms but is unable to provoke lesional processes, is different to symptoms produced by toxic doses of the same medicine.

Hahnemann also distinguished between medicines for acute disorders and chronic diseases. A discussion of chronic diseases brings us to the idea of a miasmatic similitude. From *The Organon,* we also see the distinction between natural similitude (two similar illnesses), and an artificial similitude (illness and medicines).

Eizayaga lists and discusses the following types of similitude:

- Pathogenetic, i.e., arises from experimenting with a drug on a healthy person
- According to type of illness, e.g., acute or chronic
- According to aetiology of the malady
- According to the diathesis or miasm in activity

- According to experimental or clinical experience
- According to the nature of similitude (artificial or natural)
- According to the chronology of the clinical symptoms (past symptoms taken into account only after prescriptions based on present symptoms have been tried and failed)
- According to the profound similitude of symptoms (profound mental or motivational symptoms)
- According to the potency of the medicine in relation to the patient

Totality of Symptoms

Totality of symptoms is at the heart of any discussion on method, each method having its own construct of what constitutes totality in any given case. Assembling a totality of symptoms in a case is essential; clearly we cannot reach a prescription based on one symptom.

The more symptoms we can consider, the easier it is to make a solid prescription. It would be impossible to find the right prescription for a complaint without at least a few features that define or characterise how that complaint manifests in the patient. For example, it is always a challenge to treat a vague, ill-defined headache; it's much easier to find the medicine for a patient who describes a violent occipital headache, extending to the forehead, aggravated by noise and by drinking coffee, and accompanied by excessive salivation and constipation.

Widest Totality of Symptoms

We are always searching for the widest totality of patient symptoms. This suits many patients, who are impressed with the holistic emphasis on a detailed understanding of the context of the disease.

For example, the patient above may have developed recurrent headaches. We learn that these started after the death of the patient's mother ten years ago. The patient explains, 'I never expressed grief or shed a tear after she died; I just got on with it. We were so close, especially over the last five years of her life. Her loss has left a gaping hole. I still can't really talk about it.' The best headache medicine must reflect the susceptibility of the patient and so should incorporate the patient's grief. In all likelihood, this is a significant aetiology of the complaint, and must be in the genius of the medicine.

Widest Meaningful Totality of Symptoms

However, this preference for the widest totality of symptoms can be taken to absurd extremes. If I have just accidentally hit my thumb with a hammer, I don't expect the homeopath to be asking about my family medical history. The totality of symptoms must be meaningful or appropriate to what is being treated. Meaningful totality also implies some quality of depth: if our totality is too large for what is being treated, it will include symptoms that are not relevant, which will likely result in an inaccurate prescription. If our totality is too small, there is a possibility that the medicine will be too superficial.

Widest Meaningful Totality of Characteristic Symptoms

However, not only must our symptoms be meaningful to the disease, they must also be characteristic. Hahnemann refers to this in Aphorism 153, which is the foundation of a successful prescription.

The obviousness of this statement speaks to the

impossibility or ease of finding the medicine in the two cases in the following table. Case one contains only vague symptoms, whereas the symptoms in the second case are characteristic.

Case 1	Case 2
Loss of appetite	Burning eruptions
Headache	Diarrhoea at 5am
Lassitude	Craves sweets
Restless sleep	Weeping at menopause
Pain	Stool smells like decaying eggs

Classification of Symptoms

Eizayaga went on to classify symptoms according to:

- Who feels or perceives the symptoms (subjective and objective)
- Localisation (psychic, mental, organic, neurological, general, local)
- Frequency (common, pathognomonic, characteristic, peculiar, or rare)

In this last category of frequency:

- Common symptoms are found in many people or found in most medicines, such as Case 1 in the preceding table.
- Pathognomonic symptoms are fundamental and distinctive for a pathophysiological diagnosis; such as, frequent urination and increased thirst for diabetes mellitus.
- A symptom is only characteristic when a modality of aggravation or amelioration is added to the common symptom. The modality reduces the frequency of the symptom. For example, a migraine that is aggravated by

any movement or coughing, and ameliorated by external pressure.

- A symptom becomes peculiar when it possesses less frequently occurring modalities, for example, the modalities are not common, or are pathogenetically provoked by very few provers. An example is a migraine that is aggravated after drinking milk. This means that we are required to understand the relative frequency of symptoms in different diseases, and also to have an understanding of the typical limits of human variability. As Alastair Gray mentions in previous chapters, this understanding includes a subjective component. It is difficult to teach to students, who may not have seen many previous cases of the disease being treated, and so will not necessarily know what is common or uncommon.

  Symptoms may also be peculiar if they are unexpected given the pathology, for example, a patient who is bradycardic during a fever.

- A symptom is rare when very few persons or extremely few medicines (even a single medicine) produce them; such as, cheerfulness after urination.

Classification of Diseases

Eizayaga classifies diseases in the following structure:

- Functional disturbances (a disturbance of the function of a part/organ/system of the body, without any changes in structure, or known organic cause), which are further categorised into:
    - Mental and emotional; such as, anxiety, fears, excitement, irritability

- General; such as, insomnia, tiredness, lack of appetite, perspiration
- Local, internal organic sensations, tremors, contractures, pain, among others.

- Lesional diseases, which cause structural or microchemical changes in the cell. These are further divided into:
    - Lesional reversible diseases

        In the case of acute disease, reversibility may be spontaneous; whereas in chronic disease, reversal may occur after homeopathic treatment. Some diseases may start off reversible and curable, but become irreversible after a period of time.

        Eizayaga further divides this category into lesional reversible mental disease (e.g., delirium, delusions), lesional general reversible diseases (e.g., septicaemia), and lesional local reversible diseases, which can be localised (e.g., tonsillitis) or diffuse (e.g., hepatitis).

    - Lesional irreversible diseases

        These are alterations that cannot be undone, although the symptoms may be relieved. In order to act therapeutically on irreversible and incurable lesions, Eizayaga states that the patient must be given a medicine that is active in its natural state, prescribed according to a lesional similarity, individualised, covering most of the pathological symptomatology, and is to be administered in dynamised, low-material dilutions.

Layers

Eizayaga's approach is so entwined with the concept of approaching each case from a layer perspective that it is sometimes referred to as the layers method.

Each layer is to be treated individually. The success of a Kentian prescription often succeeds when the lesion and fundamental layers require the same medicine. However, when these layers require different prescriptions, the Kentian approach is less successful.

The different layers are lesional (or multiple lesions), fundamental, constitutional, and miasmatic (morbid terrain).

Lesion Layer

The lesion layer is comprised of symptoms and characteristics of the disease (local, general, and mental symptoms occurring during disease expression, and aetiological factors).

The treatment for the lesion layer is very similar to that used by most homeopaths in an acute prescription, using a Bönninghausen symptom totality (location, sensation, modality, aetiology, and concomitant symptoms). In the footnote to Aphorism 153, Hahnemann states that Bönninghausen and Jahr have done a great service to homeopathy in their publication of the characteristic symptoms of homeopathic medicines. Hahnemann is saying that this focus on the characterising dimensions of a symptom furnishes the aspects that are to be considered in finding the medicine.

Practitioners continue this focus on the different dimensions of symptom totality to this day. Teixeira (2008), in his study on treating sepsis in Intensive Care Units, states that the following is necessary to find the correct medicine for acute disease:

1. A clinical and aetiological diagnosis, with understanding of disease, pathological anatomy and biopsy
2. Study of the pathological symptoms with their corresponding modalities
3. Study of the general and mental/emotional symptoms which appear during the acute disease, with their corresponding modalities
4. Study of other causations, such as weather, microbial, trauma, iatrogenic, etc.

Research by Frei (2009) suggests that the modalities of the case are the most reliable for selecting the correct medicine, whilst mind symptoms are the least reliable.

In order to select lesional layer medicine, Eizayaga recommends the use of *all* the symptoms of the disease or clinical entity, its modalities, and its concomitants. The mental and emotional symptoms are considered important (as per Aphorism 211) and aid in individualising the acute medicine.

However, there is an important condition here, and that is that all these symptoms appeared or were exacerbated right from the beginning of the disease. In other words, they cannot be the patient's chronic symptoms that preceded the disease. This comes from Aphorism 6 of *The Organon*, with its emphasis on treating only the deviations from the patient's former healthy state. Confusing symptoms of the disease (or the particular lesion) with symptoms of the patient (fundamental or constitutional) will likely result in an inaccurate prescription.

Note that the lesional layer may include iatrogenic disease that needs to be treated; for example, by using a tautopathic prescription. Treatment of this layer may also include organ support.

The lesional layer is the only layer that allopathic medicine can treat; there are no allopathic options for treating the following layers.

Fundamental Layer

Fundamental layer symptoms include mental and general symptoms specific to the patient in the history of the disease. Change here is on a functional rather than a lesional level. This includes emotional reactions suffered by the patient: the temperamental expression that comes from adjustment to certain environments and situations (including 'never been well since' responses to trauma). This reflects the dynamic disequilibrium of the patient and so is equivalent to the measure and quality of the patient's morbid susceptibility. It is dynamic and functional.

These symptoms are sometimes called 'pathobiographical'; they precede the disease, but are necessary in order to awaken the condition. The use of the word pathobiographical indicates that disease is not simply a material process resulting in organic changes. Rather, it is influenced by the mental, emotional, and affective life of the patient, including the patient's desires and aversions, perspectives, etc. This usage is an acknowledgement of how the individual's adaptions (physically, emotionally, mentally) to environment impact health.

Symptoms on this level include disturbances of an emotional, affective and volitional type, such as anxieties, fears, diverse emotions, disturbed affections, indifference, etc. This layer also includes symptoms of general disturbances, such as of sleep, appetite, perspiration, and alterations or disturbances of the vital temperature, or of the general wellbeing with no particular organic localisation. They precede the symptoms of the disease, and reveal a pathological alteration that must be treated with the fundamental layer medicine.

Constitutional Layer

The use of the word 'constitution' in homeopathy causes much confusion, especially since the word is used differently by practically everyone who employs it. Hahnemann seldom refers to the physical constitution in *The Organon*. In Aphorism 5, he states that the 'ascertainable physical constitution of the patient (especially when the disease is chronic), his moral and intellectual character, his occupation, mode of living and habits, his social and domestic relations, his age, sexual function, etc., are to be taken into consideration.' But just how are we to do so?

Swayne (2002) refers to constitutional types as patients with patterns of habitual body function and reaction to psychosocial and environmental factors. For some homeopaths, 'constitutional medicine' merely refers to an individualised medicine for a chronic disease (Launsø & Rieper, 2005). According to Leeser (1934), all homeopathic treatment is constitutional. Vickers and Zollman (1999) define constitution as a complex picture incorporating current illness, medical history, personality, and behaviour. Such a description does not clarify which elements make up this complex picture in each individual case. Do we find agreement between different homeopaths?

There have been some attempts to validate a 152-item constitutional type questionnaire (CTQ) and to correlate this with prescriptions from practitioners (Davidson et al, 2001; van Haselen et al 2001). While there appears to be a correlation between the medicines prescribed and the result of the scale, this has not been extended to analyse any correlation with outcomes of treatment.

Some believe that constitution refers to the Hippocratic Temperaments: phlegmatic, melancholic, choleric, and sanguine (Flury, 1979). Others refer to Von Grauvogl's classification. Gnaiger-Rathmanner et al (2008) argue constitution refers to the condition of the patient (congenital and acquired) before falling ill.

There have been whole books dedicated to defining 'constitutional types' (Bailey, 1995; Coulter, 1998; Herscu, 1991).

'For some homeopaths the constitutional remedy is a sort of Holy Grail. Indeed, some practitioners believe that when one knows someone's constitutional remedy, it can be given in virtually any situation with good effect' (Souter, 2006: 242). Constitutional types can even be defined with vastly oversimplifying labels, e.g. haughty *Platina*, fastidious *Arsenicum*, untidy *Sulphur*.

When looking at Bönninghausen's and Hahnemann's cases, it is clear that prescriptions were made based on the symptoms of the disease, and not on any notion of constitution (Rohrer, 2001). Medicines were changed whenever the symptom picture changed; constitution implies something more static or fixed.

As Campbell (1981) states: 'The modern notion of constitution, it appears to me, is a confused residue of ideas, part mystical, part philosophical, part pathological, and part pharmacological. It certainly has no foundation in the simillimum principle, and any justification it has must therefore be empirical and clinical.' Considering the uniqueness of the individual in health and disease, we can see the problems inherent in the idea of constitution as something unchanging and categorisable, being applied to any state of disease (Furlenmeier, 1992).

For Eizayaga, the constitution of the individual is present at birth, and cannot be changed, and is used to treat people only in their healthy state. This definition differs from a Kentian view of constitutional medicine, which fits in more with Eizayaga's fundamental layer.

Constitutional characteristics include features with which the individual is born, or hereditary genetic characteristics such as skin colour, bone structure, size and shape of various parts of the organism, or hair and eye colour. The constitution also includes general and organic functions that move and oscillate between certain limits, such as vital heat, desire for open air, way of perspiring, way of sleeping, thirst, appetite, desires, and aversions. Unless abnormal, these are not symptoms. An individual cannot be cured of an inclination toward sweets or highly seasoned food, or a desire for cold drinks. Unless related to someone's disease, they are not pathological symptoms, and so cannot be treated.

Treatment at the constitutional level is preventive. Eizayaga describes four normal genetic constitutions expressed by four medicines: *Sulphur, Calcarea carbonica, Calcarea phosphorica,* and *Calcarea fluorica*. Other authors have added *Phosphorus, Lycopodium, Baryta carbonica,* and *Silica* to this list (de Schepper, 1999).

Miasmatic Layer

Symptoms at the miasmatic layer are related to diathesis, miasm, or soil, which is inherited, and present from birth. This differs from Hahnemann (1996) who regards miasms as acquired, not congenital. Eizayaga described this layer as the morbid terrain:

A. Psoric terrain: hyperfunction. Functional or reversible disturbances. This includes dyspeptic disturbances, anxieties; fears, eruptions, scabies, skin allergies, etc.

B. Tuberculinic terrain: psychic and organic hyperfunction with suppurations. This includes diseases such as tuberculosis, respiratory catarrh with suppuration, haemoptysis, respiratory allergy, osteoporosis, periostitis, etc.

C. Syphilitic terrain: involves intelligence and tissue destruction, mental disorders, aggressiveness, readiness to commit suicide, ulcers of all sorts, etc.

D. Sycotic terrain: perversion of feelings and of tissues. This includes benign tumours; tissue hypertrophy, decreased memory, genito-urinary disturbances and infections, and so on.

E. Cancerinic terrain: obsessively worries about petty things, fearing cancer, malignant tumours, leukaemia and other types of blood cancer.

Treatment at this level is with the corresponding nosode. Eizayaga differs from Hahnemann and others in this respect, where the treatment of chronic disease would involve a suitable similar anti-miasmatic medicine, rather than giving the specific nosode.

Prescribing

The layers are analysed (and repertorised) separately, if possible, with the goal of finding the medicine that best covers each layer. The ideal is to find a single medicine that covers the various layers of symptoms. If this is not possible but there is a homeopathic medicine that clearly covers the presenting disease state, and the patient presents with frequent or intense symptoms related to this layer, then treatment with this medicine starts and continues until the disease symptoms disappear or significantly decrease.

To complete the treatment after the disease symptoms have been removed, the medicine covering the fundamental layer, and later the constitutional layer, is prescribed (this may be the same medicine). The fundamental layer aims to remove the morbid susceptibility, while a constitutional layer prescription is made as a preventative when the patient is healthy.

If no medicine stands out which clearly covers the symptoms of the disease, and there are strong indications for a fundamental layer prescription, especially if disease symptoms are neither frequent nor severe, the fundamental medicine can be given to start the case.

Similarly, if there appears to be a heavy miasmatic loading in the case, it may be necessary to start with the nosode of the indicated miasm. Nosodes can also be used as intercurrent prescriptions (Eizayaga et al, 1996).

Eizayaga suggests that there is not a specific sequence of layer treatment. Rather, the treatment order is individualised depending on the focus, emphasis, and intensity of symptoms.

Posology

Eizayaga acknowledges that potency is confusing, and his solution to this confusion was to experiment. He was a user of plussing medicines, as per the 6th edition of *The Organon*.

After his experiments on many patients, Eizayaga concluded that:

1. There is no difference between the plus method and the high-potency single dose in functional cases
2. The plussing/succussion method using a 30c potency is superior to the unique dose. Moreover, in non-functional cases, the therapeutic results with progressive and repeated doses are better than those obtained with the single dose
3. In cases of organic lesion, the plus method has a much better effect. In very serious, organic, lesional cases, the low or medium potencies may cause remarkable recovery without major risks of an aggravation
4. The plus method does not harm the treatment, independent of whether the patient's symptoms are undergoing a full aggravation or a cure reaction
5. There is no difference between the homeopathic aggravation due to a unique dose or due to repeated doses, even when taking a medicine during the reaction

6. An additional advantage of repeating the dose is avoiding any need to use placebo
7. Dose repetition with globules does not cause the inconvenience stated in Aphorism 247
8. Treatment with progressively ascending potencies has three advantages:
    i. The patient rarely experiences disagreeable reactions
    ii. An unexpected number of patients are cured of all their ailments with only a 30c, and sometimes with a 6c
    iii. It allows the homeopath to gradually look for the simillimum potency which will cure the patient totally without aggravating the patient
9. The majority of patients who are sensitive to a medicine are sensitive to any potency

Repertory

Eizayaga regarded use and study of the repertory as being the most reliable way for the homeopath to search for the medicine. He believed that only its constant and habitual use would make the homeopath secure in prescribing.

He felt it important to mention that the repertory is a blind guide. In order to use the repertory effectively, it requires objective, impartial, and subtle observation of the symptoms of the patient's characteristic totality. If these observations are not correct, or the translation of the patient's language into repertory language is not accurate, then the results will follow the garbage in, garbage out principle.

Eizayaga published a modern version of Kent's repertory

(*El Moderno Repertorio De Kent*), and clinical homeopathic algorithms.

Eizayaga described the study of the homeopathic materia medica as the 'most ample and finished compendium of internal medicine and even of pathology.' Repertories therefore constitute a semiological guide, and should be studied systematically.

Criticisms of Eizayaga's Approach

Eizayaga has been criticised for adopting an allopathic approach to homeopathy. Firstly, this criticism argues that he advocated a focus on treatment of disease symptoms that are not individualised to the patient. It should be noted, however, that Eizayaga preferred to use the individualising and characterising symptoms of the disease in order to find the medicine. Where these symptoms are not available, it is evident from his cases that other symptoms are used, such as pathognomic symptoms, organ affinities, etc.

Secondly, critics state that this focus on disease symptoms ignores the fact that the symptoms are the end product of disease, and not the disease itself. This treatment approach has been accused of having an overly materialistic view of disease, when disease instead should be seen as a disturbance of the vital force.

Whilst this is an interesting philosophical debate, in practical terms it is largely a matter of semantics. Only the patient's symptoms can guide us to the medicine; these symptoms are how we know the disease. After all, it is in Aphorism 3 that Hahnemann states the need to adapt what is curative in medicines to what is *undoubtedly morbid* in the patient.

Case Example

Presenting Complaint
- Drippy nose - hay fever-like - recent onset
- Changeable
- < on waking > after rising
- Discharge clear, burning, sometimes excoriating
- Started initially on an airplane when coming back from holiday - change in temperature
- < cold place to hot, or from hot to cold, can be a trigger
- >not eating or drinking
- Persistent cough
- Cough follows the coryza
- Coughs until vomits, retches
- Chronic cough (30 years) occurs annually. Current episode has lasted 6 months
- < after eating or drinking
- Hacking cough - sounds 'like I have cancer, like I'm on my last legs'
- < going from a hot room to a cold room, or vice versa
- >siting, << lying down, or even slumping in chair
- Wheeze in lungs
- Cough exhausting, ribs ache, must hold chest
- >stooping < rising from bed

- < laughing, exercise, deep breathing, talking
- Expectoration creamy or yellow

Other Complaints
- Arthritis - joint stiffness
- < winter < cold weather
- >warm shower
- Soreness < continued exercise/exertion
- Stiffness > motion, keeping moving
- 'I feel like the tin man, I need to oil my body'

Medical History
- Allergies
- Hay fever
- Sinusitis
- Appendectomy
- Tonsillectomy
- Nil medication, alcohol or recreational drugs, coffee, tobacco

Family History
- Maternal side - depression, addiction
- Paternal side - myocardial infarction, stroke, Parkinson's

Generals
- < heat (→dizziness) << humidity
- Perspiration ++ esp. on upper lip and nape of neck
- Sensitive to cold weather, in winter always feels cold
- + and > sun (mood > sun)

- < 4pm-6pm
- >10am-2pm
- Sleeps on back or side
- History of nocturia - > since stopped eating meat. Now once a night
- Snoring +++
- Nil constipation or bloating
- Loose bowels from dairy
- + chips and salt (+3) + Vietnamese & Japanese food
- < farinaceous, spicy
- thirst for large quantities of room temperature water

Female
- Menopause - 5 years ago, flushes +++, strong desire for air conditioning
- < hot humid weather, hot stuffy room
- Occasional flushes now but rare
- Dysmenorrhoea when young, flooding, dark clotting blood
- Oral contraceptive pill (OCP) for 10 years
- Back pain during period
- Enjoyed pregnancies & breastfeeding - "were the best years of my life"

Mental/emotional
- Optimist
- Sensitive to sad stories, injustice, +++
- Very sensitive pain of others, empathy for helpless people. Become involved

- Sensitive to rudeness of others → anger. 'I was brought up as a shouter.' Very sympathetic. The underdog. People who have no voice. Injustice. Life is not fair. Get angry
- Perfectionist
- Death of parents made me stronger. Realised that life is very short. People matter, not things. Making the most of every day
- Nil fears/phobias
- Nil sadness ... 'you can always change things, if you want to'

Analysis

The initial approach was to take a totality of the most characteristic symptoms; the mental and emotional symptoms were taken due to their intensity. The resulting repertorisation of these guiding symptoms is as follows:

Mind, Sympathetic, compassionate

Mind, Injustice, cannot support

Mind, Horrible things, sad stories affect her profoundly

Cough and Generalities, Cold to warm and warm to cold

Causticum was selected based on its fit with these guiding symptoms, and confirmatory symptoms such as retching and gagging with the cough, cough < eating and drinking, > sitting, the changeability of the symptoms, the back pain during menses (historical symptom), aggravation from humid weather, amelioration from exposure to the sun, and perfectionistic tendencies.

At the follow-up six weeks later, the patient described an improvement in her symptoms. She thought the medicine was 'great', was feeling mentally and emotionally much better, more even in temperament, less moody, less angry, calmer, and had increased energy. Sleep was improved, and the patient reported not needing to go to the bathroom as frequently during the night.

However, her cough was unchanged. Despite the belief that with an improvement on a mental, emotional and general level, the presenting complaint would eventually improve, the desire to alleviate the patient's debilitating and lasting complaint led to consideration of a layered approach. *Causticum* can be seen as the fundamental layer medicine. The cough (lesion) requires a different medicine.

Another analysis was made of the lesion layer symptoms, this time using Bönninghausen's *Therapeutic Pocketbook*:

cough, with expectoration (106)

expectoration yellow (66)

< change of temperature (19)

< eating while (91)

< drinking, after (71)

< talking, speaking (77)

< rising from bed (79)

<lying (125)

< laughing(22)

vomiting in general (65)

retching (63)

Carbo vegetabilis was selected due to its representation

in all eleven rubrics, its high polarity ranking (Frei, 2009), and confirmation of symptoms in the materia medica. The result was an instant improvement, with the cough resolving completely in four-five days.

An overview of this case from an Eizayaga perspective is:

Lesion 1 (cough):	*Carb-v.*
Lesion 2 (arthritis):	*Rhus-t.*
Fundamental:	*Caust.*
Constitutional:	*Calc.*
Miasmatic:	*Med.*

Conclusion

The golfer has more enemies than any other athlete. He has fourteen clubs in his bag, all of them different; 18 holes to play, all of them different; and all around him is sand, trees, grass, water, wind ... In addition, the game is 50 percent mental, so his biggest enemy is himself.

- Dan Jenkins, Sportswriter

Cases that are presented during seminars and in our homeopathic journals often appear miraculous. A disease responds well to a single medicine, and does not return after a period of several years; this is the equivalent of a homeopathic hole in one. However, these cases are not common in practice for the majority of homeopaths.

In complex cases, where all the signs and symptoms do not point to a single medicine, we have to skilfully tease out what it is that needs to be cured in each case, and the most important symptoms to consider for each careful prescription.

In order to do this, it is useful to have a map or a framework with which to understand the case. When we have a map of the terrain, to continue the golfing analogy, we can understand where the rough and the lakes are, what type of club to use, and the best swing for each particular shot. When we have a map of the terrain, this becomes easier to accomplish.

Any case that benefits from understanding the complexities of the patient's journey from health to disease is best treated using an Eizayaga approach. In simple cases, where the medicine or approach is obvious - a straightforward aetiological prescription, for example, or a patient who requires a prescription simply for an acute exacerbation of a chronic disease - sorting the case into layers can overcomplicate things.

When there are many possible ways to proceed, it is useful to understand the lie of the land, and to divide what can be an abundance of symptoms into meaningful and helpful categories. This is particularly true with cases that have a rich diversity of symptoms (including different diseases of varying chronologies) in addition to physical generals and mental and emotional symptoms that may or may not be related to the presenting complaint. An Eizayaga approach can help us to navigate the often-challenging topography of chronic disease.

References and Further Reading

Bailey, P.M. (1995) *Homeopathic Psychology: Personality Profiles of the Major Constitutional Remedies*, North Atlantic Books, Berkeley, California.

Campbell, A. (1981) 'The concept of constitution in homeopathy', *British Homeopathic Journal*, 70: 183-188.

Coulter, C.R. (1998) *Portraits of Homoeopathic Medicines: Psychophysical Analyses of Selected Constitutional Types*, Quality Medical Publishing Inc., St Louis, Missouri.

Davidson, J., Fisher, P., Van Haselen, R., Woodbury, M. & Connor, K. (2001) 'Do constitutional types really exist? A further study using grade of membership analysis', *British Homeopathic Journal*, 90(3): 138-147.

Eizayaga, F.X. (1991) *Treatise on Homeopathic Medicine*, Ediciones Marecel, Buenos Aires.

Eizayaga, F.X., Eizayaga, J. & Eizayaga, F.H. (1996) 'Homeopathic treatment of bronchial asthma: retrospective study of 62 cases', *British Homeopathic Journal*, 85: 28-33.

Eizayaga, J. (2002) 'Obituary: Dr Francisco X Eizayaga', *Homeopathy*, 91: 269.

Flury, M. (1979) *Practical repertory*, in Gnaiger-Rathmanner, J., Schneider, A., Loader, B., Böhler, M., Frass, M., Singer, S.R. & Oberbaum, M. (2008) 'Petroleum: a series of 25 cases'. *Homeopathy*, 97(2): 83-88.

Frei (2009) 'Polarity analysis, a new approach to increase the precision of homeopathic prescriptions', *Homeopathy*, 98: 49-55.

Furlenmeier, M. (1992) 'The 'constitution' in homeopathy', *Zschr Klass Homöop*, 36: 180-86.

Ghegas, V. (1996) *The Classical Homeopathic Lectures of Dr Vassilis Ghegas*, Volume D, Homeo-Study v.z.w., Genk, Belgium.

Gnaiger-Rathmanner, J., Schneider, A., Loader, B., Böhler, M., Frass, M., Singer, S.R. & Oberbaum, M., (2008) 'Petroleum: a series of 25 cases', *Homeopathy*, 97(2): 83-88.

Hahnemann, S. (1922) *Organon of Medicine*, Boericke & Tafel, Philadelphia.

Hahnemann, S. (1996) *The Chronic Diseases*, B. Jain Publishers, New Delhi, India.

Herscu, P. (1991) *Homoeopathic Treatment of Children—Pediatric Constitutional Types*, North Atlantic Books, Berkeley.

Launsø. L. & Rieper, J. (2005) 'General practitioners and classical homeopaths treatment models for asthma and allergy'. *Homeopathy*, 94(1): 17-25.

Leeser, O. (1934) 'Constitution and constitutional treatment', *British Homeopathic Journal*, 24: 230–244.

Rohrer (2001) 'Certainty in finding the remedy', *Dokumenta Homoeopathica*, 21: 1-13.

Schepper, L. D. (1999) *Hahnemann Revisited: Hahnemannian Textbook of Classical Homeopathy for the Professional*, Full of Life publishing, Santa Fe, New Mexico.

Souter, K. (2006) 'Heuristics and bias in homeopathy', *Homeopathy*, 95(4): 237-244.

Swayne, J. (2002) 'The starting point: pathography', *Homeopathy*, 91(1): 22-25.

Teixeira (2008) 'Homeopathic practice in Intensive Care Units: objective semiology, symptom selection and a series of sepsis cases', *Homeopathy*, 97: 206–213.

Van Haselen, R.A., Cinar, S., Fisher, P. & Davidson, J. (2001) 'The Constitutional Type Questionnaire: Validation in the Patient Population of the Royal London Homoeopathic Hospital', *British Homeopathic Journal*, 90(3): 131–137.

Vickers, A. & Zollmann, C. (1999) 'ABC of complementary medicine', *BMJ*, 319: 1115-1118.

Winston, J. (2004) 'Uh oh, Toto. I don't think we're in Kansas any more', *Homeopathy in Practice*, January: 32-39.

Chapter 9

Keynote Prescribing

Contents

- Definitions
- Keynote Materia Medicas
- Misapplication
- History and Development of Keynote Prescribing By Gunavante & E.E. Case
- Who Devised It?
- Why Did They Devise It?
- Who Has Used It? What Does It Involve?
- The Components of the Method
- Case Examples
- Difference between Characteristic and Keynote Symptoms
- Some Cases
- Disadvantages of Keynote Prescribing
- Advantages of Keynote Prescribing

In this chapter you will:

1. Develop an understanding of the philosophical underpinnings of Keynote prescribing
2. Learn about its historical advocates
3. Grasp its relevance though casework of historical and contemporary figures
4. Familiarise yourself with its disadvantages in certain clinical situations

Chapter 9

Keynote Prescribing

Symptoms which Hahnemann called "striking, strange, peculiar and unusual" are of great value in directing our attention to a few remedies; however, by this Hahnemann did not mean Key-note prescribing. He did not ignore any symptom in making a prescription. The school led by Guernsey, Lippe and Nash has found "Key-notes" to be valuable in suggesting the most likely remedy, the accuracy of which (in relation to the remaining symptom) should be got confirmed by a reference to the Materia Medica. Dr. H.C. Allen stressed the need for the three-legged stool (at least three characteristic symptoms or key-notes) as a sound basis for the prescription (Desai 2005).

Definitions

Yasgur's Homeopathic Dictionary describes a Keynote symptom as a,

> ...leading symptom, one which is so apparent, so clear, that it suggests a small group of remedies or even a single remedy. For example, pain in the right shoulder blade points to Chelidonium. Keynotes are actually peculiar symptoms which have taken on a highly characteristic flavour and tend to point almost directly to a remedy, yet if keynotes are taken as final and the generals do not confirm them, failures often result. Many of the

great homeopathic prescribers (Lippe, Allen, Boger) were very successful keynote prescribers, but you must realize that they had keen 'totality perceptions' and thus would not allow false-positives to sway them.

This is distinguishable from an eliminative symptom. This is one which the practitioner uses to repertorize the case. They are termed eliminative as they are used to 'eliminate' remedies gradually from the case, gradually narrowing the list down to a half-dozen or fewer. Then one does further comparative work in the materia medica to select the simillimum. One looks for eliminative symptoms in the mentals, modalities or a common symptom with an unusual flavour to it. One might consider this to be a keynote symptom which is used as the first symptom for repertorization. Since it indicates just a few remedies, it serves to eliminate a large number of remedies (Yasgur 1994).

Keynote Materia Medica's

Practical information about the method, symptoms and remedies is best found in these books.

T.F. Allen A Primer of Materia Medica
W. Burt, Characteristic Materia Medica
E. Nash, Leaders in Therapeutics
H.N. Guernsey, Keynotes of the Materia Medica
A von Lippe, Keynotes of the Homoeopathic Materia Medica
A von Lippe, Keynotes and Red-Line Symptoms of the Materia Medica
C.M. Boger, Boenninghausen's Characteristics
C.M. Boger, A Synoptic Key of the Materia Medica
H.C. Allen, Keynotes and Characteristics with Comparisons
J.H. Clarke, Grand Characteristics of the Materia Medica
R. Morrison, Desktop Guide to Keynotes and Confirmatory Symptoms
S.R. Phatak, Materia Medica of Homeopathic Medicines (Taylor 2001).

Why Keynote Prescribing at All?

These texts are all important, yet perhaps the best synthesis of the technique is to be found in Taylor (2001) at www.wholehealthnow.com. It is here that we learn that the term *Keynotes* was introduced by Guernsey (1868) who underlined the term as 'suggestive and merely provisorial'. It suggested that a remedy had to be confirmed by totality. It is very important to remember this proviso. Many keynote prescribers around the world seem to forget this very basic point. Keynote is,

> the fundamental note or tone to which the whole piece is accommodated; the key-note of music finds, by analogy – through which things most remote and unlike superficially are connected in the closest relationship – its likeness everywhere (Guernsey 1868).

The reason for such a method is a pragmatic one. Homeopaths require a quick and accurate system that delivers clear solutions in clinical situations because there are just too many remedies. In addition to the number of remedies, there are so many materia medicas, and of course an overwhelming number of provings, not to mention thousands of symptoms. So many practitioners of homeopathy grounded in classical methods have moved to a more keynote style purely due to the practicalities of earning a living. Any entrepreneur looking at the business model that is classically homeopathic will wonder how it is possible to earn a living at all when you take between one and two hours to take a case, and then analyse it afterwards?

Not all homeopaths move towards keynote prescribing. For many around the world, it is the first and only way of prescribing. My friends and colleagues in India and Malaysia look at things differently. It is for as much historical and practical reasons that a different system is advocated. I have always marvelled at how my students in those places know their materia medica so well. The first time teaching in Malaysia I was actually intimidated by the students remedy knowledge, far greater than mine. What on earth could I teach them? Over time however, it has become apparent that becoming grounded in undergraduate school in keynote prescribing has its limitations. What I have noticed with my Malaysian and Indian students is that if the first or the second keynote prescription is unsuccessful, then they have very few options available to change method and find a solution for the client.

Taylor reports the same issue: 'I recall several years ago sitting down with a capable and seasoned homoeopathic practitioner, showing off my brand-new copy of Franz Vermeulen's *Concordant Materia Medica*. He looked it over briefly, handed it back, and said "I don't know what to do with the material in here - I find it overwhelming." One of the solutions that homeopaths developed to solve the problems of too many remedies and too much information was to create the repertory. The repertory was a practical tool to assist in information management in the 1800's. Keynote prescribing was another. Taylor quoting Jahr on his website describes it best:

> It was in the year 1827 when I made my debut in the practice of Homoeopathy, at a time when the only resources at our command were the Materia Medica Pura of the founder of our school and a few cures reported in Stapf's "Archiv," and in the "Praktischen Mittheilungen" (Practical Communications.)

With these scanty means we had to get along as well as we could, and, by a diligent and attentive study of the drugs with whose pathogeneses we had become acquainted at that time, familiarize ourselves with the characteristic symptoms of each drug and its special indications, in order to avail ourselves of them for therapeutic purposes in such case as might present themselves for treatment. This was no small task, which could never have been accomplished, if the Materia Medica of that time had contained the large number of drugs that are offered at the present time to the beginner in homoeopathic practice. But since the number of drugs known at that time, did not exceed sixty, and among these only twenty had been proved with exhaustive perseverance and correctness, we had it in our power to study them thoroughly without too much trouble ... At this time such a careful study of our Materia Medica is unfortunately no longer possible to the beginner in Homoeopathy. Overwhelmed by the accumulated mass of drugs and clinical observations, he scarcely knows which way to turn for at least one ray of light in the chaos spread out before him (Jahr 1867).

Misapplication

A simple glance on the internet, performing a Google search on homeopathy, or looking at Facebook these days demonstrates the frightening amount of misinformation about homeopathy. Someone somewhere posts a picture of Princess Diana with the question, 'What Remedy Did She Need?' It is banal and trivializes homeopathy.

As with any interesting or useful innovation, the use of Keynotes has been trivialized and misapplied by many, both in & since the days of Guernsey. We have all perhaps met homeopaths describing themselves as "Keynote Prescribers" - "he's a Sulfur type - hot & messy;" "I just took one look at the cracks in the corners of his mouth and gave him Nitric acid;" etc. Guernsey's inspiration is sadly trivialized by this approach, to near-uselessness. Yet some attention to what Guernsey really intended, can offer us a robust tool to add to our kit-bag of case-analysis strategies (Taylor 2001).

History and Development of Keynote Prescribing

Keynote prescribing did not start as trivial or banal. Exploring the origins of this type of prescribing lead to Henry Newell Guernsey. He was born in Rochester, Vermont in 1817, and earned his medical degree from New York University in 1842. In 1856, he moved to Philadelphia where he became professor of obstetrics at the Homeopathic Medical College of Pennsylvania (later merging with the Hahnemann Medical College in 1869). His writings include:

The Application of the Principles and

Practice of Homoeopathy to Obstetrics, and

Keynotes to the Materia Medica (Taylor 2001).

Guernsey's work on keynotes derived out of a series of lectures delivered to the students of the Hahnemann Medical College of Philadelphia between 1871 and 1873. About these lectures, he wrote:

To give the Materia Medica, with anywhere near all the symptoms of each remedy, would require at least three consecutive courses of lectures - each course to be not less than six months long.

He intended instead to teach the leading characteristics of remedies,

> to turn the student's mind, when he should engage in practice, in the direction of the proper remedy, when prescribing for the sick.

Guernsey described keynotes as,

> There is certainly that, in every case of illness, which preeminently characterizes that case or causes it to differ from every other. So in the remedy to be selected, there is or must be a combination of symptoms, a peculiar combination, characteristic or, more strikingly, key-note. Strike that and all the others are easily touched, attuned or sounded.

It is obvious then that Guernsey's *Keynotes* were nothing other than the characteristic symptoms of a remedy that correspond rather directly to the 'striking, singular, uncommon and peculiar (characteristic) signs and symptoms of disease,' that Hahnemann discusses in aphorism 153 of the *Organon*:

> In this search for a homoeopathic specific remedy, that is to say, in this comparison of the collective symptoms of the natural disease with the list of symptoms of known medicines, in order to find among these an artificial morbific agent corresponding by similarity to the disease to be cured, the more striking, singular, uncommon and peculiar (characteristic) signs and symptoms (1) of the case of disease are chiefly and most solely to be kept in view; for it is more particularly these that very similar ones in the list of symptoms of the selected medicine must correspond to, in order to constitute it the most suitable for effecting the cure.
>
> The more general and undefined symptoms: loss of appetite,

headache, debility, restless sleep, discomfort, and so forth, demand but little attention when of that vague and indefinite character, if they cannot be more accurately described, as symptoms of such a general nature are observed in almost every disease and from almost every drug (Guernsey in Taylor 2001).

The Components of the Method

Totality Again

To understand the context of keynote prescribing, we must first once again reflect on the concept of totality. One of the bewildering questions facing a homeopath is just how to determine which of the totality of symptoms are important ones. After a consultation, there may be 500 pieces of information. Which pieces are important? Totality clearly cannot mean the numeric totality. Otherwise, we would prescribe *Sulphur* in every case. In his book the *Genius of Homoeopathic Remedies*, Gunavante (1994) wrote:

> Hahnemann has referred to the "Totality" of symptoms, in Aphorism after Aphorism in the Organon, as being the guide to the simillimum. This "Totality" has been more clearly described by various masters after Hahnemann to consist of:

1. General (symptoms which refer to the patient as a whole). - The Generals comprise
(a)   the Mental generals and
(b)   the Physical generals.
2. Particulars, i.e., symptoms pertaining to parts of the body. - These are further sub-divided into
(a)   Location of the complaint,
(b)   Sensations of pain and
(c)   Modalities, i.e., conditions of aggravation or amelioration.

3. Peculiar, characteristic, uncommon, striking symptoms, some of which are described as "Keynotes" of remedies. - These peculiar symptoms pertain to the individual and not to the disease.
4. Causations (ailments from certain causes) or "Never well since" a certain illness; and
5. Concomitants, i.e. symptoms associated with the chief complaint in point of time. (Gunavante 1994).

It is important to remember that not all the symptoms in the patient or in the materia medica are of equal importance. Totality does not mean all the symptoms from A to Z of a patient. Hahnemann made this quite clear in Aph.155. "It is only the symptoms of the medicine that correspond to the symptoms of the disease that are called into play... but the other symptoms of the homoeopathic medicine, which are often very numerous, being in no way applicable to the case of the disease in question, are not called into play at all." This means that we must fit only the patient's symptoms into the remedy, we should not think that a hundred symptoms of the remedy can possibly be found in a particular patient (Gunavante 1994).

Red-line Symptoms

The implication is clear. Not all symptoms are created equally. Some are more important than others. A skilled homeopath looks like a genius to the untrained eye because they are able to distil out from a numerical mass of symptoms the one or two key crucial points in the case.

It will be seen from what follows that as one becomes a skilful prescriber he selects only a few "Red line" symptoms for arriving at the Remedy. Yet this fact does not absolve him from taking the case in detail, because it is only after analyzing a case in all its essential aspects that one can select the "few but most crucial characteristic symptoms" as guides to the remedy. Therefore, until one has taken the case well, he is not fully equipped to analyze it on his way to find the remedy. Among the various components of the totality referred to above, Hahnemann has singled out (in Aph 153) "the more striking, singular, uncommon and peculiar (characteristic) signs and symptoms (which should be) chiefly and almost solely kept in view; for it is more particularly these that very similar ones in the list of symptoms of the selected medicine must correspond to, in order to constitute it the most suitable for effecting the cure". In Aph 211 Hahnemann states: "The state of the disposition of the patient often chiefly determines the selection of the homoeopathic remedy, as being decidedly a characteristic symptom which can least of all remain concealed from the accurately observing physician". Hahnemann further narrows down the totality when he says in Aph164. "The small number of homoeopathic symptoms present in the best selected medicine is no obstacle to the cure in case where these few medicinal symptoms are chiefly of an uncommon kind and such as are peculiarly distinctive (characteristic) of the disease". This means that we can find the simillimum on the basis of a few symptoms, provided that they are peculiar and distinctive (Gunavante 1994).

Will Taylor and Meg Ryan - Practical Keynote Prescribing

Mathur (1975) gives excellent and simple of examples of practical keynote prescribing. Will Taylor (2001) gets to the heart of the matter with a great example:

> How does focused attention on a single (Keynote) symptom

differ from prescribing for single symptoms? It is of course frowned upon to focus on the name of the condition or one part of the disease when we know that the disease is interior and all encompassing.

Let's assign you the task of telling someone how to identify Meg Ryan out of the crowd at a train station. You could arm them with a list of six or ten "Meg Ryan" rubrics from the movie-star repertory:

- Stature: feet, less than 6', 5' to 5'4"
- Eyes: blue
- Hair: blond
- Hair: short
- Face: smile, nice
- Affect: feminine
- Voice: inflection, rising, on word "love" when saying "I love you."

And you might have some success. Likely, though, your instructee would come back with 57 possibilities...So how can we lend some order to the chaos of the crowd at the train station, and to Meg's variable appearance, for a ray of light to aid us in our search? Guernsey reminds us:

"There is certainly that, in every case of illness, which preeminently characterizes that case or causes it to differ from every other."

And for Meg, we can find such a Keynote characteristic: in the peculiar expressiveness of the corners of her mouth.

Will she be the only person in the train station with this characteristic? Probably not. But armed with this particularly characteristic feature to look for, our greeter will likely come back with only 4 or 5 possibilities:

- One male
- One speaking Croatian
- One lovely overweight, grey-haired woman from Michigan with pictures of her grandchildren
- One 17 year-old kid saying "whatever…"
- And one with a reasonable fit to the rubrics in the original list — Meg herself. With that smile.

We do not really have any Keynotes that are specific for a given remedy which can define a remedy in isolation. Keynotes are not specific to a remedy, but they are those symptoms where the greatest weight resides in differentiating remedies - Meg Ryan's smile, Richard Nixon's jowls…The full characterization of a remedy requires a greater totality of symptoms, and this greater totality is required to assign similitude to a case - but these Keynote symptoms are the symptoms within the totality that most strongly declare the individuality of our medicinal agents (Taylor 2001).

What are the Characteristic Features of a Keynote?

In order to determine that a symptom in a case is a true keynote it must be a strongly expressed symptom of a remedy, one that is seen strongly marked with considerable consistency in provings and in the clinical settings calling for the remedy as simillimum. In addition, a keynote must be a peculiar symptom, one not shared with many other remedies. Taylor gives the example of the symptom, 'Bearing down pain in the pelvis, as if the pelvic organs would fall out,' which can be considered a keynote for Sepia as,

1. It is strongly marked for Sepia, being seen frequently in the provings, and frequently in cases where Sepia is called for [certainly though not in all Sepia cases - but when uterine discomfort is present in a Sepia case, it is dominantly of this nature] and,
2. It is shared prominently by only a few other remedies.

These two features translate into a repertory presence of this symptom as (1) a relatively strongly marked remedy, in (2) a relatively small rubric. I wish to re-emphasize, as did Guernsey, one cannot accurately prescribe merely "on a keynote." If one were to prescribe Sepia purely on the keynote symptom of bearing-down pains of the uterus, one would give a great deal of Sepia inappropriately to patients needing Lilium tigrinum, Murex, Platina, Sabina, etc. Rather, Guernsey suggested that the Keynote be used to rapidly focus on a small constellation of remedies bearing this symptom - as a most centrally important, potentially highly characterizing feature of the case and of the remedy bearing similitude to the case (Taylor 2001).

The 'Three-legged Stool' Approach to Keynotes

Unsurprisingly, because of the inherent issues in prescribing on just one symptom many have advocated the more prudent and safer approach of keynote prescribing, but one that is nevertheless as useful and swift in the hands of a good practitioner. Kent said:

It is sometimes possible to abbreviate the anamnesis by selecting one symptom, the key to the case, but this should be seldom attempted. But it is more prudent and often convenient (and safe) to take a group of three or four essential or core symptoms.

The keynotes of Guernsey, H.C. Allen and Nash are justly popular for this same reason. There has thus been a strong urge among homoeopaths to make the process of selection of the remedy as simple as possible. However, though Guernsey justified the use of Keynotes as they indeed covered the totality, their abuse (through incorrect understanding and application) has been decried by Yingling, Kent, etc. The reason why Keynotes alone are unsafe to use is in Boger's words,

The actual differentiating factor may belong to any rubric whatsoever. Roberts makes the same point differently: "No disease can be represented by a single symptom. The character of the drug is represented not by a single effect, but by a group of effects" (Gunavante 1994).

Storming the Fortress / Achieving Break-through at the Weak Spots

Gunavante has a useful metaphor. The problem of finding the simillimum is similar to the one facing the commander at the army headquarters.

His aim is to capture the enemy's "fortress" easily, with minimum loss of his men and materials. What are the steps he takes to achieve his goal? He surveys the field of operations thoroughly (through intelligence, spies, aerial survey, scouts etc.) in order to fully and correctly understand and assess the enemy's disposition of forces, his possible tactics and possible points of attack. This is equivalent to our "Case-taking" to understand the "picture of the patient". The Commander's object in doing all this is to find "chinks" (weak spots) in the enemy's defences through which he can attack and make a comparatively easy breakthrough in the enemy's defences. For the homoeopaths these "weak spots" correspond to the "peculiar, uncommon, characteristic" symptoms of the patient. It is these that the homoeopath tries to identify. The commander makes a frontal attack, throwing all his forces in battle all along the line, only when he is unable to locate the "weak" entry points, but this is a costly process which he will resort to only if he has no other alternative. In the same way, the experienced, "battle-scarred" homoeopath resorts to the "totality of symptoms" if he is unable to identify the outstanding "peculiar and characteristic" symptoms. Once he is able to identify them, which necessarily are few in number, his path towards capturing the "fortress" (simillimum) is easy and quick, We have to understand Aph153 of the Organon (peculiar, characteristic, individualising symptoms), as well as Aph164 (the small number of peculiarly distinctive symptoms is no obstacle to cure) in the light of the foregoing explanation of the strategy and tactics of a commander at war, or of a competent homeopathic prescriber. Master prescribers have taught, through their experiences, that the whole effort boils down to identifying the few peculiarly distinctive symptoms.

'Minimum Syndrome of Maximum Value'

This is the famous quotation. The meaning of the expression 'Minimum Syndrome of the Maximum Value' is used by a number of excellent practitioners to describe their approach when searching for the simillimum. The small number of symptoms refers to the minimum syndrome. The high rank of symptoms needed in both patient and remedy refers to the maximum value of the symptoms. In his editorial for the *Homoeopathic Heritage* (May, 1989) Koppikar said in Gunavante,

> There are conditions or, what may be called "syndromes" that are characteristic of a particular condition not found in any other situation, and the same can be said of drugs: those that can produce "identifiable" pictures or syndromes....In these types of prescriptions (Bell. for scarlet fever; Verat, Camph and Cuprum for cholera; Thuja for small pox) there is indeed the Totality principle, the totality of distinguishing, identifiable symptoms. This group of symptoms goes always together to make the picture.
>
> The best illustration of this was once given by Boenninghausen - the case of a girl with toothache, agg. every evening till midnight; amel. by going outdoors. She was given Puls. with dramatic effect. As Boenninghausen predicted, the other characteristics of Puls. were also found among the symptoms of the patient, viz. thirstless, lachrymose, agg. warmth, sleeplessness before midnight, aversion to fats, slimy diarrhoea, menses late and short lasting, dysmenorrhoea. This point about how a few of the most peculiar and characteristic symptoms of a remedy permeate the entire symptomatology of that remedy has been stressed by various masters (Gunavante 1994).

Experts at Work - a Few More Examples

Weir, Paschero and Candegabe have found that the 'Minimum Syndrome of the Maximum Value' represents the vital essence of a drug. They have not clarified how this typical group is to be found for each remedy, probably because the Group may consist of any symptoms provided they are of 'Maximum Value' (high ranking in the remedy) and 'Minimum in number'. Such minimum characteristics can only come from Mental and Physical Generals, and occasionally from qualified outstanding Particulars (Gunavante 1994).

Gladwin, a student of Kent, wrote: I wrote down against each symptom all the remedies that the repertory gave. On seeing this repertory work Kent remarked, "Lot of work...." He took three or four symptoms, referred to the repertory and immediately found the remedy. He said they are symptoms of the patient. That Kent's reference to "selecting one symptom" (quoted earlier) was not just theoretical is shown by a case.

Kent gave a problem case to two of his students, Kraft and Boyce, an expert in repertory work. After a two day exercise with the repertory, Calcarea carbonica came at the top and Thuja at the bottom. Kent ran his eyes over the tabulation and selected Thuja. When the shocked pair questioned Kent, he turned up Thuja in Hering's Condensed Materia Medica and pointed out how the peculiar urethral discharge of the patient had its closest similarity to Thuja and explained that the whole case hinged on this leading characteristic of the case. He went on to explain that one must study the materia medica, and find out the red strands running through the remedies and apply this knowledge to one's cases. (Homoeopathy, the modern medicine, Oct-Dec. 1889 in Gunavante 1994).

Clarke in his monograph, *Dr. Skinner's Grand Characteristics* writes:

If practice depended entirely on books, the multiplication of these would soon make practice impossible; fortunately, there are many features of homoeopathy which tend to simplification of practice and none knew this better then Thomas Skinner. When for instance, we have a feverish patient who turns deadly pale and faints on any attempt to rise from the horizontal posture, we have no need to make an hour's search in repertories.....The patient is crying out for Aconite. That symptom is a 'grand characteristic' in the phraseology of Skinner...This term has the same meaning as Lippe's Keynotes, and Nash's 'Leaders'. All indicate a method of simplifying a practice which is often very complicated.

Nash in his Leaders in *Homoeopathic Therapeutics* and his other book *Testimony of the Clinic* has amply illustrated the advantage of a group of the most characteristic symptoms of a remedy being kept in mind in our search for the simillimum. H.C. Allen's *Keynotes and Characteristics* follows the same pattern and justly enjoys great popularity with homeopaths at all levels.

Farrington writing under the title "Use of universal symptoms" (Lesser Writings) says: The symptoms or a group of symptoms employed plainly exhibit a universal quality of a drug, as when we select Bryonia in cases worse from motion... Causticum for paretic aphonia, even if of catarrhal origin and so on.....In such cases, we are not prescribing for a single symptom; we are making use of a universal characteristic property. - To explain further, the modality "Worse from motion" is universally present in all tissues affected by exercise.....in Bryonia. Similarly, Thuja affects epithelia everywhere.....if wart is its characteristic.... it acts upon the whole 'epithelial' man. But when we prescribe for an isolated symptom (even a characteristic) we do violence to the principle of the Organon and violate common sense. Entire case depends upon "Universal characteristics"

Farrington gives some more illustrations of the "Universal characteristic symptoms" of remedies. He says that physicians, when unable to fit the "totality", have at times chosen a remedy that suits those characteristics upon which the entire disease seems to depend. For example, Collinsonia has been employed for many diseases when there is a congestion of the lower bowels with piles, or piles bleeding, feeling of sticks in the rectum, uterine affections, varices, irritable heart - which have all yielded readily to this drug, just as though they depended for their existence upon pelvic stasis (a universal characteristic of Collinsonia). Similarly, we have seen palpitation, vertigo and dyspepsia vanish under the influence of Pareira brava selected for its grand characteristic, "Must get down on all fours and strain to pass water; pains go down the thighs." So, too, Berberis relieves a host of ailments when selected for its radiating renal pains, "Pains into the hips, urine with yellow, loamy sediment." "Anisum stellatum has cured haemoptysis when selected by its key-note," "Pain at the junction of the third right rib with its cartilage." Myrtus communis has retarded phthisis when there was present sharp pain through the upper part of the left lung. Ceanothus has removed leucorrhoea when in addition there was sharp pain in the splenic region. And so on almost indefinitely. Now in all such cases there is, of course, a connection between symptoms treated as central and the others that disappear along with them, though often we are not able to detect it. It would be very useful if we try to identify these "Universal characteristics" of as many remedies as possible. For example, "constriction" as of an iron band seem to be such a feature of Cactus; constriction of heart, throat, chest, bladder, rectum, vagina (Gunavante 1994).

Analogous Parts

Farrington gives us one more hint for studying keynotes in the *Genius of Remedies*. He says,

> Just as metastases are apt to take place in tissues of similar function, so are analogous parts prone to be affected by a drug. Reasoning from such premises, Arum triphyllum, which causes rawness of the corners of the mouth, was successfully employed by Dr. B.F. Betts for a similar condition of the os uteri; and upon the same principle, drugs which disease the testicles have been used when the ovaries are affected. On the same reasoning, the author used Apis for "incompetent os." If Apis has diarrhoea "as if the anus was wide open", why could we not extend the analogy to cervix (a contiguous part), "as if it is wide open" (Gunavante 1994).

Ruling Features of the Case Reflect the 'Genius' of the Remedy

Boger in *Studies in the Philosophy of Healing* says,

> We are accustomed to find symptoms in associated groups, and guided by their peculiarities, search out the simillimum for each...The ruling feature of every case puts the stamp of some particular type, such as bilious, haemorrhagic, etc. upon it, and when we select remedies which...conform to the present type, we say that the genius of the drug corresponds to that of the disease.
>
> Here is a sample of the genius of Bryonia from the great homoeopathic physician, Dr. Margaret Tyler: "And now, to sum up if you ever get a patient with severe stitching pains, worse for the slightest movement, worse for sitting up, better for pressure,

very thirsty for long drinks of cold water, very irritable, angry, and not only angry, but with sufferings increased by being disturbed mentally or physically, white tongue, in delirium wants to go home (even when at home), busy in his dreams and in delirium with his everyday business, you can administer Bryonia and bet on the result." To sum up, it is possible for a prescriber to identify the curative remedy in a case almost immediately on the basis of just a few symptoms which are most characteristic in the patient as well as the remedy. To realise this possibility the prescriber should have a group of the outstanding characteristics of as many remedies as possible at his finger tips to the point of being able to differentiate between one remedy and another by the presence or absence of certain symptoms in one or the other (Gunavante 1994).

How do we identify the peculiar and distinguishing symptoms? Dunham says,

> The fact cannot be too often called to mind, nor too strongly insisted upon, that our most characteristic indications for the use of a drug, which presents well defined general symptoms... are derived not from its local action upon any organ or system, not from a knowledge of the particular tissues it may affect, and how it affects them, but upon the general constitutional symptoms and their conditions and concomitants. This means that it is not the local, particular symptoms, but the general - Mental and Physical General symptoms that help us (Gunavante 1994).

Erastus Case argued,

> That the symptoms of the case have been carefully taken, giving us, as expressed in the appropriate language of Hahnemann: "The outwardly reflected image of the inner nature

of the disease; that is, of the suffering vital force". We find those symptoms confusing, often conflicting, and a host in number. Some are peculiar to the constitution of the patient; some are resultant from former disease; some are functional; others are pathological, really diseased conditions of the organs; still others are sympathetic, the result of those diseased conditions; many may be due to the action of drugs already administered; some may be purely imaginary. We have been taught to give that remedy which has produced all the symptoms of the patient. It frequently happens that we cannot find a remedy whose pathogenesis contains them all. Some of you doubtless have worked out a case, as I have often done, with a repertory, and found that the symptoms led not to a single, but to several remedies, one seeming to be just as applicable as another-a disheartening result after hours of faithful study. Shall we employ the remedy which covers the greatest number of symptom-a purely numerical comparison-or can we select some special symptoms which have more weight than others in making the choice (Case 1916)?

Drysdale divides symptoms into two classes, absolute and contingent.

Absolute symptoms are those which belong to all patients suffering from the same pathological process; contingent symptoms are those which vary with the individual and are not essentially pathognomonic. He declares that "the greater the value of a symptom for the purposes of diagnosis, the less its value for the selection of the remedy".

T. F. Allen aptly divides symptoms into determining and resulting. "Determining symptoms are those which precede and determine the development of a lesion, which, when established, becomes the fountain of new and resulting symptoms. Resulting are those which are not of prime importance to the therapeutist who seeks to arrest the progress of the real malady". He concludes: 1. Some symptoms are of more value than others. 2. The most valuable to the therapeutist are the determining symptoms, both in acute and chronic diseases. Hahnemann's Organon, Paragraph 153, reads thus: "In the search for the homoeopathic specific remedy-that is, in the comparison of the total signs of the natural sickness with the lists of symptoms of available drugs in order to find among them one bearing a pathogenetic power corresponding to and resembling the disease to be cured the striking, remarkable, and peculiar (or characteristic) signs and symptoms of the case of sickness are to be especially and almost exclusively brought before the eye; for these, especially, must be very like the drug that is being searched for in the symptom lists, if this is to be most suitable for the cure. The general and indefinite symptoms, such as loss of appetite, headache, weakness, restless sleep, discomfort, et cetera, if they are not more closely defined, deserve little attention, for we find something about as indefinite in almost every sickness and caused by almost every drug". Upon comparing the teachings of Drs. Drysdale and Allen with that of Hahnemann, we find no inconsistency between them. Dr Drysdale places of highest value the contingent symptoms-those peculiar to the sick individual under consideration; Dr Allen, the determining symptoms-those individual peculiarities which precede the development of the lesion. They simply interpret and explain the words of the master without adding to the truth contained in them. Our guide in finding the remedy, then, is as follows: "The striking, remarkable, and peculiar (or characteristic) symptoms are to be especially and almost exclusively brought before the eye, for these must be very like the drug most suitable for the cure". Now we see why our earlier attempts with the repertory failed of the best results. We were placing the absolute and general symptoms alongside the characteristic as of equal value, instead of giving them a secondary place, using them to confirm the choice of remedy made from the characteristic symptoms. A careful study of the Organon should have taught us better. It may be urged that a characteristic symptom cannot be found in every case, but surely no two persons are just alike in form and feature, and the differences in the constitution, and in the disturbance of the physical economy in disease, are so great that individual peculiarities are always present. Our success will be determined in great measure by our acuteness of observation in recognizing the peculiarities of the patient, and our skill in adapting to them the appropriate medicine (Case 1916).

"Strange, rare and peculiar" symptoms often become keynotes although not all keynotes are strange symptoms, for instance, "hunger at 11 a.m." is a keynote of Sulphur but it not a "strange, rare and peculiar" symptom; the same with the 4-8 p.m. aggravation of Lycopodium, but a keynote which is also a peculiar symptom is the well known aggravation from downward motion of Borax, or "the more you belch the more you have to belch" of Ignatia, or the peculiar symptom which is also a keynote of Calc., Alum., and Nitric acid "craves indigestible things like chalk, earth and slate pencils" (Wright - Hubbard 1940).

Other Leading Proponents

Nash

Gunavante (1994) gave further examples from Nash's case work.

The great Dr. E.B. Nash reiterates the same point thus (Regional Leaders). Take a patient who had, for instance, these four leading symptoms of Arsenicum: Great prostration, excessive anguish and restlessness, burning thirst for cold water in small quantities at a time, all worse at 1 to 3 a.m. The name of the disease or the general physiological or pathological action of the drug would have nothing to do with such symptoms as these; and yet what true homoeopath is there who does not know that these symptoms are in many different diseases valuable indications for its administration?

A few examples from Tyler will further illustrate the points. "Kent gives a case of uraemic coma in a doctor's wife. Catheter showed that there was no urine in the bladder. She had the pulling sensation at the navel...In the middle of the night her husband came in great distress; she was pale as death, and breathing slowly; deeply comatose. A single powder of Plumbum high was given, and she passed urine in a couple of hours, roused up, and never had such an attack again".

"A physician while observing the patient in one of the spasms noticed that she came out of it with a succession of long-drawn sighs. He inquired if the patient had any recent mental trouble, and learned that she had lost her brother, of whom she was exceedingly fond, and for whom she mourned greatly a few weeks before. Ignatia 30 quickly cured her."

"A woman of 33 was brought into the Hospital with pyelitis, frequent heart attacks, temperature 104 of, pneumonia. For fever at noon there is only one drug in italics, Stram. The graceful spasms, the dry hot skin and the suppressed urine again suggested Stram. Stram 1M three doses four hourly; the result was dramatic...This case shows how the curative remedy was found on a very few but characteristic symptoms, not of pneumonia or pyelitis, but of that individual patient."

"This seems to have been a common method of finding the remedy with Dr. Erastus Case, and it led him to brilliant results with many remedies that would not "work out" by mere tedious repertory methods" (Different Ways of Finding the Remedy by Tyler in Gunavante 1994).

Boger

Boger says (*Studies in the Philosophy of Healing*),

The gist of the case may be featured in any one of the three parts (Constitutional, General and Peculiar). Often it is the common factor of the essential peculiarities; again it may come down through the anamnesis, hereditary predilection, etc. He throws revealing light on the "Essential peculiarities" through three cases: (1) A child had severe chills at 11 a.m. every alternate day, face very blue, followed by intense heat, then slight moisture. Natrum mur 1M - and never another chill. (2) Suppression of profuse leucorrhoea led to salpingitis, high fever. Each paroxysm of pain gradually rose to a certain pitch, then suddenly ceased. A dose of Puls. restored the discharge followed by complete recovery. (3) Subacute pneumonia with gastritis. The stomach pain always went to the side upon which she happened to turn. Two doses of Puls. 1M stopped all distress, followed by much muco-pus expectoration... complete cure. Now Boger concludes with his lesson: "These cases emphasise the necessity of discovering the essential peculiarities which crop out from time to time in every sickness" (Boger 1964).

Pulford

Gunavante (1994) describes Pulford's approach to keynotes.

The real symptom totality of the indicated drug must consist of the very few symptoms produced on the healthy human body, and not by symptoms produced in the arousing of semi-latent predispositions in that body. They must be produced by the drug itself; and those must be constant in all provers, while the others will be found to vary with different individuals, and in the same individual at different times. That makes the existing evaluation of symptoms as they appear in our repertories erroneous, as I have many times discovered......The proving drug always produces its own little pathogenetic group; it never varies, no matter who or what the individual is. This true pathogenetic group which we term the rare, strange and peculiar symptoms, outstands all the rest of the symptoms put together. And with the small pathogenesis alone you can prescribe with confidence; without it, your efforts will end only in failure. . . the rest of the symptoms are mere pointers to the drug, and not its indicators... The mass of symptoms put through the repertory do not take us to the coveted goal...The rare strange and peculiar symptoms are the only ones that mark the true individuality of the drug.

As examples of the true pathogenetic symptom totality, Pulford cites four cases:

i. A case of hepatic colic that occurred regularly every month for two years was relieved in five minutes with Acon. 30x and has remained so now for three years. Agonized tossing about, extreme fear of death, expression of anxiety and insatiable thirst led to Aconite.

ii. A case of renal calculi that has been from pillar to post for four years, was relieved at once and two calculi passed without pain in twenty four hours... no more attacks for over a year. The symptoms that led to the remedy were the flushed redness of face during the pains, pupils dilated to the limit, the pains clutching and together with the sweats coming and going rapidly. A single dose of Bell 10M did the trick.

iii. A case of diabetes (allopathically diagnosed) had resisted their treatment, and had to be placed in the hospital for observation. This was practically restored to normal in six weeks by a single dose of Cina 1M. The constant picking at the nose, paleness around the nose and mouth, cross and capricious appetite led to the remedy. No return of complaint for over two years.

iv. A case of erysipelas that had resisted all other remedies, was given Crot-tig 30x on the basis of symptoms: yellow watery stool coming out like a shot, worse immediately after eating or drinking. The result was both remarkable and permanent. Pulford concludes: Four short groups, easy to the materia medica. Yet, no case indicating any one of those drugs was ever cured that did not include its respective small primary pathogenic group, as indicated above (Gunavante 1994).

Taylor

More recently, Taylor has published a great case demonstrating the value of keynote prescribing but from a contemporary perspective.

A 38 year-old woman presented with the diagnosis of gastrointestinal reflex. She reported "risings" in the area behind the zyphoid process and lower sternum, with sour taste in the mouth, worse lying (especially at night; she would only rarely lie down at other times, but if she did, the same symptoms would appear, especially if she had recently eaten). She felt as if a good belch would relieve her symptoms, but could rarely belch, & if did, felt no relief of the seeming need to. The pressure in the zyphoid region made it difficult to breath when she was lying down. She would wake about 2 hours after retiring to bed, feeling unable to get a good breath, with diffuse unexplainable anxiety, and a gnawing hunger in the stomach. She described a constant sensation, pointing to the zyphoid process, as "it feels like I swallowed a hard-boiled egg that just stuck right here."

I took the following rubrics for her case (the number in parentheses is the number of remedies in the rubric, using the Quantum view of Synthesis vers. 8):

Here is a standard repertorization, weighted for number of symptoms x degree:

| Stomach eructations type of sour (166) |
| Stomach eructations ineffectual and incomplete (80) |
| Stomach eructations lying agg. (5) |
| Respiration difficult lying while (107) |
| Generals eating after (189) |
| Stomach egg sensation as if swallowed an (1) |
| Sleep disturbed hunger by (10) |
| Mind anxiety night midnight before (36) |

Sulphur, Lycopodium, Phosphorus, Graphites, etc. lead the numerical repertorization, but all of these are missing the most striking, peculiar, 'auffallend' symptom of the case - the sensation of a hard-boiled egg lodged behind the zyphoid.

Using Radar, a symptom such as this one can be emphasized in any one of several ways:

When this patient described the sensation of "a hard-boiled egg" lodged at the pyloric cardia, I had difficulty remaining in my seat - having long-before learned this to be one of the most outstanding Keynote symptoms of our materia medica, as a highly characteristic symptom of Abies nigra (Taylor 2001).

Although this keynote catapults Abies nigra into the lead in the analyses above, it was still necessary to confirm its similitude to the totality of symptoms of the case - albeit a totality heavily weighted by this uniquely characterizing symptom. Finding Abies nigra also in the rubrics Respiration difficult lying while, Generals eating after and Sleep disturbed hunger by confirmed the fit of this remedy to the totality of the case. I felt OK about its going missing in the other 4 rubrics taken for the case, as it is a rather "small" remedy, represented in only 97 rubrics in the Full Synthesis Repertory, compared to over 9,000 rubrics for each of the leading remedies of the straight repertorization. Reviewing the primary and clinical materia medica of Abies nigra, along with that of other leading remedies falling out of the analysis - the essential final step of case analysis - confirmed this remedy as the simillimum for the case (Taylor 2001).

Keynotes may involve single symptoms, as in the example above; but they may also involve a characteristic concomitance or alternation of symptoms that serves as a more complex keynote. Examples of this include the concomitance of rheumatic complaints, neuralgic pains, and uterine complaints of Cimicifuga; the alternation of rheumatic complaints with cardiac/endocardial symptoms of Kalmia; and the alternation of asthmatic respiration with rheumatic pain of Dulcamara. Many of these characteristic complex keynotes are recorded directly as rubrics in our repertories, e.g., Respirations asthmatic alternating with pain; rheumatic, dulc, Med, and can be incorporated into an analysis as described above for a simple keynote (Taylor 2001).

Keynotes can serve as valuable symptoms to help us discover at least 'one ray of light in the chaos spread out before us,' in finding a simillimum to match the totality of symptoms of a case. But it is crucial we use this method with prudence. When relying on keynotes in analysis however, it is important to keep foremost in one's mind that this strategy merely aids in appreciating the totality of symptoms in a rich and full way, and is not a means of side-stepping around the need to address the totality of symptoms, in each and every case.

Advantages of Keynote Prescribing

Having trawled the literature, it is clear that Keynote prescribing has some great value in:

1. Cases with striking symptoms
2. Genius epidemicus situations
3. Acute cases / emergency cases

In learning and teaching homeopathic medicine it offers a good and logic structure. There are plenty of advocates. Clarke (1925) in *Constitutional Medicine With Especial Reference to the Three Constitutions of Von Grauvogl* says,

> A further great aid to simplicity in prescribing is that advocated by Dr. Lippe and his friends. Out of the characteristic symptoms of the remedies they marked out those which they named "Key-Note symptoms". Indeed, some symptoms or conditions of symptoms are so characteristic of certain remedies that when one of them appears in a patient it is almost certain

that other symptoms of that remedy will be found in the patient too (Clarke 1925).

Guernsey (1867) in *The Application of the Principles and practice of Homeopathy to Obstetrics and the disorders peculiar to women and young children* says,

> The distinguishing characteristics, the key-notes, which form the individual and constitutional symptoms of the patient, are sensational symptoms, rather than functional derangements or structural disorganizations. And the method we pursue in relying upon these, in the absence of other indications, and of attaching very great importance to them, even where other symptoms are not wanting, is sustained by two substantial reasons. First, in many cases we can do no better, since few if any of our remedies either have or can ever be expected to have, direct pathogenetic symptoms to correspond to the innumerable ultimate forms of structural disease which we are often called upon to treat. Second, this method has been found reliable by much experience. The purely constitutional symptoms such as those of periodicity and the conditions of aggravation and amelioration ,strictly sensational symptoms, being found to constitute infallible indications in the choice of the remedy, where all other guides are wanting (Guernsey 1867).

Pulford (1936) in the *Homoeopathic Recorder, in Why do we take the case?* said,

> It is remarkable how much more simple and easy it is to rapidly "take a case" if one masters the keynote of the drug that distinguishes it from all others, together with its essential satellites. The mere asking of endless useless questions and writing page after page of symptoms is not necessary "case taking" and all too often leads one astray. And the repertory is

the last thing on earth that would help out in such a process. The repertory, alone, would lead us to fully 90 percent of mild suppressions, rather than cures (Pulford 1936).

H.C. Allen's (1931) opinion in *Keynotes and Characteristics with Comparison*) was,

> The life-work of the student of the homoeopathic Materia Medica is one of constant comparison and differentiation. He must compare the pathogenesis of a remedy with the recorded anamnesis of the patient; he must differentiate the apparently similar symptoms of two or more medicinal agents in order to select the similimum. To enable the student or practitioner to do this correctly and rapidly he must have as a basis for comparision some knowledge of the individuality of the remedy; something that is peculiar, uncommon, or sufficiently characteristic in the confirmed pathogenesis of a polychrest remedy that may be used as a pivotal point of comparison. It may be a so-called "keynote", a "characteristic," the "red strand of the rope," and central modality or principle - as the aggravation from motion of Bryonia, the amelioration from motion of Rhus, the furious, vicious delirium of Belladonna or the apathetic indifference of Phosphoric acid - some familiar landmark around which the symptoms may be arranged in the mind for comparison. Something of this kind seems indispensable to enable us to intelligently and successfully use our voluminous symptomatology. Also, if we may judge from the small number of homoeopathic physicians who rely on the single remedy in practice, and the almost constant demand for a "revision" of the Materia Medica, its study in the past, as well as at present, has not been altogether satisfactory to the majority. An attempt to render the student's task less difficult, to simplify its study, to make it both interesting and useful, to place

its mastery within the reach of every intelligent man or woman in the profession, is the apology for the addition of another monograph to our present works of reference. It is all-important that the first step in the study of homoeopathic therapeutics be correctly taken, for the pathway is then more direct and the view more comprehensive. The object of this work is to aid the student to master that which is guiding and characteristic in the individuality of each remedy and thus utilize more readily the symptomatology of the Homoeopathic Materia Medica, the most comprehensive and practical work for the cure of the sick ever given the medical profession. It is the result of years of study as student, practitioner and teacher, and is published at the earnest solicitation of many alumni of Hering College, with the hope that it may be of as much benefit to the beginner as it has been to the compiler. In the second edition preface he wrote, The original plan has been maintained, viz: to give only those symptom-guides that mark the individuality of the remedy, that the student of materia medica may use them as landmarks to master the genius of the remedial agent (Allen 1931).

Disadvantages of Keynote Prescribing

Keynote prescribing really has little value in:
1. Cases without outstanding symptoms
2. When keynote and totality approaches point out different remedies
3. When it is easily misunderstood as a shortcut

In the *Study of Materia Medica and Taking the Case* (Boger 1941) wrote:

The diagnostic and common symptoms as shaded by the general modalities from the ground colour of the picture, from which its special features portraying the individuality emerge with more or less distinctness. The focal point of the scene reveals its inherent genius with which the outlying parts must harmonize, if we wish to fully grasp its meaning. Running after key-notes while paying scant attention to the general harmony of the picture has spoiled many a case and leads to polypharmacy (Boger 1941).

Miller (1911) argued in, *On the comparative value of symptoms in the selection of the remedy,*

In opposition to this numerical method, some physicians have gone to the other extreme, and have been content to be guided in the selection of the remedy by one or two peculiar and outstanding symptoms, practically ignoring all the others, because they have overlooked the fact that - unless there be a general correspondence between the symptoms of the patient and those of the remedy - it is not reasonable to expect a cure. This so-called "keynote" system of prescribing is very attractive, as it seems so easy, and saves all the laborious comparison of competing drugs that is involved in the numerical method, and also because by means of it many brilliant cures have been made; but it is from its very nature a wrong method, and in the great majority of cases is doomed to failure, because it ranks one or two symptoms very high and practically ignores the others (Miller 1911).

The message is the same from the start. Keynote prescribing involves particular skill. There is rarely, if ever, a shortcut. It has some significant strengths, and when used well, can lead to some excellent prescriptions and results.

Further Reading

- Mathur — *Principles of Prescribing*
- Burt — *Characteristic Materia Medica*
- Guernsey — *Keynotes of the Materia Medica*
- von Lippe — *Keynotes of the Homoeopathic Materia Medica*
- von Lippe — *Keynotes and Red-Line Symptoms of the Materia Medica*
- Boger — *Boenninghausen's Characteristics*
- Boger — *A Synoptic Key of the Materia Medica*
- Allen — *Keynotes and Characteristics with Comparisons*
- Clarke — *Grand Characteristics of the Materia Medica*
- Morrison — *Desktop Guide to Keynotes and Confirmatory Symptoms*
- Phatak — *Materia Medica of Homeopathic Medicines*
- Allen — *A Primer of Materia Medica*
- Nash — *Leaders in Therapeutics*
- Case — *Some Clinical experiences of E. E. Case*
- Wright Hubbard — *Strange, rare and peculiar symptoms*

Chapter 10

Isopathy

Contents

- Definitions
- Introductions
- Practicalities
- Context
- Examples of Isopathy in Pre-Homeopathic History
- The Isopaths Hering and Lux
- The Response
- Collett
- The Controversy
- The Components of Isopathy
- Theoretical Study of Isopathy
- Cases Best Suited for This Method / Advantages
- Disadvantages
- Practical Study of Isopathy / Case Examples
- Who Uses It Today?
- Appendix (List of nosodes, Nomenclature of nosodes with Nelson, Nomenclature of nosodes by Reckeweg)

In this chapter you will:

1. Learn about the controversies surrounding this method and why it courted so much opposition

2. Identify its historical advocates

3. Understand its modern clinical value and learn contemporary clinical situations where its value in complimenting the simillimum in the case is warranted

Chapter 10

Isopathy

There are four pathies: Homoeopathy, antipathy, isopathy (so-called), and allopathy. Isopathy is the use of a nosode to relieve the condition which has produced that nosode. In my opinion, there is no such thing as isopathy. Analyze it, and isopathy becomes homoeopathy. ……..I do not think there is such a thing as isopathy. You cannot get two things alike. (Moore 1903)

The old idea that homoeopathy is nothing but treating a disease with the products of that disease is decidedly wrong. The nosode of disease is not used in the treatment of disease as homoeopathic. It is not homoeopathic to treat any disease with the products of disease. It is treating the disease, not treating the patient. It is always given for the disease itself; and when that is done they are entirely outside of homoeopathy. Hahnemann has proclaimed against it in the introduction to the Organon, in the Organon itself and in his Chronic Diseases, as foreign to homoeopathy. (Moore 1903)

Still he (Hering) admits that all these isopathic preparations cannot be regarded as absolute specifics, but only as chronic intermediate remedies, which serve, as it were, to stir up the disease, and render the reaction to the homoeopathic remedy subsequently administered more permanent and effectual. This assertion he repeats in 1836, and states that he has never succeeded in curing but only in ameliorating diseases with their own morbid products. (Dudgeon 1853)

Definitions

At its core, Isopathy has a simple definition. It comes from the Greek 'isos' meaning 'equal', and 'pathos' meaning 'same' suffering. In other words, prescribing a medicine made from the supposed causative agent. Sounds easy? Actually it can get quite complicated.

Isopathy is the use of homeopathically prepared substances responsible for the disease itself. It is not based on the principle of similarity but on sameness, on the substance being identical to the aetiological agent, the use of pollens in allergic asthma, the use of *Arsenicum* to treat arsenic poisoning. But it can also involve the use of potentised drugs to treat toxic side effects of those drugs (also called tautopathy). Moreover, it can be similar to, and an improvement of, desensatisation therapy because desensitization may result in an increased reactional capacity of the patient to allergens. Isopathy may help eliminate toxins that have accumulated in the patient. Without doubt, sometimes practitioners and students of homeopathy get confused between all of these terms, isopathy, tautopathy, nosode and sarcode.

Strict adherence to the definition of isopathy makes it fundamentally different from homeopathy. Since isodes were never proven on healthy human subjects, one does not know the full range of symptoms it can produce and no case individualization was performed. The isode was just given based on the identical nature of disease and isode (Yasgur 1994).

Introduction

My experience with isopathy was mixed. Since it made very

little sense from a philosophical perspective in my initial use in practice I avoided it, and of course used a similar remedy based on the broadest possible totality. But of course not every case has improved over the years, and at times I have found myself searching for pragmatic solutions.

A mother bought her child to see me in 2002. The child had a blister on the instep of his foot. It had come up quickly while he was playing in the garden. Inside the blister was yellow and green and black fluid, and there was a red line started to head up the leg. She told me that, 'I drove in to see my father who is a GP, a doctor and he said to take antibiotics now. He said it looks like a white tailed spider bite. I have never given my child any antibiotics and I don't want to. Can you help?' Six months previously, we had conducted a *White-tailed Spider* proving at Nature Care College in Sydney Australia. Of the myriad of symptoms that came out of that proving, there wasn't one that resembled the blister, the infection or septicaemia that seemed to be taking place. We agreed that I would prescribe but that if there was not immediate improvement within the next couple hours, she would go to the hospital and take her father's advice, and use the antibiotics. I prescribed *White-tailed Spider 30c*, and the mother rang an hour later saying that the blister had burst, the fluid had come out, and that the child slept and was still asleep. She called me the next morning. She said that he had had the sleep of the dead. She kept a watch on him all night and he awoke feeling rested, full of energy, and was back running around.

Since that experience, I have had numerous examples of using *White-tailed Spider* in similar situations. And there can be some grim situations, some of which I've been able to capture on video, because that spider bite has the domestic reputation of creating ulcers and wounds that will not heal and long after the bite of a spider. Medical scientists are reluctant to adopt the same idea because they seem to be unable to replicate those ulcers in controlled environments, giving rise to the debate about necrotizing arachnidism (syndrome of blistering and ulceration following a spider bite). Nevertheless in my own practice I've had some delightful results, and to my mind, this kind of isopathy has its place in homeopathic medicine, either in emergencies or when all other avenues have been exhausted.

Of course Hahnemann was no fan at all. In aphorism 53, he states that isopathy '...contradicts all normal human understanding and hence all experience'... He suggests that any validity is because the substance is altered by the potentisation process and therefore acts as a 'similar' rather than 'identical' substance.

Practicalities

Going into the literature, we can see that homeopaths for virtually 200 years have employed this technique. There is also auto-isopathy, a medicine made from a patient's own by-products and / or pathology, such as a person's own blood or urine potentised and given back as a medicine, a person's swab, discharge etc potentised and re-prescribed.

Some examples include:
- *Apis* for bee stings reactions
- *Lac defloratum* or other Lac remedies for milk allergy
- *Fragaria vesca* (potentised stawberry) for strawberry allergy

- Infected urine potentised and given back to client
- Vaginal discharge that is infected with Staphylococcus B potentised and prescribed as an alternative to antibiotics
- Cancer tumours potentised and represcribed following a biopsy

It seems commonplace to hear stories in the group of the community of practitioners using the following:

Wheat	Mixed pollen
Dust	Baker's yeast
Dust-mite	Cat fur
Grass (Mixed & specific)	Dog hair
Dairy	Vegemite

And of course prescriptions such as *Tuberculinum*, *Variolinum* from matter obtained from a smallpox pustule, and *Carcinosin* the nosode from a carcinoma are common (Bellavite 1995). The dosage can range from 30c daily to every other day, to once weekly to once monthly. Some case reports cite once a day for 3 days, then once a week for 3 weeks, then once a month for 3 months.

In his book *Mastering Homeopathy* John Gamble advocates a protocol for the treatment of allergies that involves prescribing a substance to which patient is allergic, along with alternating doses of Histaminum in increasing potencies (Gamble 2005). Judy Coldicott, a homeopath in the South Island of New Zealand, reports fantastic results using *Wheat* 30 for patients with wheat allergies.

Context

Isopathy may also help eliminate toxins that have accumulated in the patient. Though the principles of isopathy were being put to therapeutic use by many others and much earlier in medical history, the term 'isopathy' is credited to Joseph Wilhelm Lux, a German veterinarian, somewhere around 1831-3. His first remedy was a 30c dilution of a blood specimen from an animal with anthrax. Thus *Anthracinum* was created. In 1833 Lux wrote *Isopathik der Contagionen*. Alexis Eustaphieve wrote a very early treatise on isopathy when he published, in 1846, *Homoeopathia Revealed. A Brief Exposition of the Whole System Adapted to General Comprehension. 2nd Ed. with a Sketch of Isopathia*. Collet (1824-1909) was another early advocate of isopathy. He wrote *Isopathie, Methode Pasteur par Voie Interne*. He suggested another category of preparation, serotherapeutic isopathy or serotherapy. This consisted of homeopathic remedies of immune serum, for example Marmorek (homeopathic remedy prepared from the antituberculous serum from a patient with tuberculosis). Julian also worked in this area and wrote *Dynamized Micro-Immunotherapy* (1977). Kruger, Nebel, Roy, Munoz, Fortier-Bernoville, Brotteaux, Schmidt, Schimmel, Parrot, Speight, Vannier, Voll, Reckeweg, H.C. Allen (*The Materia Medica of the Nosodes*, 1910), O.A. Julian (*Materia Medica der Nosoden*, 1960), have all contributed (Yasgur 1994, Julian 1997).

Isopathy and Pre-Homeopathic History

There are numerous examples of isopathy in documented medical history outside of any homeopathic thought. Some are obvious and some are downright bizarre:

- The Bohimans, according to Frasschoen (The Triumph of Homoeopathy, 1908, p. 197), make an incision near the snake bite and introduce into it a pinch of the glands with venom, taken from other serpents and dried. In similar cases, some inhabitants of Columbia take in a similar case some serum in which the liver of the serpent is macerated.

- In the far East, the Chinese people use the preventive variolisation by the compulsory wearing of the dresses of a patient in full suppuration stage or by the dried pustule, preserved one year, then introduced into the nostrils (the left for boys and the right for girls, (Huard and Wong: La médecine chinoise a travers le siécles).
- In the West, Hippocrates, who was the first to write in his Traité des Lieux de l'Homme (I, 688): "Vomitus vomitu curantur" Pline (23-79, after J.C.) teaches us that: "Est limus salivae sub lingua rabiosi canis qui, datus in potu, fieri hydrophobos non patitur" (There is under the tongue of the rabid dog a slime formed by its saliva, which taken in drink, guards against rabies (Pline: Natural history, 1st century after J.C.).
- Dioscorides of Anasarbe (75 after J.C.) recommends to give to eat to a hydrophobic the liver of the dog which has bitten and even grilled earthworms for the treatment of worms (Dioscorides: Materia Medica, 1st century after J. C.) said that there where is the disease, there is also the remedy. He recommends to crush the scorpion where it has bitten to eat the flesh of the viper which has bitten (Aetius-Opera medica, tr. by Cornarius, 5th century after J.C.)
- Paracelsus (1493-1541), wrote 'The similars cure the similars, the scorpion cures the scorpion, mercury cures mercury. The poison is mortal for man except, if in the organism there is another poison with which it may fight, in which case the patient regains his health' (Paracelsus: Compendium

philosophae, 1568). With this aim in view he uses very weak doses of the poison in question.

- In his "Archidoxes", he recommends the fell Tauris for the hepatic cirrhosis, and the extract of the spleen for the "'obstruction" of the spleen. He indicates blood serum to stop the hemorrhages and equally preconises the therapeutic utilisation of opotherapic products. In the 16th century, Oswal Crollius advises the utilisation of an isopathy; in his treatise "Signatures and Correspondences" (Crollius in La Royale chemin, tr. by M. Boulene, Paris, 1633) he writes: "To stop the overflowing of menstruation of women, it is necessary to take 3 or 4 drops of the same blood, always choosing the most clear and let the patient drink it, without her knowing and there is no doubt it will stop the overflow. The rat bite is cured by the powder made of the same rat after having burnt it. The scorpion carry their cure as well as all animals, and it is a fact that in the "Provence" (province) they have the custom to crush the scorpion between two stones and apply it on the bite and by this means the illness goes whence it has come". Thus, according to Jérome Cardan "Omne similia similibus confirmatur" in (Ars curandi, Parva, 1566).

- Fludd, nicknamed the Researcher Jesuit of Ireland, treats the phthisis with the dilution of the sputum of the patient. In his Philosophia Myosaica (Robert Fludd: Philosiphia Myosaica, Goudae, 1638, sheet 149, col. 2), writes 'But do we not see generally the similar of which the nature has but modified by putrifaction (Spagyric method of preparation) has a particular noxious effect for the similar.' Thus the worms eliminated by the organism, dried and powdered and given internally, destroy the worms. The sputum of a patient suffering from Phthisis cures after appropriate preparation

(Spagyric method of preparation) phthisis. The spleen of man having undergone a particular preparation (spagyric method of preparation) is a remedy against enlarged spleen. The stone formed in the bladder and in the kidney cure and dissolve the stone (Hunewald and Reirfer-Historique de l'Isopathy, L'Hom. moderne, 1936, No. 4, p. 255).

- Anthanasius Kircher in the work: Magna sive de arterial magnetica writes 'The poisonings in general are cured by their proper counterpoisons. Thus the bite of the spider will be cured by the application of a spider, the biting of a scorpion by the application of the scorpion, the poison of a rabid dog is drawn out of the body by the furs of the same dog'. In the treatise of poisons (Kircher: In mundus subterranius, Amsterdam, 1645) he affirms: 'Ubi morbus, ibi etiam medicamentum morbo illis oppotunum' (There where is the disease, there also is the proper remedy of the disease).

- In the 17th century, Lady Montague, wife of the English ambassador at Constantinople, got her child vaccinated by the extract of variolic pus (R. Tichner: Das Werden der Homoeopathic, 1950, p. 20). Prof. Phillipus Nettr of Venise (R. Ticher-ibid) (Ph. Netter Fundamenta medicinae theor. argentor, 1718, v. 2, p. 646) advised the dry pus of a plague bubo for the treatment of plague.

- Francis Home of Edinburg, used the blood of the patient suffering from measles against that disease (in R. Tichner-ibid) (Homoeo medical facts and Experiments, London 1754). Adrian La Bruyere published in 1734 a thesis "De curatione per similia" on the use of galenic Simili (R. Tichner-ibid). The vaccination against pox preconised by Jenner in 1798 is taken up again under another form of the vaccine method of the Chinese (Julian 1997).

And there's more still:

- Some methods of isopathy used in Old China (pus out of fistulas to "kill the fistular worm," or diluted excrements against dysentery, etc.; the old medical expression for this kind of treatment being; i-tu-kong- tu, which means the poison is also the antidote). (Galatzer 1949 Eight years in china (N. Galatzer).

- The lungs of the fox were recommended for asthmatics by Dioscorides, Xenocrates, Galen, Serapion, Paulus Aegineta, and by many other writers, down indeed to the most modern times, for we find them still a favourite remedy for the like affection in the earlier editions of the Pharmacopoeia Londinensis. Dioscorides: advised the brains of a cock to be given in haemorrhage from the meninges, whilst Galen says that the brains of a camel are a cure for epilepsy. Paracelsus also might be pressed into the service of isopathy……….. his disciple, Oswald Croll, believed and taught that the sound organs of certain animals were useful in the diseases of those organs in man. About two hundred years ago Dr. Durey revived the treatment of hydrophobia recommended by Dioscorides, of giving the liver of the rabid animal to those bitten by it. Ten persons having been bitten by a mad wolf, and nine of these having died, the wolf was captured and killed, and its liver, after being washed with wine and dried in the oven, was given to the tenth person who had been bitten. He consumed the whole liver in three days, and remained free from the disease (Dudgeon 1853).

Advocates

Hering

Hering brought into common homeopathic use some remedies made from snakes, rabid dogs, the pus of the itch, and of course, was responsible for bringing into homeopathic materia medica, a huge amount of new and well-proven remedies (Nebel in Julian 1985). His experiments on himself and others were herculean. In 1833, Hering wrote a long paper, wherein he extols the efficacy of the prepared itch-matter, which he now calls psorine. He called it,

> ...equal to our very strongest medicines in power; that it has a great power of producing eruptions; that it is one of the most efficacious means for restoring the lost or weakened action of the skin; that it is the most important remedy in every form of scabies, and that it is a prophylactic against infection with itch. He mentions leucorrhoeal matter as being curative of leucorrhoea, gleet-matter of gleet, phthisine of phthisis, ascardine of children's vermicular diseases. He suggests that the seeds of plants potentised may possibly be the means of eradicated and destroying such plants, and that insects potentised may be capable of destroying the life of their own species; and then he exclaims what a blessing this discovery will prove to farmers in getting rid of weeds, and to housewives in freeing their houses and children from vermin (Dudgeon 1853).

Constantine Hering was born on the 1st January 1800 at Oschatz, a small town of Saxony situated between Dresden and Leipzig, not that far from Hahnemann's whereabouts. His father Carl Gottlieb was an organist and composer of songs for children, but Constantine found mathematics and natural sciences. From 1811 to 1817 he followed classical studies in the College Littan. Wishing to study surgery, he went to Dresden then to Leipzig, and became the assistant of the Surgeon Robbi. Asked by the publisher Baumgartener to write a book exposing a complete refutation of homeopathy, Robbi gave the task to Hering. He began to study the works of Hahnemann, and finally convinced, declared himself a fan of this heretical medicine. Disapproved by Robbi and his professors, Hering however upheld his doctorate thesis (1826) taking the side of homeopathy. The following year he went to Surinam in the company of the natural scientist Weinhold. He remained six years in Surinam practising homeopathic medicine and working on his book containing works on natural history. After the publication of this book in the Archives of Stapf, the court of Saxony ordered him to stop researching and practising homeopathy. Contrarily he resigned and continued his work. Soon after he completed his study on *Lachesis,* and his first ideas on the uses of homeopathic remedies prepared from excretions or from pathological secretions, which he named 'nosodes'. In 1835, he went to Philadelphia and soon founded the 'Academy of North America for the Medical Art by Homeopathy' at Allentown, the first institution for the teaching of homeopathy in the world. In 1848 that school was transferred to Philadelphia (Homoeopathic Medical College of Pennsylvania). He taught materia medica and the theory. He also taught in the 'Hahnemann Medical College' from 1867. Hering died in 1880 leaving as his legacy the prolific *Guiding Symptoms* and the *Domestic Physician.*

Lux

The second isopath of significance was the veterinary doctor

Johan Joseph Wilhelm Lux. Very little is known about him, but according to J. Brusch (*Uber Homoeopathie in/der veterinaermedizin* 1934) he was born in 1776 at Oppeln in Silesie in Germany. His father was a small businessman and also a veterinary doctor. He studied at Berlin and was destined to become a vet. In 1803, he continued his study of medicine and natural sciences at Leipzig. He received his doctorate in medicine in 1805, and in 1806, was appointed professor of veterinary sciences in the University. In 1800, he published an article in which he concluded strongly, 'The veterinary doctor is the most important person of the state'. He also published:

Characteristics of the Epidemic of Bovides. (1803)

Translation of Tolnay: Arteris Veterinaire, Compendium pathologicum. (1808)

Study on the Teaching of Marechal Ferr and, Leipzig. (1809)

Justice of Shepherds its Relation to the State. (1815)

Popular Study on the Domestic, Animals. (1819)

From 1820, Lux began to become familiar with the writings of Hahnemann and applied it in veterinary medicine, and his successes brought him an immediate reputation. From that time, he became an ardent advocate. While he may have been a fan of Hahnemann, it was not mutual however. He founded many homeopathic societies, and from 1830, published the first periodical on veterinary medicine, entitled *Zooiasis* (or the Homoeopathic cure destined to animals, Kollmann Leipzig) in which he dedicated the 1st volume to Hahnemann with the inscription, 'You are the Sun which rises in the horizon of diseased animals, and as such, I place you among the veterinaries in the temple of Aesculapius of whom you represent the foundation stone.' Hahnemann's mistrust of Lux had previously been evident. Lux wrote to Hahnemann on October 14th, 1832, 'I ask to be allowed to dedicate to you the first volume of my treatment of animal diseases with homeopathy, so as to be able to say openly from the beginning that you also have demolished that enormous wall which separates animal and human therapy, and have established a simpler and more natural treatment of animals. I hope that the Veterinary surgeon will cause you less annoyance, and that they will soon, together with the physicians, make known throughout all zones, the outcome of your research.' Hahnemann only remarks on the letter, 'Not answered', perhaps because Lux was a member of the Leipzig local Society of Homoeopathic Physicians, whom Hahnemann attacked so vigorously nine days later in the "Leipsic Tageblatt" (Haehl 1922).

Hahnemann saw isopathy being used by close colleagues, such as Gross, and by those accumulating fame elsewhere, such as Hering, but he himself rejected it wholesale. Hahnemann wrote to Bönninghausen, 'I agree with your opinion on the blind use of so-called isopathic, and other unproved remedies, and we cannot protest loudly enough against them.'

An example was in 1831, where Zibrik in Hungary asked him in writing for a homeopathic remedy against 'glanders and anthrax'. Not yet knowing any homeopathic means against these epidemics, Hahnemann's reply was negative. Still there is a suggestion that he advised the 30th dilution of a drop of the nasal mucous of an animal attacked by glanders, and to give it to all the animals suffering from that disease. Thus he created the stock of *Anthracinum* then *Malleinum* (Julian 1997). In 1833, Lux published his results in a small pamphlet entitled *Isopathik der contagionen* or 'all the diseases carry in them the means of their cure'.

The Response to Isopathy

The ideas of Hering and Lux found immediate support amongst homeopaths. Surprisingly it was Stapf, founder of the *Archive für die Homoeopathische Heilkunst*, in 1822 who turned out to be a proponent. But he did find a difference between nosodes prepared from the contagion of contagious diseases and the others, for which he specified using stocks coming out of the patients themselves (which later on became known as auto-isopathy). Gustav Wilhelm Gross, another one of Hahnemann's favourites and contemporaries, used the 30th dilution of sanious juice of gangrened spleen (according to the specific localisation of anthrax of animals). Gross seems to have become at once deeply enamoured of the isopathic theory.

Dudgeon attributes Gross with saying,

> the simile is not exactly the right thing, and that for some time he has been convinced that oequalia oequalibus or the isopathic principle is the correct one, and that similia similibus or the homoeopathic principle is only a makeshift or indifferent apology for the other. Gross's isopathy consisted mainly in giving vaccinine in natural small-pox, and in recommending it as a prophylactic against the small-pox in place of cow-pox inoculation. He also recounts how that one day, having inflicted on himself a small wound, the idea occurred to him to potentise his blood. He moistened a globule with his blood, and put it into a bottle with 10,000 fresh globules, and likewise shook them together energetically for a quarter of an hour. He administered

a globule of this second bottle to a lady who suffered from congestions to the head and chest, and it cured her. The same curative result was obtained from this medicine in the case of a young man troubled with haemoptysis, with similar symptoms of congestion to the head and chest. These days sportsmen receive injections of their own potentised blood to assist in accelerating recovery. We read in Dudgeon, that the blood of common pigeons, wood-pigeons, and turtle-doves is recommended to be injected into the eyes to remove extravasated blood caused by a blow. He further alleges that the blood of domestic fowls stops haemorrhages of the membranes of the brain, and that the blood of kids mingled with vinegar cures haemoptysis (Dudgeon 1853).

It can't have been easy for Hahnemann. While his ideas about his new system of medicine were evolving, he also saw it being poorly practiced all around. His views clearly changed about isopathy. At first he was openminded, but later turned hostile. In the 5th edition of Organon (1833) he writes, 'one may admit in fact a fourth method of using medicines against diseases; the "isopathic method", the method of treating a disease by the same miasm that has produced it.'

Nevertheless, soon it was being used as far away as Russia. A letter by Jolly, a dentist of Constantinople, written to Hahnemann on the 24th of December 1835, relates that Theuille a homeopathic doctor of Moscow came 'to study and isopathise' the plague and obtained numerous cases of cure using the 30th dilution prepared out of the serous exudation plague bubos, (in archive of homoeopathic medicine, 1837, v. 6, p. 289 and Bibliothéque homoeopathique of Genèva, 1836, VII, p. 102).

Herrmann, Genke and Griesselich all wrote about the use of

isopathy in those early years. They were dealing with diseases such as measles, scarlatina, variola syphilis, sycosis, psora, anthrax, hydrophobia, and were looking for practical ways to relieve suffering. Helbing, Rau of Giessen, Moritz Muller and Herrmann, published about their practical experience. Hermann in 1848 wrote *True Isopathy;* or, on the *Employment of the Organ of Healthy Animals as Remedies in Diseases of the same Organs in the Human Subject.* Dudgeon argued (1853):

> Isopathic agents should, in my opinion, be strictly limited to really infectious morbid products, and when possible the morbid product of the patient himself should be employed, but when that cannot be procured, I see no serious objection to the administration of the morbid product taken from another individual. Thus varioline, vaccinine, morbilline, etc., may be employed at the commencement of the respective diseases of which they are the morbid product and the contagious principle.

Dudgeon gave historical precedent as the fundamental reason for his adoption of the method.

> Dioscorides, Galen, Paulus Aegineta, and others, make mention of various excrementitious matters useful for the cure of diseases, among which we find the dung of dogs, children, wolves, sheep, oxen, pigeons, fowls, storks, mice, starlings, and crocodiles; the urine of men, boys, mules, goats, and camels; again we find such delectable remedies prescribed by the wisdom of our ancestors as bugs, lizards, carth worms, locusts, serpents' slough, the blood of various animals, spider's web, soot, burnt hair, sweat, etc., and these delicacies were given in palpable quantities with their full natural flavour attached to them, not frittered away by infinitesimal dilution into the colourless and insipid preparations of our modern isopathists. If, then, our

opponents will insist on raking up the infinitesimal dirt that some unacknowledged, self-styled homoeopathists have chosen to introduce into our previously pure Materia Medica, we are prepared to meet them on their own Materia Medica to raise a stench under their nostrils that shall for ever make them repent of having begun the combat with such foul weapons. (Dudgeon 1853).

Collet and Others

After the death of Hahnemann, the use of Isopathy continued on both sides of the Atlantic. Hering continued his use of it in America and published a monograph on *Lyssin* (or *Hydrophobinum*) in the *North American Journal of Homoeopathy* of 1870. The same year, Swan published in the *New Organon* two cases of tuberculosis cured by *Tuberculinum* (ex-Phthisine of Hering and Lux) prepared from the suppurated tubercular cavity. Burnett utilised *Bacillinum* and published his experience of five years in the treatment of tuberculosis (Burnett 1880). This was five years before Koch. Drysdale introduced *Pyrogenium* in typhus and in septic conditions. Swan recommended *Erysypalinum* and *Diphtherinum* (*Homoeopathic Physician* 1892). Clarke (*Homoeopathic World*, 1891) published an analytical pathogenesis culled from all the cases observed up to that time by the allopathic doctors relating to the action of '*Tuberculine*' on the tubercular patients, and also on the non-tubercular patients.

But it was a Dominican priest from France that took the idea further. Father Denys Collet (1824–1909) was another early advocate of isopathy. He wrote *Isopathie, Methode Pasteur par Voie Interne* in 1898 at age 74. He suggested another category of preparation, serotherapeutic isopathy or serotherapy. This consisted of homeopathic remedies of immune serum. An example was *Marmorek* (antituberculous serum from a patient with tuberculosis). Collet, was born in Frazi, France. Rediscovering Isopathy himself, it is reported that he prevented an epidemic of small-pox at Flanigny in 1871 using a dilution of 4CH of '*vaccin*' (*Vaccinum*). He acted as a physician of a small convent and treated his community by isopathic method.

For Collett there were three methods of cure: Allopathy, Homeopathy and Isopathy, each one of which was valuable to select in function of the clinical indications. And Collet distinguishes three kinds of Isopathies:

1. "*Pure isopathy which takes the products of secretion of a patient as medicinal agent to cure the same disease.*
2. *The organic isopathy (at present our organotherapy) and*
3. *Scrotherapic isopathy*" (*dilution of hyper-immune serum*).

In the 20th century, Julian's *Materia Medica of the Nosodes* is the significant publication in relationship to Isopathy. He describes the work of Kruger of Nimes, Nebel, Gallivardin, Jousset. Before then in 1910, the book of H.C. Allen, *The Materia Medica of the Nosodes* explored the subject. Allen described the indications of *Medorrhinum* and *Psorinum*. And furthermore Léon Vannier in 1912 wrote the review *l'Homoeopathie fransaise* in which from the first number he discusses the use of Isopathy which he renamed 'Isothirapie' (Julian 1985).

The Controversy

Clearly the idea of isopathy encountered its opposition, most notably it came from Hahnemann. This was as much a policy decision. Slack allopaths dabbling in the new method of homeopathy were looking for quick fixes to complex chronic diseases. It must have been hard for him to watch lazy allopathic homeopaths giving nosodes without discrimination or understanding.

Hahnemann's view was unequivocal.

It is on such examples of domestic practice that Mr. M. Lux founds his so-called mode of cure by identicals and idem, which he calls Isopathy, which some eccentric-minded persons have already adopted as the non plus ultra of a therapeutic method, without knowing how they could carry it out. But if we examine these instances attentively we find that they do not bear out these views. The purely physical powers differ in the nature of their action on the living organism from those of a dynamic medicinal kind. Heat or cold of the air that surrounds us, or of the water, or of our food and drink occasion (as heat and cold) of themselves no absolute injury to a healthy body; heat and cold are in their alternations essential to the maintenance of healthy life, consequently they are not of themselves medicine. Heat and cold, therefore, act as curative agents in affections of the body, not by virtue of their essential nature (not, therefore, as cold and heat per se, not as things hurtful in themselves, as are the drugs, rhubarb, china, ..etc., even in the smallest doses), but only by virtue of their greater or smaller quantity, that is, according to their degrees of temperature, just as (to take an example from purely physical powers) a great weight of lead will bruise my hand painfully, not by virtue of its essential nature as lead, for a thin plate of lead would not bruise me, but in consequence of its quantity and massive weight. If, then, cold or heat be serviceable in bodily ailments like frost- bites or burns, they are so solely on account of their degree of temperature, just as they only indict injury on the healthy body by their extreme degrees of temperature.

Thus we find in these examples of successful domestic practice, that it is not the prolonged application of the degree of cold in which the limb was frozen that restores it isopathically (it would thereby be rendered quite lifeless and dead), but a degree of cold that only approximates to that (homoeopathy), and which gradually rises to a comfortable temperature, as frozen sour crout laid upon the frost-bitten hand in the temperature of the room soon melts, gradually growing warmer from 32 or 33 (Fahr.) to the temperature of the room, supposing that to be only 55, and thus the limb is recovered by physical homoeopathy. In like manner, a hand scalded with boiling water would not be cured isopathically by the application of boiling water, but only by a somewhat lower temperature, as, for, example, by holding it in a vessel containing a fluid heated to 160, which becomes every minute less hot, and finally descends to the temperature of the room, whereupon the scalded part is restored by homoeopathy. Water in the act of freezing cannot draw cut the frest isopathically from potatoes and apples, but this is effected by water only near the freezing-point. So, to give another example from physical action, the injury resulting from a blow on the forehead with a hard substance (a painful lump) is soon diminished in pain and swelling by pressing on the spot for a considerable time with the ball of the thumb, strongly at first, and then gradually less forcibly, homoeopathically, but not by an equally hard blow with an equally hard body, which would increase the evil isopathically. The examples of cures by isopathy given in the book alluded to - muscular contractions in human beings and spinal paralysis in a dog, which had been caused by a chill, being rapidly cured by cold bathing - these events are falsely explained by isopathy. What are called sufferings from a chill are only nominally connected with cold, and often arise, in the bodies of those predisposed to them, even from a draught of wind which was not at all cold. Moreover, the manifold effects of a cold bath on the living organism, in health and disease, cannot be reduced to such a simple formula as to warrant the construction of a system of such pretentions! That serpents' bites, as is there stated, are most certainly cured by portions of the serpents, must remain a mere fable of a former age, until such an improbable assertion is authenticated by indubitable observations and experiences, which it certainly never will be. That, in fine, the saliva of a mad dog given to a patient labouring under hydrophobia (in Russia), is said to have cured him that "is said" would not seduce any conscientious physician to imitate such a hazardous experiment, or to construct a so-called isopathic system, so dangerous and so highly improbable in its extended application, as has been done (not by the modest author of the pamphlet entitled The Isopathy of Contagions, Leipzic: Kollmann, but) by its eccentric supporters, especially Dr. Gross (v. Allg. hom. Ztg., p. 72), who vaunts this isopathy (oequalia oequalibus) as the only proper therapeutic rule, and sees nothing in the similia similibus but an indifferent substitute for it; ungratefully enough, as he is entirely indebted to the simila similibus for all his fame and fortune. The experienced cook holds his hand, which he has scalded, at a certain distance from the fire, and does not heed the increase of pain that takes place at first, as he knows from experience that he can thereby in a very short time, often in a few minutes, convert the burnt part into healthy painless skin. (Hahnemann 1922).

In the foot note to aphorism 56 (6th edition of Organon), he says,

Isopathy

A third mode of employing medicines in diseases has been attempted to be created by means of Isopathy, as it is called - that is to say, a method of curing a given disease by the same contagious principle that produces it. But even granting this could be done, yet, after all, seeing that the virus is given to the patient highly potentized, and consequently, in an altered condition the cure is effected only by opposing a simillimum to a simillimum. To attempt to cure by means of the very same morbific potency (per idem) contradicts all normal human understanding and hence all experience. Those who first brought Isopathy to notice, probably thought of the benefit which mankind received from cowpox vaccination by which the vaccinated individual is protected against future smallpox infection and as it were cured in advance. But both, cowpox and smallpox are only similar, in no way the same disease. In many respects they differ, namely in the more rapid course and mildness of cowpox and especially in this, that it is never contagious to man by mere nearness. Universal vaccination put an end to all epidemics of that deadly fearful smallpox to such an extent that the present generation does no longer possess a clear conception of the former frightful smallpox plague. Moreover, in this way, undoubtedly, certain diseases peculiar to animals may give us remedies and medicinal potencies for very similar important human diseases and thus happily enlarge our stock of homoeopathic remedies. But to use a human morbific matter (a Psorin taken from the itch in man) as a remedy for the same human itch or for evils arisen therefrom is-? Nothing can result from this but trouble and aggravation of the disease. (Hahnemann 1922).

In addition, in the introduction of the Organon he writes the following remarks on Isopathy,

The antipsoric medicines treated of in the following volumes contain no so-called isopathic remedies, because their pure effects, even those of the potentized itch-miasm (psorin.) are a long way from being sufficiently proved to enable us to make a sure homoeopathic use of them. I say homoeopathic, for the prepared itch-matter does not remain idem, even if given to the patient from whom it was taken, because, if it is to him good, it can only do so in a potentized state, seeing that crude itch-matter, which he has in him already, being an idem, has no action on him? The preparation that develops its power (potentization) changes and modifies it, just as gold leaf, after being potentized, is no longer crude (leaf) gold without action on the human body, but at every stage of its potentization is more and more modified and altered. (Hahnemann 1922).

Potentized and modified in this way, the itch-matter (psorin) for administration is no longer idem with the curde original itch-matter, but only a simillimum. For between idem and simillimum there is, for those who can reflect, nothing intermediate; or, in other words, between idem and simile only simillimum can exist. Isopathic and aequale are misleading terms, which, if they can mean anything trustworthy, can only mean simillimum because they are not idem (Hahnemann 1922).

Other authors quickly fell in and towed the line. Allen wrote in the publisher's preface,

Concerning the character of this book, Nosodes, it may be said that Dr. Allen first, last and all the time, regarded these drugs as homoeopathic, and not as isopathic, remedies; that they were to be proved as homoeopathic remedies and prescribed according to the totality of the symptoms (H.C. Allen 1910).

Swan in *Isopathy and Homoeopathy* (Swan 1872) wrote.

...the rapidity of a cure of small-pox few years since, which followed the administration of Variolinum, high, led to the consideration of the question whether Isopathy was not in reality Homoeopathy, the remedy becoming by potentization, a simile to the drug, a like, and yet not the same (Swan 1872).

Dewey in his lecture on *Diphtherinum* wrote,

Dr. Samuel Swan of New York, very aptly put forth the difference between Isopathy and Homoeopathy thus: "Isopathy would give raw cucumbers to a person made sick by eating cucumbers and would make him worse. Homoeopathy would give him Cucumis in a high potency and not only cure the patient but also enable him to eat cucumbers with no untoward symptoms." All down the line of homoeopathic literature we will find many examples of this. We will mention a few: In 1867 Adolf Lippe had a case of chronic poisoning by cane sugar (in other words a super sensitiveness to this substance). He removed it completely by Saccharum officinalis. (Hahn. Mo. Oct. 1867.) A case of Quininism cured by Cinchona sulphuricum high. (Organon Vol. iii p. 208.) The susceptibility to parsley can be cured by Petroselinum 30, says Dr. James W. Ward, one of our best and most careful observers. Asthma from eating scallops cured by Pectin, which in a high potency cured permanently. Asthma due to susceptibility to the proteid substance in eggs, cured by repeated doses of Egg White. Boericke's Materia Medica p. 491. I have personally cured many cases of hay fever due to the rag-weed by Ambrosia artemisiaefolia in potency. The pharmaceutical houses of today are making much capital out of the pollen extracts of the various hay fever producing plants. Right along this line of thought come such remedies as Hydrophobinum for rabies, advocated in Homoeopathy when Pasteur was but 8 years old! Anthracinum for anthrax. Tuberculinum for tuberculinum, Pertussin for whooping cough, etc. The hypersensitiveness to Rhus poisoning has been removed many times by the use of Rhus toxicodendron, and why it does not relieve in all cases is simply owing to a difference in sensitiveness in different people and to the many varieties of the plant (Dewey 1934).

In his lecture on *Tuberculinum bovinum*, Kent put it as follows,

> I do not use Tub. merely because it is a nosode; that is, a product of the disease and for the results of the disease. This I fear is too much the prevailing thought in using nosodes. In certain places it prevails and is taught that anything relating to syphilis must be treated with Syph; that anything relating to gonorrhoea must be treated with Med; anything psoric must be treated with Psor, and anything that relates to tuberculosis must be treated with TUB. That will go out of use some day; it is mere isopathy and it is an unsound doctrine. It is not the better idea of Homoeopathy (Kent 1904).

And later he said it this way,

> What is contagion, as understood, and what is cure, but the irresistible appropriation of some unknowable energy applied by accident or intelligence. We have seen that Rhus cures the patient of his sensitiveness to Rhus as well long after as before he was poisoned by it. This is not Isopathy, as it was not Rhus that was cured, but the patient, and is was simply pointed out to the intelligent physician by the accidental poisoning wherein Rhus was pointed to as one of the medicines that he is sensitive to; it being fully understood that the patient is always highly sensitive to his needed medicine. This, therefore, is but a centering of a

complex of symptoms in a homoeopathic problem (Kent 1926).

Gross, attacked by Hahnemann because of his leaning towards isopathy, made known in his solemn public declaration.

That the idea never entered my head of encroaching in any way on the highest principle of healing, although I have arrived at the conviction that it is really possible to heal isopathically. Isopathy is only a further extension and perfection of homoeopathy. Without the latter, we should never have attained the former. Therefore long live homoeopathy! (Haehl 1922).

Lippe's view was,

Now there comes a new departure. Unproved but highly diluted nosodes with new laws, supplementary to the sole universal therapeutic law of the similars, are paraded before the homoeopathic school. It was hoped that a paper by Dr. P. P. Wells, published in this journal for August, on "Unproved Remedies," would be sufficient to put at rest this new departure, but if we so believed, we were in error. Lux was the father of isopathy, and based his healing method on the principle "AEqualia aequalibus curantur." The modern isopathists claim it to be a law of cure that the products of a disease taken from one individual, when highly potentized, will cure the same disease in other individuals. Under this newly revived law, Tuberculinum will cure tuberculosis, Cariesin will cure caries, Syphilinum will cure syphilis. They also claim that highly potentized cucumber will cure the ill effects from eating cucumbers and eradicate any long-standing idiosyncrasy. In proof of these claims we are offered facts in the shape of related cures with unproved but highly potentized isopathic remedies, and are asked "what will you do with these facts?" Why, accept them of course for what they are worth, but we do not accept the deductions these isopathists would draw from these facts, remembering well the accepted axiom that "Facts alone prove nothing." All these facts prove is that these isopathic remedies have an effect on the human organism.

Such was the situation when Cullen, in his Materia Medica, dwelt on Cinchona and the reported cures of intermittent fever by this drug. But when he accepted the facts as he found them, i. e., that Cinchona had cured some cases of intermittent fever and failed to cure other cases, he did not claim it to be a specific, but very sensibly asked the question then unsolved, under what circumstances it would cure cases of intermittent fever? Hahnemann solved the question by proving, first on himself and later on others, the sickmaking properties of the drug. Our isopathists are now just in the same position Cullen found himself at the end of the last century; they find that products of diseases have medicinal properties, and that is all. Among all the best known and best proved products of a disease stands first and foremost Psorinum. Would it not be preposterous to claim that Psorinum could cure all cases of the itch? Has it cured any such cases? And what will become of the law, aequalia aequalibus curantur if Psorinum has failed to cure all, or many, or any cases of the itch? Psorinum was proved, and will forever remain an important curative agent, when properly applied under the law of the similars; so may probably all other products of disease become valuable curative agents after exhaustive provings have been made. If isopathy, as it is now attempted to be foisted on Homoeopathy, were a true method of healing the sick it would be necessary to show that it possessed universal applicability. What would an isopathist do for hooping cough, or hysteria, or the great host of nervous diseases? What then, if "AEqualia aequalibus curantur" is not of universal applicability? What then if "Similia similibus curantur" has been found to be of universal applicability for the cure of the sick? The one, a failure, can surely not be foisted on the other which has fully been tried and is a success. And now for an illustration to show that the deductive method adopted by the isopathists is a fallacy, and that the only reliable method is the strictly inductive method of Hahnemann (von Lippe 1881).

And von Lippe further states,

From times immemorial have men of undoubted learning vainly searched for specific remedies for specific diseases. It could not be otherwise as their very first proposition, the existence of specific diseases, is a fatal error, an error first and last. From times immemorial diseases have continually changed their nature and forms. What at present appears to correspond with the genus epidemicus, the various phenomena which appear to be strongly expressed in all forms of the now prevailing disease, will no longer be characteristic accompaniments of this same disease, probably three months hence. From times immemorial persons suffering at the same place and at the same time from epidemic diseases were all afflicted similarly, but not alike; while there existed an apparent great similarity between the afflicted, the close observer readily discerned a great difference between the symptoms of the similarly-sick. These close observers were Hahnemann and his disciples, and as illustration we may be allowed to refer to some very frequently indicated remedies in the Asiatic Cholera. While some cases corresponded with the characteristic sick-making properties (ascertained from provings on the healthy) of Camphor, other cases corresponded with Veratrum or Cuprum or Arsenic, etc. Each of these remedies had its characteristics, and became thereby and therefore a curative agent under the law of the similars. Pasteur, as well as Koch and others, profess to have found the germs of infectious diseases, and believing that they have found these germs, they come to the conclusion, following their deductive method of reasoning, that they also know how to stamp out these diseases. When, heretofore, an infectious disease broke out in a certain locality, there were necessarily several conditions present, allowing the germs to develop themselves and their infectious character; after a certain time the germs, now having rapidly multiplied, were found to become harmless, as persons long exposed to their influences remained well, having no susceptibility to that specific poison; then, what became of these multiplied germs? Can chemistry or any other exact science explain? No more than they can explain why A, B and C became ill when exposed to these poisonous germs, and why D, E and F were not at all affected by the same influences. If, after a long lapse of time, an epidemic breaks out where it formerly raged, is not that new epidemic invariably very different from the former one? If we are accustomed to individualize, it is hardly to be expected that we should even think of accepting such positive generalizations as are offered us by these scientists, certainly we should not accept them as therapeutic guides (von Lippe 1882).

Wesselhoeft had his opinion also.

We ought to make a distinction between nosodes and isopathy. It is a great mistake to give a nosode for the disease from which it is derived on isopathic grounds. We do not give Psorinum for the itch, but it cures the consequences of the itch when indicated by the symptoms (Wesselhoeft 1888).

Roberts didn't hold back. Isopathy was not homeopathy.

We must keep this distinction ever before us. Isopathy is identity; homoeopathy rests its whole case on the similarity, and in the degree of its perfection we may be sure of the results. We cannot be accused of combating symptoms; rather, we are guided by symptoms in combating disease. The law of cure, similia similibus curentur, is as fundamental as any law in nature. It is a law of universal adaptability to human sickness; it ranks in the field of medicine with Newton's law of gravitation in the field of astronomy. This is the only general law for the cure of the physical and mental ills of man; it is the only method of healing that depends, as a whole, upon one general principle, and it is the only method of healing that has continued to withstand the pressure of time and changing circumstances. It is a law of nature, discovered by following the thread of inductive reasoning, and proven to be true by countless tests (Roberts 1936).

In the late 20th century, there has been no shortage of opinion either. Ghegas writes,

Any serious illness can leave behind a miasma that has to be taken away before further treatment can follow. It is better to do this in a homoeopathic way and not isopathically (e.g. with Measles 200K). A young girl displays the complete image of Calcarea carbonica. A year ago the child had measles and since then she has had problems with reduced sight. To remove the measles miasm it is absolutely necessary to start with Pulsatilla here, and not with Calcarea carbonica (K 276: vision dim measles, after). E.g. When a child, after going through measles, has become aggressive and violent, uses dirty words and plays with the genitals without shame, it is absolutely necessary to start with Hyoscyamus to remove the measles-miasm (Ghegas 1994).

With respect to teaching and studying materia medica, Saine writes,

> I teach materia medica in a traditional way. The history of homeopathy is based on basic principles and these are basically unchanged. As soon as Hahnemann mentioned these principles, you started to have some branches. You had one in 1828, isopathy. They said, the cure to all diseases is not giving the similar, but is to give the same: isopathy. Do you know anybody that practices isopathy today? It doesn't exist much. Isopathy came, died and later on, at about 1880 it came back again. It came in cycles. And it died again and it came again in 1930, in France and it is dead again. But homeopathy is still there (Saine 1999).

And the elder Sankaran writes the following on nosodes,

> Soon after Hahnemann propounded the similia principle which states that diseases could be treated by drugs which are most similar in their effects, it was realised that the most similar is only slightly removed from the completely similar or the identical substance (Idem). Naturally, efforts were made to utilise the identical morbific agent in the treatment of diseases, which led to the method of treatment known as Isopathy. Nosodes have been compared to vaccines and even called oral vaccines. Boger writes: "When our late confrere, Dr. H.C. Allen, pointed to the nosodes as the most important of remedies in arousing reaction, he did the greatest thing of his busy life." Coleman says, "Vaccine therapy has found its way into general medicine of today. It is only a modification of the method taught by Xenocrates and introduced later thorough the homoeopathic school by Dr. Lux in 1823 under the name of Isopathy. Hering, Swan, Burnett and others did much along this line..." Hubbard thinks that the practice of homoeopathic pediatrics cannot develop its best

results without the frequent use of the basic nosodes (Sankaran 1996).

Refining the Method

Opposition has not stopped many from turning it into an art form and created a significant classification for its employment. Julian (1997) classified isopathy as,

1. Nosodotherapics or Nosodes

Nosodes are homoeopathic preparations obtained from microbe cultures, from viruses, pathological secretions and excretions.

2. Isotherapics

These are medicines prepared according to the homoeopathic pharmacopraxis, coming from the patients themselves or supplied by the patients themselves. Thus one distinguishes:

Auto-Isotherapics	Humoral products, secretions or excretions coming from the patient (blood, urines, secretions and excretions which are pathogenical)
Microbian-auto-isotherapics	Microbes isolated from the patient by culture on the appropriate ground
Exo-Isotherapics	Allergenotherapics, which are somewhat particular isopathics, because it is the question of Allergens, detergents, pesticides, insecticides, allergising medicines etc
Organotherapics	As has already been mentioned, dynamised and diluted organotherapics have seen light after the beginning of Isopathy of Lux, with J.F. Hermann of Ausburg. Still the word 'Sarcode' is sometimes used for the dynamised micro-organotherapics or according to Tetau and Cl. Bergeret-diluted and dynamised organotherapy
Hormontherapy	Particular mode of diluted and dynamised organotherapy

He has also made a study of homeopathic clinical pathology of hormone, parathyroid, thyreotropic hormone; of folliculostimuline (Julian 1997).

Advantages and Some Extraordinary Examples

Julian (1997) argued that the indication of a nosode according to long experience of Hahnemannian homeopaths is legitimate in the following five circumstances:

1. When a well selected remedy have given some effects, but these do not continue or do not persist, or the beneficial action stops.
2. When the disease relapses continually, although ameliorated with every dose of the medicine: repeated coryza, hay-fever, periodic return of some affections. If it is the question of pulmonary affections which relapse constantly, one will more willing give Tuberculinum for example; if it is the question of mucous secretion, one should think of Medorrhinum; in the presence of a tumefication, tissular proliferation one should think of Syphilinum etc.
3. When there has been suppression in consequence of an abortive treatment: Suppression of an eruption, of a discharge, of sweat, of menses and when the indicated remedy does not act.
4. When a patient presents the characteristic symptoms of their pathogenesis, i.e. to say their experimentation on healthy man, as Homoeopathy requires it for the application of every remedy. It is the homoeopathic indications of Nosode,˙
5. Finally according to the anamnesis of the patient, if he presents only in part of the pathogenesis of Nosode, or when

a patient has suffered of a microbian infection, as for example old Scarlatina, diphtheria, measles, syphils, tuberculosis etc... which one may find in the personal antecedents of a patient who does not progress any more.

The following is a selection of great examples from the literature.

It is true, the most suitable homoeopathic remedies afforded me relief; the incarceration of calculi in the ureter especially was relieved by Nux; but they were unable to put a stop to the formation of calculi; this result was only attained by the preparation of Calc. Ren (Anshutz 1900).

A brown-haired youth of sixteen years has broad flat warts scattered over his hands and fingers. Several careful prescriptions have been made for them, with no beneficial results. 1892, Nov. 26. Verrucinum 50m Skinner, one powder. Dec. 22. The warts have grown larger, no new ones. Verrucinum 50m Skinner, in solution, four doses in one day. 1893, Jan. 23. The warts seemed dry and hard for several days, but are now lusty as ever. Verrucinum cm Skinner, one powder. Sept. 9. The warts decreased in size and have all disappeared excepting the largest and oldest, which is now growing. Verrucinum cm Skinner, one powder. That finished the cure (Case 1916).

Calculi bili and Fel. tauri: isopathic remedies, very helpful in cases of jaundice, loss of appetite, diarrhoea (Barker 1940).

Dr. J.S. M. Chaffee describes a case of rattle snake poisoning which he cured with Crotalus on Isopathic principle. "I was to see James Wright, aged 54 years, who, while binding wheat, was bitten on third finger of right hand by a rattle snake. I found him bleeding from the bitten finger, and from eyes, nose, ears, mouth, rectum and urethra, pulse 110, small, wiry; respiration 40; temperature 105; haggard expression; whole body bathed in hot perspiration; delirium. This patient had had the regular routine treatment of whisky, quinine, and carbonate of ammonia for ninety-six hours, when the attendants withdrew and pronounced the case beyond the reach of medical aid. A marked characteristic symptom was a mouldy smell of breath, with scarlet red tongue, and difficult swallowing. Great sensitiveness of the skin of right half of the body, so much so that the slightest touch would produce twitching of muscles of that side. I prescribed Crotalus hor., 30th trituration, 30 gr. in four ounces of water, a teaspoonful every hour until my return visit, twenty-four hours later, when I found marked improvement. Temperature normal; pulse full, soft and regular, delirium gone; saliva and urine slightly tinged with blood; appetite returning, he having asked for food for the first time since the accident (Choudhuri 1929).

Some patients who had responded to Carcinosin but whose improvement only lasted for a short time have derived benefit from auto-isopathy. I give a single dose of Pharyngeal Mucus 30CH (Foubister 1967).

Grimmer cited many examples,

1. Homoeopathic potencies of cancerous fluids have been made for a long time: Epitheliomine (extract of epithelioma), Scirrhinum (extract of scirrhus), Carcinosine (extract of any cancer). The results obtained have been inconstant and variable ...
2. Attempts have been made to isolate one or more cancer organisms and to prescribe them in homoeopathic dilutions. That the isolated organisms may perhaps be only witnesses

or saprophytes or profiteers in the tumor, rather than its deep and real cause, is not the question. It is not less true than in certain case products of this kind show themselves to be efficacious. It is to M. Nebel that we owe our Micrococcin (Doyen's Micrococcus in the 30th, 200th and higher) and to Joseph Roy his Oscillococcin. The latter often acts with great benefit in those predisposed to cancer but it is dangerous and can aggravate the confirmed cancer cases, even according to the author. On the other hand, Micrococcin has often a really beneficial action, if not durable, at least temporary and distinct, on the weight and general condition. The optimal potency would seem to be the 200th. It is not necessary to repeat it more often than once every two or three months. Before that the patient ought to be well drained. He ought to receive regularly also at ten, fifteen or twenty day intervals his constitutional remedy.

3. Dr. Nebel uses especially in cancer potencies of his Onkomyxa (preferably the 4th, subcutaneously).

4. The employment of potencies of blood in cancer or pre-cancer cases has been thought of; following Roger. Dr. Joseph Roy, the first in France, used individual blood isotherapy. J. Roy has now abandoned this practice, finding it dangerous and of only transient action. In my opinion the truth is perhaps here in a golden mean; believe neither in a marvellous therapeutic action of a miraculous panacea or in the converse. It is certain that one ought to be very cautious about using potencies of blood from cancer cases. Aggravations are to be feared. We have also been witnesses, however, to beautiful ameliorations. It would be necessary to be able to isolate form the blood the really homoeopathic

principle which is capable of curative action; a principle which ought to be restrained, neutralized unfortunately by other substances, other forces.

5. Clinical experience is the only method capable of judging the results of this method and not, in our opinion, philosophical concepts, which were conceived à priori.
6. Since then J. Roy has preferred to use isotherapy of young and healthy blood, of which we have no personal experience. Now it would seem to veer more towards organotherapy. In the same sense, Guild has previously used serum-vaccines with variable results.
7. Rubens-Duval had the idea of using globulin extracts from cancers. This is his proteinotherapy described by himself in this revue. His results are very encouraging and impressive and the indicated dilutions are distinctly homoeopathic.
8. Following many authors. Cuvier and Carrere have recently re-attacked the question of treatment with tumor extracts and have some very interesting results. (Grimmer and Bernoville 1965)

A modern perspective without any clinical verification comes from Eyre using mobile phone radiation.

The proving was started in January 1999. For well over the past year or two it was becoming increasingly obvious from press and TV coverage that concerns were growing over the possible dangers of using mobile phones, whilst the mobile phone companies and others with vested interests all assured us that they were totally safe. Suddenly, nobody could live without a mobile phone! It became the essential item for all teenagers, and top of the list for Christmas presents that year. Go to any public place - shops, buses, trains, even the refuge of the local pub -

and sure enough, those conversations would spring up from every corner. Suddenly all our private business became public, and the rest of us became expert eavesdroppers. Meanwhile, it seemed like every day a new article appeared in newspapers and magazines, or a television programme, warning of the dangers, and describing the ever-increasing range of symptoms experienced by users. It seemed an obvious choice for a proving (Eyre 1999).

Conclusion

The prescribing technique adopted by homeopaths over the years has ranged from a single dose of a high potency remedy to an injection on a daily basis. And then there is everything in between. Ignored by many practitioners, many choose to use it as a last resort and there are many reported cases responding favourably to isopathy and auto-isopathy.

These days, with so many patients sensitive or allergic to many foods, chemicals, and household products, every homeopath has seen the ever-increasing incidences of patients with these complaints. Many respond beautifully to conventional homeopathic treatment, but many don't. Isopathy remains a viable option in cases with unclear characteristic symptoms.

Further Reading

- Haehl — *Samuel Hahnemann His Life and Work*
- Julian — *Materia Medica of Nosodes with Repertory*
- Anshutz — *New Old and Forgotten Remedies*
- Barker — *Gallstones*

- Choudhuri — *A Study on Materia Medica*
- Foubister — *The Carcinosin Drug Picture*
- Grimmer — *Homoeopathic Treatment of Cancer*
- Case — *Some Clinical experiences of E. E. Case*
- Nebel — *Contribution to the history of Isopathy*
- Burnett — *Five years experience in the new cure of Consumption*
- Sankaran — *The Elements of Homoeopathy*

Appendix

List of Nosodes (Julian 1997).

Albinum: Albin (albino) Graecum Album. White excrements of constipated dog being ill of intestines (of dogs constipated being ill of intestines).

Alveolinum: Pus of dental alveola.

Anthracinum: Anthrakinum.

Ascaridinum: (Ascaris vermiculars L) Vermiculus totos vivas.

Balanorrhinum: Mucilageneous fluid which in Gonorrhoea is separated from glands of the glans penis.

Boviluinum: Mucous fluid that flows from nose and throat of buffaloes during pest.

Brossulinum: Syphilinum Brossulinum-pus of venerian ulcer.

Bupodopurinum: Mucous secretion of the mouth of buffaloes who are ill from epizootic claudication (scorbutic disease of the mouth).

Carcinominum: Secretion taken out of the cancer of armpit.

Cariasinum: Purulent matter of bone carries.

Ceruminum: Cerumen.

Cholelithinum: Biliary calculus.

Coenurinum Ovium: Cerebral hydatide (Coenurus cerebralis).

Condylominum: Total condyloma.

Coryzinum: Catarrhal mucosity.

Coryzinum Equorum: Mucous of the lachrymal fistula.

Dysenterinum: Anal secretion of dysentric mucous.

Emphyeminum: Pus of a pulmonary vomit.

Enteropurinum: Enterohelcosinum, ichorous pus of stools.

Enterosyringum: Fistula of "Boyau-culier".

Gonorrhinum: Spermatic liquid.

Helinum: Foot corn.

Herculinum: Foam from the mouth during epilepsy.

Herpinum: Dry and humid pustules of herpes.

Hippoestrinum: Larva of ox-fly found in great quantity in the stomach of horses in the form of bunches.
Hipposudorinum Humidum: Sweat of horse.
Hipposudorinum Siccum: Dust adhered to the sweat of horse.
Hippozaeninum: Pus or mucous secreted through the nostrils of horses suffering from humid morve.
Humaninum: Human stool.
Hydrophobinum: Saliva of rabies.
Influenzinum: Grippum.
Karkininum: The Karkininum is distinguished from those of glans penis and from those of lips, nose and uterus. Ichorous pus or humors taken out of these cancers.
Kynoluinum: Yellow mucus secreted through the nostrils and the eyes in the disease of dog which is called canine paste.
Kynotaeninum: Tenia of dogs.
Kynotorrhinum: Pus from the ear of a dog.
Lachryminum: Tears.
Laryngophtisinum: Purulent secretion of trachitis.
Leucorrhinum: Whites (White flour).
Lippitudinum: Pituitary fluid, coming out of the eyes of men in opthalmia.
Lumbricinum: Ascaris lumbricoides.
Maculahepatinum: Hepatic maculae.
Mastocarcinominum: Pus of breast cancer.
Medorrhinum: Mucous secreted from urethra in syphilitic gonorrhoea.
Meletinum: Black matters in bloody vomitings.
Metrorrhaginum
Morbillinum
Nephroposteminum: Pus of kidney abscess.
Nephrolithinum: Kidney stone.
Odontosyringinum: Purulent matter secreted from the fistula of the teeth.
Oipodopurinum: Purulent matter secreted by the hoofs of ruminants in the epizootic claudication or the sisense that destroys the hoofs.
Otorrhinum Hominum: Purulent liquid that flows out of the ears of men. Otorrhinum of deaf persons is to be distinguished from that of non-deaf persons, and Otorrhinum of ill men from Otorrhinum of scarlatina.

Isopathy

Ozaeninum: Humours of ozena related to carries.
Parotidipurinum: Humors of parotid secretion after an angina or an inflammation of the parotid.
Pneumolithicum: Lung stone.
Pneumophtisinum: Pus of purulent phthysis.
Podoclavinum: Corns of the sole.
Polipinum Narinum: Polypus of nose.
Prosopopurinum: Purulent matter of cutaneous pustules of the face.
Pyoninum Bobonum: Humours of bubo, that of venerian bubos and that of non-venerian bubos are to be distinguished.
Pyoninum Oculorum: Purulent matters secreted from opthalmic eyes; that of cornea, and that of syphilitic cornea are to be distinguished.
Ragadinum: Raghades.
Scabiesinum: Psorinum hominum.
Scarlatinum
Scrofulinum
Sudorinum Phthisicum: Liquidfied sweats of phthisic patients.
Sycosinum: Venerian wart of men.
Sudorinum Pedum: Foot sweat.
Tinaenum: Crusts.
Ureninum: Sediment of urine of patients suffering from intermittent fever.
Urolithinum
Variolinum: Purulent matter of the lymph of pustules of variola of vaccinated men Varicellinum (Julian 1997)
Nomenclature of nosodes with Nelson, London (Julian 1997)
Actinomyces 30
Adenoidum 3-200
Adenoma prostrate, non-malignant 3-30
Anthracinum 6-50M
Antityphoid and Paratyphoid (T.A. B.C.) 6-50M
Arteriosclerosis 3-200
Aviaire (see Tuberculinum aviaire)
B.C. G. vaccine 3-30
Baccillinum testiculatum (see Tub. Test)

Bacillinum (Bacillinum Burness) 6-CM
Bacillinum and Influenzinum 12-IM
Bacillus coli 6-IM
Bacillus diphtheria (see Dipht. Bac.)
Bacillus dispar 6-30
Bacillus Friedlander see Friedlander)
Bacillus pyocyanaeus (Pseudomonas acruquinosa) 3-30
Bacillus tetani (Tetanus) 6-30
Bacillus typhimurinum 30
Bacillus Welchii 30
Bilharzia 6
Botulinum 30-IM
Bowel Nosodes (see separate leaflets)
Brucella abortus 3-200
Brucella melitensis 3-200
Calculi biliary 6-1M
Calculus renalis 6-200
Calculus renalis (phosphatic) 6-200/10M/CM
Calculus renalis (uric) 200
Cancer Serum Koch (Glyoxalide) 6-200
Carcinoma (bowel) 12-30
Carcinoma (rectum) 6-30
Carcinoma Co. (bowel) (C. Intest Co.) 12-200
Carcinoma Co. (K) 12-200
Carcinoma adeno (colon) 12-30
Carcinoma adeno (stomach) 12-1M
Carcinoma adeno (bladder) (C. adeno. vesica) 12-30
Carcinoma adeno papillary (ovary) 12-30
Carcinoma adeno papillary (uterus) 12-30
Carcinoma Scirrhus (breast) C. Scir Mam. 12-200
Carcinoma Scirrhus (stomach) 12-30
Carcinoma squamous (lung) 12-30
Carcinosinum 30-CM
Cataract (immature) 6-30

Cataract (mature) 6-30
Cattle ringworm (Trychophyton) 6-30
Chicken pox (see Variola)
Cholera 6-30
Coqueleuchin (see Pertussin)
Deformans (Micrococcus deformans) 30
Cysticercosis 6-200
Denys (Tub. Denys) 12-1M
Diphtheria antitoxin (maceration) 6-200
Diphtheria antitoxin (trit.) 6-200
Diphtheria bacillus 6-200
Diphtheric membrane (maceration) 6-200
Diphtherinum (membrane trit.) 6-CM
Sclerosin (disseminated) 9-30
Distemperinum (canine) 12-CM
Dysmenorrhoea (polyvalent) 6-30
E. Coli 3-30
Empyemia 200
Enterococcinum 6-200
Epithelia syphilitica 30-CM
Epivax (see Hard pad living virus)
Erysipelas 30
Feline hepatitis 6-30
Fox lung (see Pulmo vulpis)
Fowl pox virus 6-30
Friedlander (Bacillus Friedlander) 6-30
German measles (see Rubeola)
Glanders 30
Glandular fever 8x-30
Glinicum (see Medorrhinum)
Glyoxalide (see, Cancer Serum Koch)
Gonococcin (see Medorrhinum)
Hemolytic streptococcus (see, Strept. Hem.)
Hard pad (eyes) 6-30

Hard pad (nose) 6-30
Hepatitis, cat (see Feline hepatitis)
Hepato luesinum 8-200
Herper zoster 6-1M
Hippomanes (Horse serum) 8-200
Nippozaeninum 6-200/10M
Hydrophobinum (Lyssin) 6-10M/CM
Influenza A England/43/472 6-30
Influenza virus A (Asia) 1957 6-200
Influenza virus A 2 (Hong Kong) 1968 6-200
Influenza virus B (Hong Kong) S-72 2x-30
Influenza virus A (Port Chalmars) 1973 2x-200
Influenzg virus A (Scotland) 1974 2x-30
Influenza haemophilis 6x-30
Influenzin-antitoxin 200
Influenza catarrhalis 200
Influenza meningoeoccus 200
Influenzin serum 200
Influenzinum 12-10M-CM
Influenzinum virus A 6-200
Influenzinum virus B 6-200
Influenzinum virus AB 6-200
Lepropsy 3-30
Louping ill vaccine 3-30
Luesinum, Lueticum (see Syphilinum)
Lyssin (see Hydrophobinum)
Malandrinum 30-CM
Malta fever (see Melitotoxinum)
Marmoreck 12-1M
Measles (see Morbillinum)
Measles vaccine 6-30
Medorrhinum (Gonococcin) 6-CM/MM
Melitotoxin (see Brucella Melitensis)
Meningococcus 30-200

Isopathy

Micrococcin 30
Micrococcus catarrhalis 12-200
Micrococcus neoformans 10M-CM
Mongol nosode (Nosode M) 6-200
Morbillinum 30-CM
Mucobacter Mersch 6-200
Mumps (see Parotidinum)
Myxomatosis 6-30
O.A. N. (hip) 6-200
O.A. N. (Osteo arthritic nosode, Osteo-arthritic synovial fluid) 6-1M
Oncolico nosode 30
Oryptococcus linguae pilosac 3-6
Osseinum 6-12
Paratyphoid A 6-200
Paratyphoid B 6-200
Parotid gland 3-200
Parotidinum (Mumps) Ourlainum 30-200
Pertussin (coqueluchin) 12-CM
Pertusis vaccin (whooping cough) 6-30
Pestinum 30-200
Pneumococcus 12-50M
Pneumonia virus pig. (see Virus Pneumonia)
Polio (mixed) 30-200
Polio vaccin (Polyomyalitis vaccin) 12-30
Polio vaccin (S.A. I) 6-30
Polio vaccin (S.A. II) 6-200
Poliomyelitis oral vaccin (Sabin) 6-30
Polypus nasalis 30-00
Psorinum 6-CM
Pyrogenium (Sepsin) 6-CM
Quadruple nosode (Bacillinum, Influenzinu, Pneumococcus and Streptococcus) 30-200
Rachi-Luesinum 8-200

R.A. N. (Rheumatoid arthritic nosode) 6-30
Renal calculus (see Calculus renalis)
Rosen (see Tuberculinum Rosen)
Rous Sarcoma (Sarcoma) 6-30
Rubela (German measles) 6-200
Rubela virus vaccin 1970 6-30
Salmonellosis (Calf vaccin Dublin) 3-30
Scarlatininum 12-CM
Scirrhinum 6-CM
Sepsin (see Pyrogenum)
Serum anti-leptospera 6-30
Small pox pustule (see Variolinum)
Small pox vaccin (see Vaccininum)
Staphilococcinum 6-CM Stophilococcinum abdominalis 30-10M
Staphylococcus albus 6-30
Staphylococcus aureus 6-30/10M/CM
Staphylococcus haemolyticus aureus 6-200
Streptococcus 12-10M
Streptococcus haemolyticus viridans 6-30
Streptococcus longus viridans 6-30 Streptococcus lubesis 6-30
Stredtococcus viridans (Influenza 1970) 3-30
Streptococcus rheumaticus 3-200
Streptococcus viridans cardiacus 30-1M
Swine erysipelus 6-30
Lyphilinum (Lueticum, suesinum, brossulinum) 6-CM/MM
T.A. B. (Typhoid paratyphoid A and B) 6-200
T.A. B.C. (see Antityphoid and paratyphoid)
Tetanus antitoxin 6-30
Vetanus bacillus (see Bacillus tetani)
Tetanus toxin 6-CM
Tetanus toxoid 6-30
T.K. (see Tuberculinum Koch)
T.B. (see Tuberculinum Koch Exotoxin)
Tonsilinum (infected) 6-30

Trichomonas vaginalis 6-30
Tuberculinum aviaire 15-1M
Tuberculinum bovinum 6-CM/MM
Tuberculinum Denys (see Denys)
Tuberculinum Kent 1M-CM
Tuberculinum Koch 6-1M
Tuberculinum Koch Exotoxin (T.R.) 6-CM
Tuberculinum Rosen 6-100
Tuberculinum Spengler 6-200
Tuberculinum testiculatus 30-1M
Typhoidinum 6-200
Vaccininum 3-10M
Varicella 6-200
Variolinum 12-CM
Vincent's Angina 6-30
Virus pneumonia pig 6-30
Whooping cough (see Pertussin and Pertusis)
Yellow fever 6-30
Some explanations concerning the use of this list. Most of the remedies can be procured "in normal Gammut." A normal gammut consists in the real Hahnemannian dilutions (done by hand) as below: 0, 1X, 3X, 4X, 6X (CH), 8X, (4CH), 6, 9, 12, 15, 30, 200, 1M (M or 1000), 50M (50,000), CM (100,000) but the latter are not prepared by hand according to the Hahnemannian method.
Explanation 1X-CM indicated that it is the question of a complete gammut i.e. , to say from 10 (1X) upto 100,000. 2X-30/10M, the bar/indicates on interruption in the gammut i.e. to say after the 30th CH, the immediate high dilution is 10,000 (10M). The names in capital letters after the name of a remedy indicate the name or general spelling; thus "Achilea millefolium (Millefolium) (see Millefolium) (Julian 1997).
Nomenclature of nosodes with heel, according to H.H. Reckeweg (Julian 1997)
Anthracinum-Injeel+forte (D 15), D 20, D 30, D 200 (+Einzelpotenz D 10).
Bacillinum-Injeel+forte (D 15), D 20, D 30, D 200 (+Einzelpotenz D 15).
Bact. coli-Injeel+forte (D 6), D 12, D 30, D 200 (+ Einzelpotenz D 5).
Bact. lacis-aerog-Injeel+forte (D 6), D 12, D 30, D 200 (+inzelpotenz D 5).
Bact. protcus-Injeel+forte (D 6), D 12, D 30, D 200 (+Einzelpotenz D 5).
Bact. pyocian-Injeel+forte (D 6), D 12, D 30, D 200 (+Einzelpotenz D 5).

Bruc. Abort-Bang-Injeel+forte (D 6), D 10, D 30, D 200 (+Einzelpotenz D 5).

Carcinominum-Injeel+forte (D 15), D 20, D 200(+Einzelpotenz D 200).

Carc. hepat. metastat-Injeel+forte (D 6), D 10, D 30, D 200.

Carc. laryngis-Nosodes-Injeel+forte (D 6), D 10, D 30, D 200.

Carc. Mammae-Injeel+forte (D 6), D 10, D 30, D 200.

Carc. Urin (nur in D 200 liefebar).

Cozasackie-Virus-Injeel+forte (D 10), D 15, D 30, D 200 (+Einzelpotenz D 7, D 8).

Diptherinum-Injeel+forte (D 10), D 18, D 30, D 200.

Grippe-Nosode-Injeel+forte (D 6), D 10, D 30, D 200.

Hydrophobinum-Injeel+forte vide Lyssinum-Injeel.

Influenzinum-Injeel vide Grippe-Nosode-Injeel.

Klebs, pneum-Injeel+forte (D 6), D 12, D 30, D 200.

Luesinum-Injeel+forte (D 10), D 15, D 30, D 200, D 1000 (+Einzelpotenz D 7, D 8).

Lyssinum-Injeel+forte (D 12), D 15, D 30, D 200 (auch als Hydrophobinum bez.).

Medorrhinum-Injeel+forte (D 10), D 12, D 30, D 200 (+Einzelpotenz D 1000).

Paracoli-Injeel+forte (D 10), D 15, D 30, D 200.

Paratyphoidinum B-Injeel see Salmon, paratyphi B-Injeel.

Pertussis-Nosode-Injeel+forte (D 6), D 10, D 30, D 200.

Pneumococcinum-Injeel vide Klabs. neum-Injeel + forte.

Polymyetitis-Nosode-Injeel+forte (D 15), D 20, D 30, D 200, D 400.

Psorinum-Injeel+forte (D 9), D 12, D 30, 200 (+Einzelpotenz D 6), Eiter aus Kraetzpusteln.

Pyrogenium-Injeel+forte (D 8), D 12. D 30, D 200 (+Einzelpotenz D 5, D 6).

Salmon-Paratyfi-B-Injeel+forte (D 6), D 10. D 30, D 200.

Salmon-typhi-Injeel+forte (D 6), D 12, D 30, D 200.

Scarlatinum-Injeel+forte (D 6), D 12, D 30, D 200 (+Einzelpotenz D 5).

Staphylococcus-Injeel+forte (D 6), D 12, D 30, D 200 (+Einzelpotenz D 5).

Strept. hemolyt-Injeel+forte (D 6), D 12, D 30, D 200 (+Einzelpotenz D 5).

Syphilinum-Injeel+forte vide Luesinum Injeel.

Tetanus-Antitoxin-Injeel+forte (D 6), D 12, D 30, D 200 (+Einzelpotenz D 200).

Tuberculinum-Injeel+forte (D 8), D 12, D 30, D 200 (+Einzelpotenz D 100, D 10,000).

Vaccininum-Injeel+forte (D 8), D 20, D 30, D 200 (+Einzelpotenzen D 200). Variolinum-Injeel+forte (D 15), D 20, D 30 D 200 (+Einzelpotenzen, D 15, D 200, D 1000, D 10,000) (Julian 1997).

Chapter 11

Tautopathy

Contents

- Definition
- What Exactly is the Method
- Why Do We Need It
- Review of the Literature
- Application of Tautopathy
- The Pill, Naprosyn, Cortisone and Vaccinations
- Intercurrent Prescribing
- Case Examples
- Who Uses it Today and Research
- Limitations
- Provings and Tautopathy
- Homeopathic Provings of Allopathic Drugs

In this chapter you will:
1. Explore the different interpretations of Tautopathy
2. Identify the reasons for its controversial position in homeopathic medicine
3. Explore its positive and negative application in the historical literature and modern practice
4. Familiarise yourself with many of the modern Tautopathic options

Chapter 11
Tautopathy

Among chronic diseases we must still, alas! reckon those so commonly met with, artificially produced in allopathic treatment by the prolonged use of violent heroic medicines in large and increasing doses, by the abuse of calomel, corrosive sublimate, mercurial ointment, nitrate of silver, iodine and its ointments, opium, valerian, cinchona bark and quinine, foxglove, prussic acid, sulphur and sulphuric acid, perennial purgative ... setons, ... etc., whereby the vital energy is sometimes weakened to an unmerciful extent, sometimes, if it do not succumb, gradually abnormally deranged (by each substance in a peculiar manner) in such a way that, in order to maintain life against these inimical and destructive attacks, it must produce a revolution in the organism, and either deprive some part of its irritability and sensibility, or exalt these to an excessive degree, cause dilatation or contraction, relaxation or induration or even total destruction of certain parts, and develop faulty organic alterations here and there in the interior or the exterior(cripple the body internally or externally), in order to preserve the organism from complete destruction of life by the ever-renewed, hostile assaults of such destructive forces. (Aphorism 74 Hahnemann 1922).

These inroads on human health effected by the allopathic non-healing art (more particularly in recent times) are of all chronic diseases the most deplorable, the most incurable; and I regret to add that it is apparently impossible to discover or to hit upon any remedies for their cure when they have reached any considerable height. (Aphorism 75 Hahnemann 1922).

Only for natural diseases has the beneficent Deity granted us, in Homoeopathy, the means of affording relief; but those devastations and maimings of the human organism exteriorly and interiorly, effected by years, frequently, of the unsparing exercise of a false art with its hurtful drugs and treatment, must be remedied by the vital force itself (appropriate aid being given for the eradication of any chronic miasm that may happen to be lurking in the background), if it has not already been too much weakened by such mischievous acts, and can devote several years to this huge operation undisturbed. A human healing art, for the restoration to the normal state of those innumerable abnormal conditions so often produced by the allopathic non-healing art, there is not and cannot be. (Aphorism 76 Hahnemann 1922)

Definition

Yasgur defines Tautopathy as a form of isotherapy in his Homeopathic Dictionary.

Tautopathy involves using a homeopathically-prepared allopathic medicine in order to counteract side-effects caused by that particular allopathic medication, e.g. giving homeopathic DPT to counter the ill-effects produced by the DPT vaccine or giving homeopathic Valium to counter the ill-effects produced by Valium. To carry this one step further, some practitioners feel it necessary to treat the allopathically-dosed patient in this manner before commencing homeopathic treatment (Yasgur 1994).

What Exactly Is the Method?

We are living in toxic times; the air we breathe; the food we eat; the water we drink. You have to have a post-doctoral qualification in nutrition to be able to understand the labelling on the back of a product in a supermarket. You don't know for sure just what it is that you're taking into your body. Has there ever been a time in human history where our organs of elimination have been under such pressure? Livers and kidneys bear the brunt of humanity's fascination with altering that which is natural. In order to make a buck, in order to grow things quicker, in order to do things cheaper, manufacturing companies use human beings and animals for that matter as guinea pigs, even guinea pigs. The long-term consequences of this onslaught of toxicity are unknown. It seems to be no surprise that cancer rates continue to spiral, chronic diseases become harder to treat and often emerge out of the blue in our patients.

Ian Watson identifies 'tautopathy' as a variation of isopathy, the only real difference really being that the remedy is made of a potentised drug or toxin with which the patient has previously been poisoned. And for him, tautopathy has had significant successful application as an adjunct rather than a replacement for homeopathic treatment (Watson 1991).

From a purely aetiological perspective, if the patient's health has never been well since taking some sort of drug, or since receiving some vaccination, and no clearly identifiable medicine based on the totality of characteristic symptoms is identifiable, then this is a legitimate place to start treatment. Some homeopaths use other methods to detoxify the patient. Vannier advocated the use of organ remedies. So many patients have reported that they are not well since a particular medication or vaccination. Industrial poisonings, modern industrial diseases, vaccination in either childhood or for the purposes of travelling have all been reported as the reason that 'I am no longer healthy'.

Watson says that the ill effects of taking drugs toxin and other treatments can be antidoted by remedy based upon the symptoms of the patient. For example, *Pulsatilla* is known to be a leading remedy for patients who have suffered from taking too much iron, and of course, *Nux vomica* is commonly used for narcotics or alcohol, and *Thuja* for any ill effects from vaccination. Watson's book has some great examples (Watson 1991).

Why Do We Need It?

One of the daily problems that homeopaths face is the cumulative effects that new chemicals, drugs, vaccines and anaesthetics have on the human body. And of course, it is not uncommon for patients who are unwell, and especially the elderly, to be on several, sometimes dozens of simultaneous forms of medication (Watson 1991). Great results have been achieved in cases where drugs or toxins were the direct cause of the patient's problem.

There is nothing more frustrating. The patient has clearly defined characteristics. They clearly indicate a known homeopathic remedy. You prescribe it, and nothing happens. You try a different potency of the same remedy, and then try plan B, plan C and plan D. There is no good reason that homeopathy, so effective in so many situations, would not be effective in this case.

One of the things that we can postulate is that the 21st century visit to the homeopath is conducted in significantly different conditions of 200 years ago when Hahnemann was writing the *Organon of Medicine*; our bodies are the same but our diseases are not. In addition, both recreational and conventional drugs and medications are taken in the extreme, which is not to say that patients were not heavily medicated or taking recreational drugs in Hahnemann's day either. Snuff, tobacco, and beer were all commonplace in his time, not to mention opium or for that matter, laudenum. After all, human beings have been taking medication, addicted to and smoking drugs, altering their states of health since time immemorial. We can assume that by the time young adults heading towards middle age take stock of their lives and health, they will have been exposed to, and perhaps deliberately poisoned themselves with a level of toxicity unprecedented in human history. Their livers and kidneys, and the other filtering systems of their bodies have been exposed to pollutants, and food additives on a scale that is again unprecedented even if they don't drink or smoke, or partake in stimulants.

In fact, there is a significant difference from Hahnemann's time. From a historical perspective, there was no such thing as psychological medications. There were barbaric treatments, but not the suppressive or heavy medications that our patients are commonly taking at this end of the 21st century: Prozac, Effexor, Zantac, barbituates, suppressants, antidepressants, antianxiety medications. It is not uncommon these days to have patients who are expressing some sort of anxiety that have been medicated with some anti-epileptic medication from an overzealous conventional practitioner. What's the effect of all of this medication? Is there a consequence to all of this?

My own perspective of practising in the city as opposed to a quiet rural or regional environment has changed my thinking on these matters. There are times that it is entirely appropriate to deal with this level of toxicity and these obstacles in a purely pragmatic way to make some headway with a patient. It is not the highest idea of cure by any means. This is not getting to the centre of the case. However, it provides opportunity for some small immediate relief for the suffering client, and quite possibly a way to gain some traction, perhaps a bit of momentum, and restoring that patient back to health.

Delving into the literature, this is not a new issue by any means. In India Patel, Chatterjee and P Sankaran have all written on the subject.

Review of the Literature

With such strong medicines and with such abuse of allopathic medicine it makes some sense. One oncologist told me that cancer patients do not die of cancer but more probably with high doses of chemotherapy and its side effects. "Iatrogenesis, from the Greek Iatros (Doctor), literally means "Doctor- induced". It refers to any illness, injury or fatality that is the result of medical intervention, ranging from incorrect diagnosis or inappropriate treatment to harmful drug interaction, misinterpretation of a laboratory test or a fatal reaction to an injection of penicillin or other medication."…"Adverse side effects and dangerous interaction between drugs are probably the most common type of iatrogenic illness. To my knowledge there are no drugs without some side effects. Overuse of antibiotics is epidemic in some hospitals and clinics." The tragic doctor errors are not exposed to public as many Multi-national pharmaceutical firms are involved and great many important people in Government and profession are also involved. Combination of Antibiotics and other drugs have created a lot of complications in therapeutic approach.... I do not know where it will end but my mind is clear that patients all over the world will become so oversensitive to allopathic drugs that they will reject to take synthetic or any drug and would like to go for Nature - cure or Homeopathy. If you see the trend in U.S.A., U.K. and European countries the time has come that patients demand alternative systems of treatment than allopathy (Patel 1988).

Tautopathy (Tauto-same) is a method of curing or removing bad or side effects of drugs by iso-intoxication, i.e., curing by means of the identical harmful agent in potentised form. Tautopathic drugs have two advantages. They can be proved according to Homeopathic "Proving" and can be assimilated in Homeopathic Materia Medica and can be given to antidote the bad-effects of crude or offending and harmful identical agents... not the least do I want to go away from Homeopathic principles but just I want to remove some "obstacles to recovery in each case" which are coming up in the way of Homeopathy in Modern "Wonder drugs" era. "Tautopathy is indirect Homeopathy. It is Homeopathy minus actual proving of the drugs on healthy provers. It is used on the basis of (i) Causative factor (abuse of the corresponding drug) and (ii) The symptoms produced as side effects of the abused drug." (Dr J.N. Kanjilal) "Tautopathic drugs have nothing to do with allopathy on the following grounds (i) they are used on the basis of symptoms produced by the crude drug on diseased persons (unhealthy provers) (ii) they are prepared strictly in the process of homeopathic pharmaceutical discipline (iii) they are used in potencies." (Dr J.N. Kanjilal) "The key to correct diagnosis and good therapy rests for the most part in well documented history, never slighting the review of system and history, of drug intake." The effectiveness of the antibiotics and other scheduled drugs, their adverse reactions on the human system apart, has attracted the attention of Homoeopathic Research Organisations and Pharmacists in India and abroad which have successfully potentised quite a number of them for use in homoeopathy. These are called Tautopathic drugs. Although only a few of them such as Pencillin, Chloromycetin, Streptomycin, have been partially "proved", they have been found useful (i) to counter the side-effects of the same drugs and (ii) to control the diseases for which such drugs are administered in crude form. This has opened up a new vista to handle difficult cases homoeopathically and should be fully exploited (Chatterjee 1988).

The work of R P Patel of India in this connection is, indeed, commendable. It will be very useful if such modern anti-TB drugs as Ethambutol, Refampicin, Isonazid are potentised and made available for their therapeutic use in homoeopathy. In the absence of proper and complete proving, it is only their clinical uses and published results from such uses that go a long way to enable the homoeopathic practitioners to prescribe these remedies in appropriate cases. Homoeopathic practice of present day has to take into account not only disease miasms but drug miasms as well. And, in this context, a knowledge of diseases, modern medicines, their uses and side-effects as embodied in the text books on Clinical Pharmacology is an inescapable necessity for successful homoeopathic practice. The tautopathic drugs have provided the necessary thrust in this direction (Chatterjee 1988).

P Sankaran wrote,

Recently the method of curing or removing the ill-effects (toxic or allergic) of crude drugs by the administration of the identical substances in potentized form has become popular. Mr. Dudley Everitt has coined the term Tautopathy for this therapy and Ramanlal Patel has written extensively about it (Sankaran 1996).

And now we come to a major or serious interference with the natural process of cure and that is drugging. Many modern drugs are very powerful, powerful enough to subvert the normal harmonious functioning of the body. They may not only interfere with and prevent the action of the carefully chosen remedy but they may even produce various side-effects which may be toxic, allergic or of any other kind. A recent issue of the Practitioner of London had devoted nearly a hundred and thirty six pages to the toxic manifestations of various modern drugs. A separate group of diseases known as Iatrogenic diseases (i.e. disease caused by physicians or medicines) is now recognised and described. Proctitis caused by the use of antibiotics and liquid paraffin, the nerve deafness caused by Dihydrostreptomycin, various changes in the body due to the prolonged use of cortisone are some examples.

Turner says, "This use of sprays, applications, mouth washes and gargles may be the reason why some cases fail to respond readily to what seems to be the indicated remedy."

Modern homoeopaths remark that after the patient has taken cortisone the homoeopathic remedy does not act well. Stokes says that habit-forming drugs also interfere with the action of our remedies. Downer gives illustrative cases and says that first the road must be cleared of drugs that are hindering the true line of cure and then the indicated remedy must be given.

That these drugs seriously interfere with and prevent a cure is known to the homoeopathic physicians. But fortunately for us, the same drugs, in potency seem to have the power of antidoting and nullifying the ill-effects of the massive drugging. Such treatment called Tautopathy was mentioned by Dudley Everitt and later on described by Ramanlal Patel. There is also a large amount of self-medication. People take all sorts of medicines that are being advertised but do not care to inform the doctor about this.

Again as Foubister says, the use of an anaesthetic may subvert the harmonious functioning of the organism. So he suggests that it is always wiser to enquire for a history of operations and the undue after-effects of any anaesthetic applied therein. Where the anaesthetic is clearly known, e.g. Chloroform or Ether, a potency of the same may clear up the ill-effects. The use of vaccines and sera can seriously interfere with the action of the indicated remedies. For after-effects of serum Boger recommends Anthracinum, Psorinum or Sulphur and Hayes suggests Phos (Sankaran 1996).

Stuart Close was adamant about its use.

How small the list of natural diseases is may be seen by observing primitive peoples. Psora, Syphilis and Sycosis in their various manifestations, have been augmented and perpetuated almost as much by the fearful drugs used to combat them, as by any inherent tendency in themselves. Crude drugs not only stir up and render more active these great miasms, but set up their own morbid processes, which may be quite as bad as the original disease. Any drug capable of curing Syphilis is capable of setting up a process in the human organism as bad as Syphilis, under certain conditions.

Boenninghausen, Hering, Guernsey, Swan, and many others,

have advised giving a dose of the high potency of a drug known to have been abused, and the effects of which constituted a part of the case as shown by the symptoms. This advice has been strenuously condemned by others, who in their fear of routinism, or from excessive conservatism in general, have regarded it as a heresy. These objectors would never use the same drug, but only similar drugs for antidotal purposes. To them, knowledge that a drug had been abused was sufficient to cut that drug absolutely from the list of available medicines to be used in the treatment of the case. Thence came the lists of "antidotes" in our materia medicas, consisting of a varying number of drugs mentioned as bearing some antidotal relation to certain symptoms, or groups of symptoms, produced by the drug abused. These were selected partly from clinical observations, and partly from their similarity, known by comparison of symptoms. These workers were content to base their treatment of drug diseases upon similars, often of a very low degree. Hence their failure, and the dogma of the incurability of drug diseases. The conception that there existed a simillimum, or absolute equal to a group of symptoms known to have been produced by a drug, and that simillimum the high potency of the drug itself, had never entered their minds. Accepting as true the law of Similars and the law of Potentiation, there can logically be only one simillimum to the effects of any drug or morbid agent whatever, and that is the high potency of the drug itself. The most that any other drug can be is a simile. This must be perfectly evident to any one who will reflect upon it. The last infinitesimal degree between simile and idem, between simility and identity, between similar and the same, is expressed by the term Simillimum. It is synonymous with Equal, but is not identical. Nothing can be so similar to the actual drug abused, and yet not be the same thing, as a high potency of the drug itself.

Potentiation changes the form but not the essential nature of the drug.

In what is called natural disease we may find the simillimum, but we cannot be certain of it beforehand, because we cannot know with certainty what agent produced the symptoms. The best we can do may result in finding only a simile. Fortunately similes are also curatives, in proportion to the degree of similarity. But the simillimum, having the highest degree of simility short of absolute identity, is the equal or perfect curative.

In a case depending upon a drug miasm, however, it is different. We find a certain disease condition in the patient, represented by symptoms. The symptoms correspond to the symptoms of a certain drug. By careful inquiry we trace them back to the use of that drug in crude form or in massive doses. Under the homoeopathic law we have found the Simillimum, and in giving the high potency of that drug we are making the highest known application of that law. Under these conditions no other remedy will so quickly remove the symptoms and cure the case. No other drug or agent could produce or cure the same condition or symptoms. This is self-evident, and properly conducted experience confirms it. That drugs act unconditionally is evidently untrue, for it leaves out of consideration entirely the fundamental principle and condition of all vital activity, namely, Susceptibility. Not every person, patient or prover, is susceptible to every drug in crude form. This is too well known to need illustration. Under the law of correspondence or similars, a person is normally susceptible only to those drugs whose characteristic symptoms, especially the mental symptoms, correspond to his own characteristic symptoms or traits as an individual. To all others he offers a resistance which is effectual up to the point of actual breaking down and overwhelming of the life force by massive and poisonous doses. When this occurs an artificial or morbid susceptibility is set up which becomes itself the basis of treatment.

A patient may have used many drugs during his lifetime and been actually impressed or injured by very few of them. Those to which he was susceptible at the time of use, or those so abused as to destroy his normal resisting power and set up an artificial susceptibility, will be made known by the presence of symptoms which will be disclosed by a careful examination and study of the case. They cannot be known in any other way. Some symptoms of the drug or drugs involved in the case will be found by the careful examiner, and these must be the subject of careful consideration. To give a high potency of a drug which has been abused, under the conditions already stated, is not Isopathy, as some have objected. It is Homoeopathy, pure and simple, as shown by Hahnemann in his remarks upon the use of Psorinum. (See Chronic Diseases, page 152, Tafel's translation). Referring to Isopathy and the homoeopathic use of potentiated Psorinum (Close 1898).

The homeopathic literature is full of voiced concerns at the damage caused by suppressive medications. Patel collated a significant number in his 1988 work.

Before the era of Antibiotics and Sulphonamides, it was already the practice to influence and check infection by non-specific therapy" (Thampan and Bergschmidt). And with that the resistance of the body against disease was created first in the body.

Disturbances in the intestinal bacterial flora have been observed during antibiotic treatment predominantly after the oral administration of Broad-Spectrum antibiotics" (Thampan and Bergschmidt). Neurologic disturbances have been described in prolonged treatment with streptomycin and dihydrostreptomycin such as are often necessary in tuberculosis. Streptomycin may cause disturbances of equilibrium while dihydrostreptomycin may cause auditory disturbances. (Thampan and Bergschmidt)

A higher rate of relapse has been observed, when the introduction of chloramphenical is done in the treatment of typhoid" (Laporte and Fritel, Vorlaender and Schnutz)

But as regards the resistance of the body, it has been noted that antibiotics unfavourably influence the defence mechanisms in the human body, a fact which has been confirmed also by animal experiments. It was found that the administration of Penicillin in healthy individuals causes a decrease in leucocyte counts. (Galnsslen and Lehmann).

I was amazed at the toxic possibilities after the exhibition of the sulpha drugs and penicillin- confusional psychosis, anuria, epilepsy, glossitis- infact, the ultimate results seem rather unpredictable and one wonders what the patient may have to pay for the gains achieved. The antibiotic's action is a directly lethal one over the other bacteria and the abrupt change in the bacterial flora, of the respiratory and alimentary tracts is likely to have consequences which we cannot at present foresee. How far the patient's normal defence mechanisms are modified by the use of Sulpha drugs and antibiotics remains to be seen. (Sir John Weir).

A number of reports on fungus diseases following antibiotic treatment, especially with broad-spectrum antibiotics were lately published (Scelchow Nikoluski, Hosenann). Special interest has been roused by fungus infection due to Morilia Allsicans. This normal harmless fungus may, during treatment with antibiotics spread in the whole body and systemic fungus disease may end fatally. The British medical journal in 1952 warned that the use of the wonder drug streptomycin may have to be abandoned because it is too dangerous. The journal said the drug can have serious poisonous effects on the 'eighth nerve' causing giddiness and deafness and may even upset a patient sense of balance permanently. The drug is used frequently to combat tuberculosis but in the majority of cases patients become resistant to the drug and remain so indefinitely. Rarely does it occur to the prescriber that the 'complication' is but the symptomatic reflection of the drug or drugs he has previously given. I say, rarely, for sometimes he does seem to have faint glimpses of such a truth, as when tetanus, trismus or acute Bright's disease speedily follow vaccination, or when haemorrhage in lungs, kidneys or retina quickly supervenes upon the administration of massive doses of Quinine or when he happens to recognise one of the "puzzling eruptions" said to be caused by one or more drugs.

Hepatic disorders due to chlorpromazine (Thorazine) are reported at the rate of 1 to 50 cases to 3 in 71. Viscosity of bile is increased: an obstructive type of jaundice develops as biliary canaliculi are plugged. Although some patients die, most recover on cessation of therapy. Similar changes may be brought about by therapy with theouracel, methimazole, arsphenamine and methyltestasterene."

Toxic hepatitis with inflammatory infiltration and liver cell damages is caused by many drugs, including Phenylbutazone and phenacerylurea (Phenurone). O.D. Quarterly reports that sulfapyridine is causing stone in the kidney and urinary tract. The science News letter reports that Dr Mekenzie of Johns Hopkins has discovered that the Sulpha drugs are causing enlargement of the thyroid."

Peptic ulcer is common during treatment with ACTH and cortisone. Even in healthy individuals, ACTH raises the concentration of Hydrochloric acid and pepsin in the gastric juice and reduces the viscosity and amount of mucus."

Peptic ulcer and migration of prostatic cancer to the breast are known side effects of therapeutic hormones. Metastasis to the breast may occur when oestrogen is given for prostatic carcinoma. The hormone causes gynaecomastia by increasing vascularity and growth of loose textured fibrous tissue."

Perforation and haemorrhage from peptic ulcer is common after Rauwolfia Serpentina" according to Dr W.O. West, from the Department of Internal Medicine, Charleston Memorial Hospital, Charleston. Further he said, "Peptic ulcer occurrence, recurrences and complications associated with the administration of Rauwolfia Serpentina probably contribute another to the evergrowing list of diseases of Medical progress"

Dr L.C. Cope, Physician at the Post-Graduate Medical School of London has said "Cortisone and Corticotrophin do not cure, they merely suppress some manifestation of disease."

Fungus infections, Staphylococcin enteritis or vitamin deficiency may occur if the natural balance of gastro-intestinal organisms is upset by antibacterial agents."

Antihypertensive agents have various undesirable effects, 'Hexamenthorium' in long courses may bring an acute interstitial pulmonary fibrosis and progressive dyspnoea that is fatal in thirty days." Disturbances are initiated by hydralazine hydrochloride (A presoline) in as many as 10 per cent of persons who receive an average of 640 mg. daily for one year. Symptoms of rheumatoid arthritis, lupus erythematosis, serum sickness or collagen disease may develop. Chills, migratory joint pain and myalgia occur, sedimentation rate ascends and haemoglobin falls. Arthritis follows and with continued administration, fever, prostration, effusions in body cavities, rash, splenomegaly and lymphadenopathy." (Modern Medicine- Man-made disease) It is true that if the use of crude drugs could be entirely done away with, the sum of human ills would be greatly reduced, or as wise and witty Dr. Olivers Wendell once said "If all the drugs in the world could be dumped into the sea, it would be better for mankind and the worse for the fishes."

Medicine is far from having decreased human sufferings as much as it endeavours to make us believe. Indeed, the number of deaths from infectious diseases has greatly diminished. But we still must die and we die in a much larger proportion from degenerative diseases. The years of life which we have gained by the suppression of diphtheria, small pox, typhoid fever etc. are paid for by the long sufferings and the lingering deaths caused by chronic affections and especially by cancer, diabetes and heart disease............Although modern hygiene has made human existence far safer, longer and more pleasant, disease have not been mastered. They have simply changed in nature" writes Dr. Alexis Carrel, the famous scientist in "Man, the Unknown."

Dr Benehtrit holds the opinion that "Vaccines and sera are principally responsible for the increase of those two really dangerous diseases, cancer and heart disease ... I have been for a long time a serologist and I know what I am talking about." "Belief in serum therapy rests on a foundation of sand." (Sir Almorth Wright)

Humanity today is drug ridden as never before in history. "It is my personal opinion that vaccination enforced on the public for the last two or three generations are responsible for the enormous increase in Allergic conditions in children and adults- a costly and painful price to pay for the protection against Small- pox, whooping cough, typhoid fever, typhus and many other diseases." (Dr Roger Schmidt- U.S.A)

The last taken drug affords the best medication for the next prescription." (Dr Hering). And mind well Nux. Vomica at present cannot afford, to antidote the present powerful chemical 'wonder drugs'. If you prescribe to every patient who comes from allopathic brothers, Nux. Vomica 6, 30 or 200, you are wasting your time in 90% of cases (Patel 1988).

P Sankaran (1996) wrote,

When the homoeopathic doctor has given much time and labour to taking the case history which is the first great essential in every good prescription, and then devoted more time and labour to repertory study and research through the Materia Medica, he cannot afford to have such a prescription spoiled or interfered with by some foolish external action of the patient, which may nullify the expected results of all the physician's painstaking efforts and leave both physician and patient disappointed and discouraged. With these facts in mind, it behoves the physician to instruct his patient emphatically that he must refrain from taking all other drugs such as pain killers, cathartics, camphor or menthol in any form." He also gives a long list of substances such as dentrifices, mouth washes, gargles, nose drops, face creams, soaps, processed foods, chlorinated and flouridated water, etc., which can interfere with the action of the homoeopathic remedy.

Grimmer writes that the four best antidotes to the coal tar

drugs like Aspirin are Arnica, Carbo veg., Lachesis and Mag. phos. to be given according to the symptoms present in each individual case. Grimmer writes further, "One more important source of interference with the homoeopathic remedy is the widespread use of sera and vaccines as protective agents against acute disease. The reaction to these products of diseases is often lasting in its effect and leaves the victims of this practice sick and suffering."

Grimmer writes, "The most pernicious of these interruptables is the aluminium toxin that enters the human system by way of aluminium cooking utensils and by water polluted with aluminium chloride which is used to soften hard water. This toxin acts much like one of the miasms and it must be eradicated from the system before a cure of the patient is possible. The most certain, rapid antidote for it is Cadmium oxide in potency, and of course the source of intake of the toxin must be discontinued. After the poison is removed by the Cadmium oxide, the remaining symptoms and conditions of the patient may be successfully attacked by the remedy that is indicated by the totality of remaining symptoms."

He also says, "(when aluminium vessels have been used for cooking), many times even the indicated remedies seemingly will not act until at least a single dose of Cadmium has been given."

Le Hunte Cooper in a well-documented paper describes the wide variety of symptoms and conditions that the use of aluminium cooking vessels can produce in sensitive people (Sankaran 1996).

Application of Tautopathy

A lot of these examples relate to medical practices from the middle of the last century. But in addition, we have to consider the contemporary use of allopathic medications given the changing landscape of drugs to which modern patients have been exposed.

The Pill, Naprosyn and Cortisone and Vaccinations

We are often left wondering why some of our prescriptions fail. It's a stressful business. We need the correct (or at the very least a close) medicine, the correct potency, and the correct administration. And the reality is that there could be an obstacle in the way of that remedy's action.

A relevant case in point is the contraceptive pill. We are now into the third generation of women, a tiny blip in human history, where the effects of the Pill are starting to become known. Of course, these things are normalised now to a huge extent.

In publications such as *The Pill: are you sure it's for you?* (*Bennett and Pope 2008),* the authors argue that the psychological and physiological effects of these generations of medication are just starting to become known. It is argued that male fertility levels, over masculinity in women and over femininity in men are all possible and real effects of suppressive medication. The Pill, theoretically devised to give women the choice as to whether they have a family, has also come at the price of allowing women to be completely sexually available to men at all times. In my own clinic over the years, I have regularly prescribed on the ill effects of this medication, and as a consequence, in my dispensary I have every potency of Folliculinum, Depopravera, and each of the specific pills such as Diane, Triphasal 28, Micro-gynae etc. In particular one-sided cases, I discovered that this is a far better way to get some movement towards a cure in cases without characteristic symptoms.

Ian Watson's cases of treating patients using Naprosyn, and P Sankarans experience of using cortisone in potency, demonstrate good results. Search out their published cases. And when it comes to vaccinations, many homeopaths use MMR and BCG to counter the effects of adults and children who have been badly affected, with symptoms such as fatigue, through to symptoms resembling rheumatoid arthritis, general malaise and various types of pain and fibromyalgia. Again Watson (1991) provides some great examples; cases of underdevelopment or stuttering that were cured with a homeopathic potency of the drug that poisoned them. The link between glue ear and DPT is established, and the tautopathic use of remedies in conjunction with accurate similars is an established clinical option.

Intercurrent Prescribing

Watson (1991) also provides great examples of the use of the potentised drug as an intercurrent remedy. Again, this is the situation where a well indicated remedy fails. Perhaps a drug or some toxin previously ingested is preventing the homeopathic remedy from acting fully. Watson uses the example of a woman with eczema and *Calcarea carbonica* was indicated, then she quickly relapsed. On the basis that she had been given penicillin previously, she was prescribed *Penicillin* in potentised form, and it led to significant improvement. It is the same with cortisone when it has been injected into the joints. After a few doses of *Cortisone* 200, it either produced a marked improvement in the condition or enabled further treatment to progress unhindered (Watson 1991). Further examples are those patients that have had numerous x-rays and failed to respond, or patients that have had chemotherapy or radiation exposure.

Case Examples (Patel 1988)

Child age 6-1/2 months. Weight 12 lbs. Temperature 102 degree. Cough and vomiting for 3-4 times. Child was losing weight. Stomatitis. Mother said 'His belly is going thinner and thinner. On examination; chest rales- both sides at the bases. The child was under treatment of a M.B.B.S. (Allopathic) Doctor for 10 days. Was given some mixture plus tablets (Cibazol).

1st day: I gave Ant. Tart. 30 one dose- 6 hourly.

2nd day: Cough was painful. The child was crying when it was to start. Fever –less, only for two hours. Ant. Tart 30, 3 doses. Six hourly.

3rd day: No further progress.

4th day: No progress. Sulphathiazole 30 was given, one dose. 2 grains in powder fom.

5th day: temperature rose up during night and continued upto morning. Cough, motion in morning. Stomatitis, vomiting once. Sac. Lac.

6th day: cough ameliorated. No temperature. No vomiting. No crying.

Child was better and was asking for milk. Motion in the morning- Sac. Lac.

7th day: slight cough without any trouble- General improvement seen. Sac. Lac

10th day: No cough. No temperature. Mother said 'He is alright.' Sac. Lac.

12th day: Weight 13 lbs.

13th day: Calc. Phos 3x two grain per dose, two times for 8 days (Patel 1988).

Mr. K.V.S. Age 65 yrs. Had severe cough 3 months ago, was X- Rayed. Diagnosed- Pulmonary Tuberculosis. He was given Streptomycin Injection- nearly 50; followed br reaction,- Rash all over the body with burning sensation. Allergic to Ethambulot. Given Garamycin but developed oedema all over the body with black discoloration on the body, itching and burning. Redness of eyes with pain. Had blocking of ears with vertigo during Streptomycin injections. Skin peels off. Gas trouble. Fainting- twice. Cough, persistent at night. Evening rise of temperature. Family history: Sister- Tuberculosis. Hot blooded, worse night. Depressed, sad, fear of disease, desire for company.

3-2-84- Streptomycin 30, morning & evening for 15 days.

18-2-84- All reactions subsided. Pain and swelling of breast. Ars. Iodide 0/3 and it was continued for one year.

22-4-85- No complaints (Patel 1988).

Mr. N.R.B. Age 19 yrs. Redness of Eyes- especially right eye after using Terramycin ointment for conjunctivitis- 2 yrs ago. Takes internal allopathic medicines including steroids then. There is relief but no cure. It recurs again and again with redness and itching, at times. Slight vision defect with right eye noticed recently on reading, if left eye is closed. Photophobia-in bright sunlight. Strain in rt. Eye if writing continuously. Appetite normal, cold attack occasionally. Hot blooded. Desires bath. Better by sleep. Company aversion, Consolation better, weeps.

12-12-86- Terramycin 30c, Morning and Evening for 15 days

27-12-86- Feels >. Irritation in rt. Eye. Kali iodide 0/3, Morning & Evening for 15 days.

14-2-87- Came with dimness of eyes, had jaundice, mild pain with slight redness. Terramycin 30, Morning & Evening for 30 days.

12-6-87- No complaints-No medication (Patel 1988).

Who Uses It Today and Research

Overwhelmingly, it is in eliminating toxins from the body that this method has had documented success. Watson advocates lower potencies, similar to the traditional French style of prescribing, 4C, 5C, 7C, 9C, 15C etc.

Significant research needs to be undertaken in this area alone. It is interesting that some institutions are attempting to demonstrate the efficacy of homeopathy by conducting trials utilizing isopathy and tautopathy. Poisoning seeds with arsenic and then treating them with a homeopathic potency of *Arsenicum album* before then measuring growth rates is one way to trial the efficacy of the infinitesimal dose. Such research at the University of Bern in Switzerland, and Endeavour College of Natural Health in Australia, can only assist in creating more compelling evidence of efficacy in the conventional evidence hierarchy. Variations on this type of research involving humans is also taking place around the world.

Nevertheless empirical evidence is strong, and anecdotal evidence confirms that tautopathic prescribing is widely used and widely effective. It is used to detoxify the body. It is therefore also useful in weaning people off orthodox allopathic medication where appropriate. Tranquillisers and steroids are notoriously hard to withdraw from, and again, when there are no clear characteristic symptoms leading to a prescription based on a larger totality, tautopathic prescribing is useful and appropriate. Watson uses the example of *Prednisone 30c* to assist the withdrawal process over a period of time. Given perhaps twice weekly, this could gradually reduce the dose of the drug over weeks and months or even longer. A patient is weaned onto the homeopathic remedy, and weaned off the allopathic medication in this way.

Limitations

The most obvious limitation of the method lies in case management. How is this to be taught? The assertion that taking a tautopathic remedy twice a week as in the previous example sounds fine on paper, but what about the management issues? Exactly how does one gauge the action of a remedy prescribed for a chronic condition when an intercurrent tautopathic remedy is laid on top of the previous remedy's action?

Provings and Tautopathy

It has been argued from day one that this style of prescribing is not genuinely homeopathic because the medications have had no provings. From this perspective, it is a well-made point. However, from another perspective Tautopathy becomes very valid when viewed from the patient's eyes. If a patient gets better using this method of prescribing, then who cares? If, as it is argued and demonstrated, that cases where the indicated remedy fails, then begin to improve after the prescription of a tautopathic remedy, then the clinical significance of that improvement cannot be ignored. It also ignores the fact that a great many of these drugs have in fact been proved to some degree lending further weight to the push for their legitimacy in the method tool kit of contemporary homeopathic prescribers.

Further Reading

- Foubister   *Constitutional effects of anaesthesia*
- Patel   *What is Tautopathy*
- Chatterjee   *Fundamentals of Homoeopathy and Valuable Hints for Practice*
- Sankaran   *The Elements of Homoeopathy*
- Close   *Homoeopathy and Drug Miasms*

Appendix

Homeopathic Provings of Allopathic Drugs

Acide acetyl salicylique (acetyl salicylic acid)
- Outrepuich C.
- 1987.
- no further information.

Acide gamma-aminobutyrique (gamma aminobutyric acid)
- Souk-Aloun P.
- 1 self-proving, 1 simple-blind proving with 2 provers (1 woman).
- 30CH
- 1989; 1 month.
- unpublished.

Ciclosporine (cyclosporin, ciclosporin)
- Souk-Aloun P.
- 1 self-proving,1 simple-blind proving with 5 provers (4 women).
- 1990; 1 month.
- Souk-Aloun P., Proving exploratoire de Ciclosporine 30CH. Homéopathie française 1992; N°1: 22-24.

Chloramphénicol
- Julian O.A.
- Hahnemann's method; 16 provers (3 women).
- 3DH, 7CH, 30CH, placebo.
- 1970.
- Julian O.A. . Dictionnaire de matière médicale homéopathique.

Chlorpromazine

- Julian O.A.
- Hahnemann's method, 23 provers of the " Société médicale de biothérapie ".
- 5CH, 7CH, 9CH, 15CH, 30CH, placebo.
- 1968.
- Julian O.A. . Dictionnaire de matière médicale homéopathique.

(Chlorpromazine was proved one first time by the Dr N.P. Pai in 1963, 16 provers, 30CH).

Crésol (cresylolum)

- Julian O.A.
- Hahnemann's method; 5 provers (2 women), 1 dog.
- 5CH, 7CH, 9CH.
- 1958.
- Julian O.A. . Dictionnaire de matière médicale homéopathique.

Diazépam

- Souk-Aloun Phou, Sarméo Anne.
- 1 self-proving, 1 simple-blind proving with 1 woman prover.
- 30CH.
- 1992; 1 month.
- Souk-Aloun P., Sarméo A., Proving exploratoire du Diazépam 30CH. Homéopathie européenne 1993; n°6: 25-26.

Interferon alpha

- Souk-Aloun P.
- 1 self-proving, 1 matched set proving with 7 provers (4 women).
- 30CH.
- 1989; 1 month.
- unpublished.

Lévomépromazine

- Julian O.A. .
- Hahnemann's method; 16 provers (7 women).
- 3DH, 7CH, 9CH, 15CH, 30CH, placebo.

- 1968.
- Julian O.A.. Dictionnaire de matière médicale homéopathique.

Thiopropérazine (majeptil)
- Julian O.A..
- Hahnemann's method; 37 provers.
- 3DH, 7CH, 30CH, placebo.
- 1976.
- Julian O.A.. Dictionnaire de matière médicale homéopathique.

Méthysergide
- Julian O.A..
- Hahnemann's method; 27 provers (6 women).
- 3DH, 7CH, 30CH, placebo.
- 1976.
- Julian O.A.. Dictionnaire de matière médicale homéopathique.

Naloxone
- Guemonprez M., Traisnel M., Boniface M.
- double-blind ; 40 provers.
- 1982.
- Julian O.A.. Dictionnaire de matière médicale homéopathique.

Oxprénolol
- B. Long, D. Froment, P. Cayrel, C. Pepey, P. Souk-Aloun.
- self-provings, double-blind provings with control subjects, 17 provers (9 women) having take Oxprénolol.
- 5CH, 15CH, 30CH.
- 1986; over 2 months.
- Long B., Souk-Aloun P., Froment D., Pathogénésie de l'Oxprénolol. Revue Belge d'Homoéopathie 1987; 2: 49-69. Long B., Souk-Aloun P., Froment D., Cayrel P. Expérimentation de l'Oxprénolol dynamisé. Cahiers de Biothérapie 1987; 93: 35-45. Long B., Souk-Aloun P., Froment D., Cayrel P., Données expérimentales de l'Oxprénolol dynamisé. Cahiers de biothérapie 1987; 97: 73-77. Souk-Aloun P., Pepey C., Long B.. Pathogénésie de 2 bêta-bloquants: Propranolol et Oxprénolol. Homéopathie française 1990; N°2: 42-48.

Penicillinum

- Guermonprez M.
- self-proving, 11 provers (3 women).
- 7CH, 9CH.
- 1950.
- Julian O.A.. Dictionnaire de matière médicale homéopathique.

Propranolol

- Souk-Aloun P., Pepey C., Long B., Deries N.,Jobert J., Mabilon J.L. .
- first proving with the 20 physicians provers of " Groupe Mercurius ", double blind, randomisation, 10 control subjects take placebo, 10 provers (4 women) take 30CH; 1987. Second proving with the 20 provers of the " Ecole H.H. du Dauphiné-Savoie " and the " Association Benoit-Mure ", matched set of 10 validated provers (3 women); 30CH; 1989
- 30CH.
- 1987, 1989; over 1 month for each proving.
- Groupe Mercurius, Proving du Propranolol. Bulletin semestriel du Groupe

Mercurius 1987; N°1: 10-23. Souk-Aloun P., Pepey C., Long B.. Pathogénésie de 2 bêta-bloquants: Propranolol et Oxprénolol. Homéopathie française 1990; N°2: 42-48. Souk-Aloun P., Pepey C.. Pathogénésie du Propranolol. Revue belge d'Homoéopathie 1989; N°2.

Maléate de perhexiline (pexid)

- Julian O.A.
- Hahnemann's method; 32 provers (6 women).
- 1975.
- Julian O.A. Dictionnaire de matière médicale homéopathique.

Réserpine

- Julian O.A.
- Hahnemann's method; 13 provers; with animal proving (mice, guinea pigs).
- 3DH, 5CH, 7CH, 9CH, 15CH, 30CH.
- 1964.
- Julian O.A. Dictionnaire de matière médicale homéopathique. (Souk 1993).

Chapter 12

Organ Prescribing, Organopathy and Burnett

Contents

- Introduction
- Background
- Affinity, Organ Prescribing, Organopathy, Supporting the Organs
- Specificity of Seat
- Locality
- The Limitations of the 'Totality of Symptoms'
- Drilling Deeper: Burnett's Influences
- Rademacher and the Organ Remedies
- Burnett's Cases
- Burnett's Use of Potency
- The Organ Remedies
- Random Gems from Burnett, Rademacher and Others
- Nosodes
- For and Against
- Computers and Burnett
- The Full List of Burnett's Works
- Conclusion

In this chapter you will:

1. Realise the practical value of this method
2. Identify opportunities in modern practice to apply the method
3. Understand how Burnett bridged the herbal, allopathic and homeopathic traditions with his advocacy of organ support
4. Learn the clinical options for individualised organ support
5. Learn the theoreticial underpinnings and foundations of the method

Chapter 12
Organ Prescribing, Organopathy and Burnett

The medical profession at large condemn homeopathy – they know nothing about it. There was a time when I also condemned it – I also knew nothing about it; but now, having studied it and practised it, my airy contempt has given place to humble-minded thankfulness, and I maintain that homeopathy – real scientific homeopathy – is the most mighty weapon against any disease known to mankind (Best of Burnett).

When drugs affect certain parts of the economy specifically, the general fact is the one elaborated by the great and greatly vilified Paracelsus, and it constituted the backbone of his practice. Remedies owning this quality were his Appropriata. That is, they are appropriated by the organs they respectively and specifically influence, much as we may suppose the kidneys seize upon the particles in the blood to form what is then known as urine. Grounded on this basis, the medical practice of Paracelsus was not only in advance of the common medical practice of his own now distant day, but actually much in advance of the orthodox medical practice of the time that now is (Burnett Curability of Tumours 1898).

No, I could not be a homoeopath; I would try the thing at the bedside, prove it to be a sham, and expose it to an admiring profession (Burnett Fifty Reasons 1888).

Introduction

Organopathy cannot be spoken about without a glance at the life, times and work of James Compton Burnett (1840-1901). He is the bridge between ideas present in natural medicine that long predated Hahnemann and homeopathic medicine as we know it today. With his friends and colleagues who formed the Cooper Club, Robert Thomas Cooper, Thomas Skinner and John Henry Clarke, he shaped homeopathy in the UK for a century.

He is one of the characters of homeopathic medicine. Described as 'burley', there are some striking and startling parallels with Hahnemann. Burnett studied medicine in Vienna, married twice and had 13 children. Hahnemann also studied medicine in Vienna, married twice and had 13 children. Both were rejected by university authorities because of their pro-homeopathy stance; Burnett being rejected because of his thesis. Both had to deal with significant conflict and were especially harsh on pseudo-homeopaths.

Background

Good source of information on Burnett are in Morrell (2000) and Taylor (*www.wholehealthnow.com* 2001a). He was born in Redlynch, near Salisbury, Wiltshire England in 1840. There is little in the historical record between that and his attending medical school in Vienna in 1865, where he remained two additional years studying anatomy. The tuition was free and later on he was proud of the fact that he had graduated from Hahnemann's old school in 1869.

Passing through a brilliant examination in anatomy, lasting one hour and a half, the professor shook hands with him, saying that he had never examined a student with so brilliant and thorough a knowledge of anatomy (Morrell 2000).

This knowledge of anatomy comprised one of the crucial facets in his ability to bridge the Organotherapy of Rademacher and Paracelcus and the homeopathy of Hahnemnann. Burnett returned to Britain, enrolled at Glasgow University and graduated in 1872. Converted to homeopathy through his friend Alfred Hawkes, he completed an internship for his degree at Barnhill Parochial Hospital and Asylum in Glasgow in 1876.

His original thesis was rejected for being overly homeopathic but a second one was accepted in 1876. The details of his conversion to Homeopathy can be found in *Fifty Reasons for Being a Homoeopath;* after a study of Aconite in a fever ward he began treating some of the children with a few drops of the mother tincture in a large bottle of water for their chills and fever and was amazed at the rapid response. The nurses called it 'Dr Burnett's Fever Bottle'.

He studied further homeopathy in Liverpool under Drysdale and Berridge, at first very secretively for fear of reprisals from allopathic colleagues. Faced with such hostility, Burnett's decision to explore homeopathy was a brave one. But rather than being an apologetic proponent of homeopathy, he was quite aggressive, combative and quarrelsome and he practised with the 'single-minded passion and zeal necessary to overcome such adversity.' In 1874 he began private practice in Chester and was treating patients in a dispensary owned by a homeopathic chemist, Edward Thomas, whose daughter he married in 1874. There were six children but Agnes died in childbirth in 1882. There was a second marriage and seven more children later.

Burnett ran two busy medical practices in London. In 1879, a few months before becoming editor of the *Homoeopathic World*, he moved to London where he developed a thriving medical homeopathic practice, as well as developing a very full program of research, such as provings, delivering medical papers to the Homoeopathic Society, contributing to medical journals, and publishing his books.

Affinity, Organ Prescribing, Organopathy, Supporting the Organs

So Burnett's approach to homeopathy was richly informed by his dual skills in anatomy, and understanding of the work of Paracelsus, Rademacher and Fludd. He had a firm grip on pathology and pathophysiology as it was understood at the time but he was not willing to let go of this understanding in applying homeopathic principles. He felt that if a greater understanding of the disease process could be obtained, then it should be incorporated into our homeopathic work.

He argued that a person could be treated through the organs with 'organopathy' and on this basis he mainly used the low potencies and tinctures. He also employed what came to be called *'the ladder of remedies'*, zigzagging his way through the symptoms of a case taking out a single symptom at a time. The 'ladder' consisted of:

> ...a series of different medicines prescribed at different potencies and subtly adjusted to the needs of a particular case.

The trickiest problems pleased him most, and the quirkier the solution, the better it suited him (Morrell 2000).

It was Hughes' book, *A Manual of Pharmacodynamics*, the first authoritative homeopathic textbook published in English that also shaped his homeopathic ideas. On the one hand a fundamentalist and a purist, Hughes resented all attempts to tamper with his own interpretations of what he perceived as the truth laid down by Hahnemann. On the other hand, he resented the empirical or individual approach to clinical symptoms. From his case books it seems that Burnett was a little more pragmatic than Hughes, and argued that often the outer pathological symptoms were so gross that he could not see the causal simillimum. As a result, he utilised a systematic approach in which he treated a patient by clearing up the symptom picture to the point where the simillimum could be prescribed.

To that end, when he was unable to identify a clear totality of symptoms, Burnett used herbal medicines, nosodes or organ specific remedies to begin a case before prescribing on a larger totality. Some of the results were breathtaking.

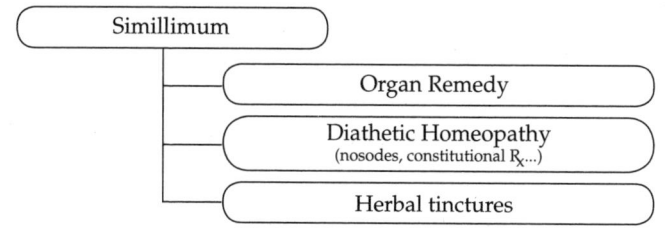

```
Simillimum
    ├── Organ Remedy
    ├── Diathetic Homeopathy
    │   (nosodes, constitutional Rx...)
    └── Herbal tinctures
```

Specificity of Seat

To Burnett the idea of Rademacher's organ remedies,

was not unholistic and anti-Hahnemannian heresy as it was seen by purists at the time, but a profoundly insightful and pragmatic reality which could be harnessed into practice. It enriched homeopathy when used well. Likewise, he had great respect for the plant and mineral remedies of Paracelsus, and also for the old plant remedies of English herbalism (Morrell 2000).

Therefore Rademacher's principles, plus his understanding of Paracelsus, supported his empirical observations enabled Burnett to argue that the physical organs were the seat of disease, often creating symptoms seen and felt elsewhere in the body 'through sympathetic affections of the strangest nature'. As with Hahnemann, Rademacher did not seek the nature of these diseases in the 'invisible interior of the organism', but rather identified them by similitude to their remedial substance - a Celandine liver disease, a Carduus mariae liver disease, etc. - in other words a true homeopathic diagnosis in the Hahnemann / Bönninghausen tradition. Remedies were selected based on their affinity for the organ in which the disease was thought to reside, and differentiated further on the basis of the genus of the disease.

For Burnett, Drysdale's concept of 'specificity of seat' made perfect sense, and he used this term and concept liberally in his writings. However specificity of seat of a remedy and the Organopathic concept of organ-specific remedies for diseases 'of the organs' seemed to stand in conflict with the homeopathic understanding of disease originating in the dynamic plane, and of remedies acting on the dynamis, rather than on specific tissues of the body. There was strong criticism. But Burnett rationalized it in this way in *Diseases of the Liver* (Taylor (2001a).

That the organ in the organism does indeed possess not

only autonomy but hegemony, i.e. the organ is an independent state in itself and in and on the organism exercises an important influence (Burnett, Diseases of the Liver).

The medicinal disease of *Lycopodium* was explained in this way. Those natural diseases bearing similarity to *Lycopodium*, exist in the dynamis, and not really in the gut, the liver, or the right side of the body; yet these dynamic diseases preferentially *manifest* in these tissues. It would be difficult to describe *Lycopodium* without referring to its *specificity of seat* in the gut, the biliary tree and the right side of the body. It would be difficult to prescribe this remedy in a case where disharmony was not expressed in these localities.

Or take *Ledum, Rhododendron,* and *Kalmia,* three members of the botanical family Ericaceae. These remedies display a strong specificity of seat for rheumatic affections of the joints, synovial tissues and connective tissues of the body, seen in the prominence of symptoms in the Head Pain, Back, Extremities and Extremities Pain sections of the repertory (Taylor 2011).

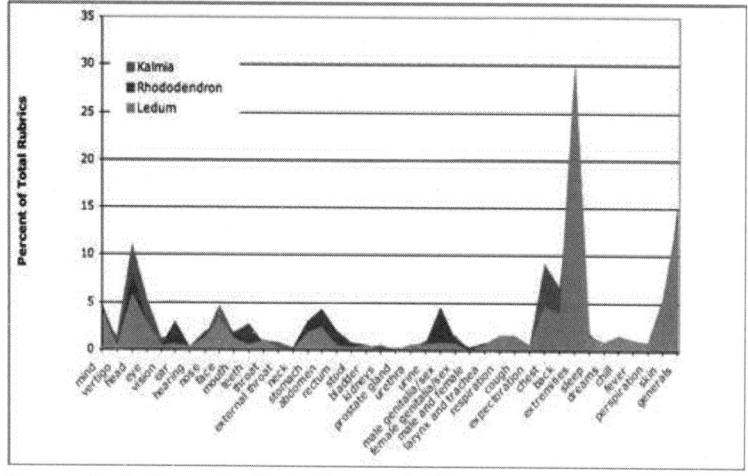

Source: RadarOpus, *Synthesis Treasure Edition 2009,* Frederik Schroyens. Design: Marci Mearns

Or consider *Uva-ursi, Oxydendron, Epigea* and *Chimaphilla*, four other members of the botanical family Ericaceae. For these remedies, a strong specificity of seat is demonstrated for the urinary tract, with a preponderance of symptoms in the Bladder, Kidney, Prostate, Urethra and Urine sections of the Repertory. These rubric extractions are inspired from Will Taylor's articles in the *www.wholehealthnow* website. They demonstrate various remedy organ affinities, from straightforward rubric extractions from Radar Opus.

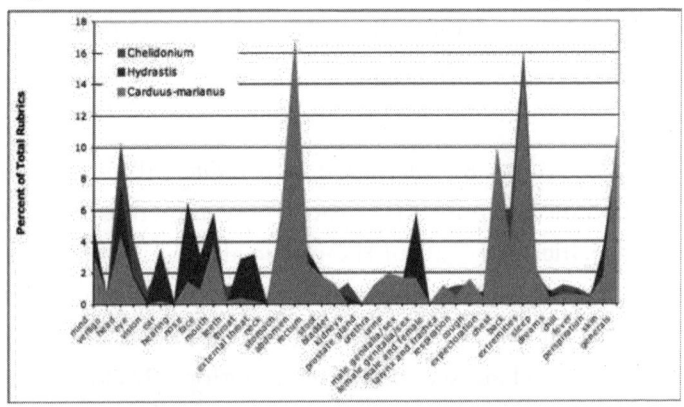

Source: RadarOpus, Synthesis Treasure Edition 2009, Frederik Schroyens. Design: Marci Mearns

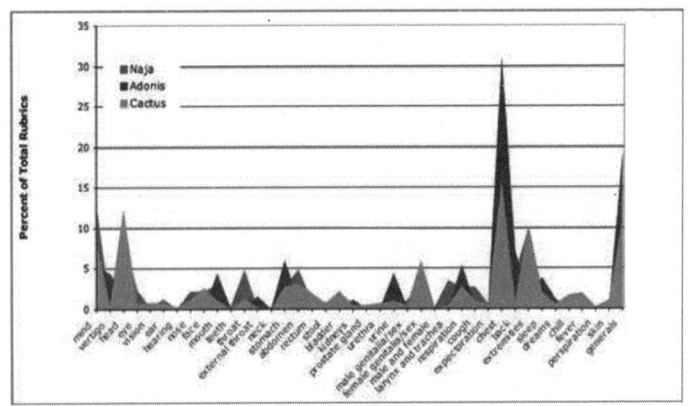

Source: RadarOpus, Synthesis Treasure Edition 2009, Frederik Schroyens. Design: Marci Mearns

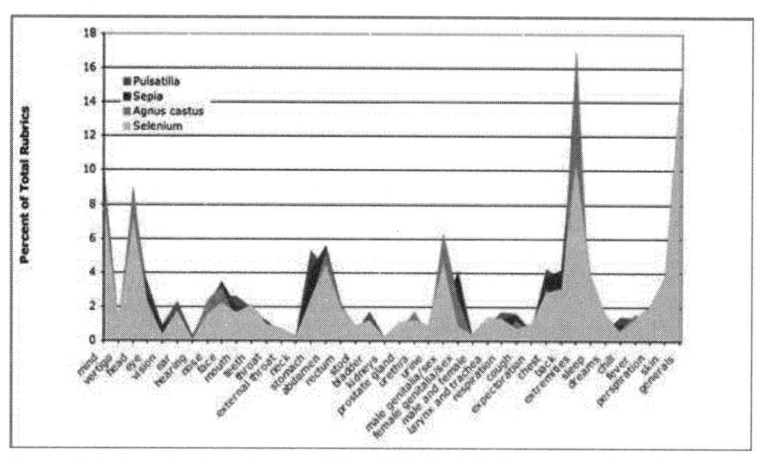

Source: RadarOpus, Synthesis Treasure Edition 2009, Frederik Schroyens. Design: Marci Mearns

Locality

Provings demonstrate, experience teaches us and simple rubric extractions show us that remedies have affinities for parts of the body. Lycopodium is described as a 'liver' remedy, and Naja a 'valve' remedy. In the proving of mosquito in 2002 in Sydney a startling proportion of symptoms were located in the lips. This is a statistical reality from the provings and from the results in the clinic. But the significance of this emphasis on Locality is that the simillimum needs to cover the whole pathology of the case, not merely match the superficial symptom-expression. Taylor expands,

> Hahnemann's aphorism 7 '... it must be the symptoms alone by which the disease demands and can point to the appropriate medicine for its relief ...'

This is not to suggest that these remedies act directly *on* or *through* those tissues - but rather that the disharmonies with which these remedies are associated manifest preferentially in these localities. And this allows us to have a purely homeopathic perspective on Burnett's "organ remedies". *Chelidonium* is not really a remedy that acts on the body *through the liver*, but a remedy whose dynamic disharmony expresses preferentially in (whose specificity of seat is in) the liver and biliary tree. In his *Diseases of the Spleen*, Burnett suggested so much when, he wrote:

I am not maintaining that treating an organ affection by an organ remedy after the manner of Hohenheim, Rademacher and their respective co-doctrinaires, will stand as a medical system in itself, but that it is eminently workable, and is largely of the nature of elementary homoeopathy, is, in fact, specificity of seat…

Rademacher's organopathy (that an otherwise able modern writer appropriates with child-like naivete) is no more and no less than the homoeopathic specificity of seat, with just a dash of a mystic psychic something in the several organs; if we set aside this little particular soul for each organ, it is only local affinity, or elective affinity. And it is quite true in nature, and the mind that cannot, or will not, recognize it, is wanting in catholicity of perception; and in practice will often go a mile when three paces would have reached the goal. Whatever else *Cantharis* may be, it is first and foremost a kidney medicine; whatever else *Digitalis* may be, it is primarily a heart medicine; and let *Belladonna* be what it may, it is before all things an artery medicine, and just in this sense *Ceanothus americanus* is a spleen medicine."

In this manner, Burnett characterized groups of remedies he considered to bear 'specificity of seat' in a variety of organs and tissues in the body. His 'liver remedies' included *Chelidonium, Carduus mariae, Leptandra virginica, Cholesterinum, Myrica cerifera, Chelone glabra, Quassia, Crocus sativus* and *Podophyllum*. Burnett's

'Spleen remedies' included *Ceanothus americanus, Squilla maritima, Quercus, Juniperus communis, Oleum succinum, Conium maculatum, Magnesium tartaricum, Rubia tinctorum* and *Urtica urens*.

The significance of this emphasis on Locality is that the similliumum needs to cover the pathology of the case, not just match the superficial symptom expression. This is not at variance with Hahnemann's aphorism 7 ('... it must be the symptoms alone by which the disease demands and can point to the appropriate medicine for its relief ...'). Rather, it demands only that we fully observe the signs and symptoms of disease in the case at hand. In Burnett's words,

Homoeopathy may be said to be based upon organopathy, for a drug to cure the heart of its disease specifically must necessarily affect the heart in some manner. But the homoeopath specializes, and says further: The drug that is to cure the heart must affect the heart, certainly - that is one of the foundations of our whole therapeutic edifice, but that is not enough; the nosological organopathy and the therapeutic organopathy must be and are similar. And in as much as we can know disease only by its subjective and objective symptoms (its language), it follows that the two organopathies must be symptomatically alike ...

...but to be curative the natural disease of the organ (nosological organopathy) must be like in expression to the therapeutic organopathy or drug-action. (Burnett, Diseases of the Spleen) "Experience teaches me that if we are to avoid false issues in treatment we must start with diagnosing, if possible, where the malady is primarily located. At any rate, I find this the shortest way to curing. If this be neglected we not infrequently cover and cure the symptoms, leaving the malady itself more or less untouched. (Burnett in Taylor 2001a)

A close reading of his works therefore identifies these theoretical underpinnings to the practical application of his homeopathy. So for Burnett,

1. The organ in the organism does possess not only 'autonomy but also hegemony', i.e. the organ is an independent state in itself and in and on the organism exercises an important influence.
2. Imbalance in the organ results in disease of the organism.
3. That the organ-to-organ homoeopathy of Paracelcus is a scientific fact (Burnett Diseases of the Liver in Taylor 2001a).

With this premise, a diagnosis is needed from "recognition of the primary seat of the disease". Each organ can be made ill by the organism, but, in its turn, it can make the organism ill. Then as the strength of the chain is that of its *weakest link*, similarly, the value of a person's life may be equal to that of his *weakest vital organ*; here the particular vital organ is equal in importance to that of the entire organism. Thus when treating the organism, it is important to relieve the weakest organ first.

Burnett did not claim originality of the concept of 'organopathy', but attributes it to Paracelsus (in Medicina paracelsica), and then rediscovered by Rademacher in the early 19th century. Remedies owning a quality to affect certain parts of the body specifically are its *Appropriata* (Burnett 1893).

In order to understand the nuance expressed here, and to understand the argument that what Burnett was suggesting and practicing was fully in keeping with the principles of homeopathy and not allopathic. Burnett was in constant conflict with homeopaths at the time who that heard or read his ideas and dismissed them as a bastardisation of homeopathy (Taylor 2001a).

The Limitations of the 'Totality of Symptoms'

Will Taylor describes it well (2001a). Burnett took the law of similars as the fundamental guide for his treatment but he had a flexible attitude towards its application because he felt Hahnemann was too rigid in imposing the totality of characteristic symptoms as the only means for making a prescription. This is not to far from the radical shake up proposed by Scholten and Sankaran more recently. Even though there were different kinds of similarity. Burnett felt some were of greater value than others so he classified similarity into three categories:

1. Pathologic simillimum where the drug matched the actual disease process.
2. Simple symptomatic simillimum which corresponded to the totality of characteristic symptoms, and
3. Simple simile, a remedy that had a limited and superficial similarity to a number of symptoms.

For a cure to occur, the following four types of action must be taken into consideration, and are central to Burnett's ideas:

What is It?	Considerations
1. The Seat of Action	
This refers to matching the centre/origin of the disease and the action of the remedy. The location must be attended to and covered by the prescription. Matching the symptomatology itself is often insufficient to cure a disease, but matching the *seat* is of the utmost importance.	Firstly the *Seat of Action*. How do drugs affect certain organs? A homoeopath considers a remedy by comparing symptoms of disease and symptoms of the drug. The drug that corresponds nearest to the manifestations of the disease (picture) is chosen as remedy. The Organopath however considers the morbid anatomy of drug action and its resemblance with the anatomy of the disease (drug picture). The drug that causes a certain pattern in a specific organ is chosen as remedy for similar disease picture. These two concepts are subjectively and objectively similar. *By comparing the symptoms of the disease and of the* *drug that symptomatically corresponds nearest to the manifestations of the disease, that drug is the presumptive remedy for the case..."* (Burnett, *Curability of Tumours*) For example, on a morbid anatomy level, the effect of Phosphorus on the lungs causes pulmonary lesions like those found in pneumonia and phthisis (pulmonary TB). The organopath cannot choose which remedy to use in pulmonary disease unless they have clinical knowledge of the disease and the effect of Phosphorus on the lung tissue. The morbid anatomy of phosphorism resembles the morbid anatomy of the disease. This is where Burnett's thorough knowledge of anatomy is really noted.

2. The Kind of Action	
What is it?	**Considerations**
This refers to how remedies affect certain organs parts specifically and what is the quality of such action e.g. inflammation of the stomach and ulceration of the stomach may produce two very similar subjective symptom pictures i.e. vomiting, pain, nausea, sweating etc. Burnett contends that if we know the patient's pathology and have an equally good understanding of our medicines true pathogenic qualities then the choice becomes easier.	Symptoms of a drug and symptoms of the disease must be like one another *"A remedy must not only affect the same part as the disease by special elective affinity, but the symptoms of drug and the symptoms of disease must be like one another..."*. Symptomatic degrees of the kind of action are varied and extensive.
3. The Range of Action	
This refers to the action from end to end of the affection. It is not enough to work out the homeopathic equation *symptomatically*. What is the cause/origin of the disease? If a pneumonia is caused by a nail getting into the lung and causes distress of breathing, cough, bloody expectoration etc. *phosphorus* is selected by the symptomatology and relieves the 'nail pneumonia'. However the *causation* of the nail is not removed and the *phosphorus* will not cure because the *range* of action is not matched.	The *Range of Action* is to be observed, taking into consideration what part (or depth) of the disease will the drug affect? In the example of Phosphorus, it will cure the symptoms of pneumonia, but it will not destroy the bacterium that caused it, so therein lies the range of action of Phosphorus. Here a new remedy can now be chosen due to removal of symptoms (pneumonia symptoms) and the next layer is found accordingly based on "new" symptoms, or the next layer of disease.
4. The Stop – Spot of Action	
This refers to that spot in the morbid process beyond which a remedy cannot go. Burnett illustrated the importance of identifying the stop-spot by a case of congestion of the brain. The symptomatology suggested *Belladonna*, it gave relief to the patient in repeated attacks – but it failed and the patient died (Curability of Tumours p.7-14)	This is that spot in the morbid process beyond which the remedy cannot reach further. Consideration into this is important because it can mean the difference between cure and psuedo-cure. Constant removal of the symptoms by a remedy that has reached a stop spot will not cure a patient. Using the example of Phosphorus, its stop spot is where the bacteria is left and must be removed by another means because the Phosphorus does not have the capability to do so (Taylor 2001a).

"To really cure a disease, one must affect the same or similar part as the disease; it must affect it in a similar manner and moreover the range of drug action must be co-extensive with the disease action"

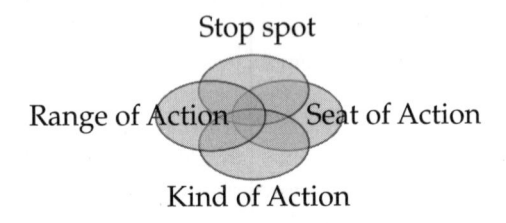

Stop spot

Range of Action — Seat of Action

Kind of Action

Drilling Deeper: Burnett's Influences

Drysdale

Drysdale (1816-1890) had qualified at Edinburgh and spent several years in European medical schools before settling in Liverpool, where his successes in the cholera epidemic of 1849 had so 'roused the envy of his allopathic colleagues' that he was forthwith 'expelled from the Liverpool Medical Institute' (Clarke's Life of Burnett, 1902). Richard Hughes wrote, in *A Manual of Pharmacodynamics*:

> Dr. Drysdale also has laid much stress on what he calls "specificity of seat," connecting it with the special irritability displayed by the various parts for their natural stimuli and for causes of disease, and extending it to the minutest localities or nerve-branches which have anything independent and special about them (Taylor 2001a).

Scheussler

Morrell (2000) says of Wilhelm Schuessler (1821-1898) that he is, often dismissed as a failed homeopath, polypharmacist, traitor to Hahnemann, and mongrel low-dilutionist. He studied in Berlin and Paris, founded the 'biochemic system', an ideological offshoot of homeopathy, which concentrates on cellular activity only and ignores mental symptoms and generals, and thus comes close to the pathology of low potency homeopaths like Hughes. He published the *New Treatment of Disease, Abridged Therapeutics Founded upon Histology and Cellular Pathology* giving the indications for the application of the inorganic cell salts and indications of the underlying conditions of morbid states of tissues, the 'biochemic method' of treating disease. This was also articulated in *The Biochemical Treatment of Disease, and Biochemic Pocket Guide* and the *Tissue Salts* in 1875. Typical of the period, his cell salts were prepared in 3x or 6x potencies.

Rademacher and the Organ Remedies

Another influence on Burnett was Johann Gottfried Rademacher (1772-1850) born in Germany. He was an observer, follower and admirer of Paracelsus but was not a homeopath. His main work was *The Universal and Organ Remedies*, published in Berlin, 2 volumes of 800 pages each in 1841. The full title of his work was *Rechtfertigung der von den Gelehrten misskannten, verstandes rechten Erfahringsheillehre der alten scheidenkunstigen Geheimarzte, und treue Mittheilung des Ergebnisses einer 25-jahrigen Erprobung dieser Lehre am Krankenbette* – 'Justification of the empiric medical practice of the old alchemistic physician, misjudged by the learned, yet perfectly rational ...'. Rademacher based his work on his own empirical observations, which he supported by the writings of Theophrastus Bombast von Hohenheim (Paracelsus), the 16th-century Swiss alchemist and physician. Many of Rademacher's remedies were introduced to homeopathic practice, or saw homeopathic applications inspired by their organopathic uses via Burnett. His work looked at the idea of correspondences and signatures between organs and the disease states of the body and argued that by treating organs one was able to treat the disease.

The reason why homoeopathy swallowed up organopathy lies in the fact that homoeopathy is organopathy and something else besides, viz.: the differentiating law of similars (Burnett 1898).

Rademacher was a practitioner in the small city of Goch on the Rhine. He never believed fully in Hahnemann's ideas, but instead adopted the doctrines of Paracelsus, making clinical experiments in search of specifics. About 1840 he published his *Vindication by Experience of the Ancient Chymical Physician's Art of Healing, misapprehended by the Learned, with Truthful Results of Clinical Tests made during a Practice of twenty-five Years.* He argued that

(1) There were three primordial diseases of the whole organism and which may be cured by three universal remedies, Natrum nitricum, Cuprum and Ferrum.

(2) There were primordial diseases of single organs which may be cured by organic remedies, and he designated certain remedies for each respective organ, e.g., pulmonary remedies, stomach remedies, kidney remedies, etc. If the consensual diseases of organs last a long time they become changed into primordial diseases and require the specific organic remedies. A universal and a disease of a single organ may exist at the same time, in which case the cure must be

effected by a universal in connection with an organic remedy (Puhlman 1880, Tyler 1927, Yasgur 1994).

Burnett's Cases

A case from Burnett's *Diseases of the Spleen* quoted in Taylor (2001a) provides an excellent illustration:

> ... I was at the house of a patient in London, the wife of a general officer and the conversation fell upon the general's heart affection, and also upon that of their char-woman. I learned that the lady of the house took a certain interest in her charwoman because she had seen better days and had an invalid husband depending on her labor more or less.
>
> This charwoman was, it was said, suffering from an incurable disease of the heart, causing her terrible distress; on rising in the morning she would have to fight for her breath, so that it would take her often three-quarters of an hour to get dressed, having to pause and rest from the dyspnoea and its effects, nevertheless she persisted in thus getting up and dressing, and did as much charing as she could get. Her pride would not allow her to beg of her friends. Such was the story, and I really felt curious to see the charwoman, and promised to do what I could, though from the account given me by the general's wife, I certainly thought it quite a hopeless case.
>
> Calling a few days later, I saw the lady and the charwoman, and having duly examined the latter, I promised to cure her! She was to come to my city rooms, and report herself every fortnight. On returning from the bedroom to the drawing room, the general's wife accused me of cruelty in thus raising the poor old woman's hopes "when," exclaimed she, "you must know it is impossible."

I tried to explain that it was a case of enlarged spleen, and not the heart disease at all, that the charwoman was suffering from, and that the palpitations and fightings for breath were the mechanical sequels of the splenic engorgement, but my patient evidently did not believe it, for she wound up by saying, '.As you will treat her for nothing, I hope you may succeed, and it is very kind of you, but you must know that the poor woman has been under various doctors, and all have declared it incurable heart disease, and I merely wanted you to tell me of something to relieve and ease the poor old thing."

This was towards the middle of October. A careful physical examination showed that the heart-sounds were normal, but there was much beating visible in the neck, arid the heart's action was labored. In the left hypochondrium there was a mass corresponding to the position of the spleen, and a dull percussion note was elicited not only in the left hypochondrium, but also in the right, and all across the epigastrium, or pit of the stomach, from side to side.

The following notes were put down at the time: "Heart-sounds, normal; apex beat, exaggerated; splenetic dullness extending up to the left mamma; the whole region very tender, so much so that she cannot bear her clothes or any other pressure." The prescription was: Ceanothus Americanus 1x 3ij, five drops in water three times a day.

November 14. Has been taking the Ceanothus five weeks today, and has taken altogether three bottles of it, viz., 3vj. It has nearly stopped the pain in the left side, which had lasted for quite twenty-five years. This pain came on suddenly, especially if she drank anything cold. She would get an indescribable pain under the left ribs, and she would have to fight for breath, and the dyspnoea would be so severe that it could be heard in the next room, frightening everybody. She had ague thirty years ago in Northamptonshire. Repeat.

November 29. Not much pain left; the cold feeling still there, but nothing as it was. Repeat.

December 20. Has the pain in the left side, but very little; has not had any of those attacks of fighting for breath; she can walk better, and the side is much smaller, which she knows from her dress. In her own opinion she is less in the waist by two inches. Before taking the medicine, for very many years she was compelled to pause in the morning when dressing, and lie down on account of the beating of the heart, but this has all gone; on examining by palpation and percussion I find the dullness diminished by four inches in the perpendicular, and by about the same from side to side.

However, there is still some tenderness on pressure, and the swelled spleen can still be felt towards the median line and inferiorly. She can now do her work (charing) very much better. R. Tr. Ceanoth-Am. 1, four drops in water three times a day.

January 10. The pain is gone; has now no pain in walking, and she is a great deal stronger and better. The coldness in the pit of the stomach has gone. Repeat.

February 7. In the left hypochondrium there is now nothing abnormal; the old ague-cake has disappeared, there being no dull percussion note. Her own conception of the size of that portion of the enlarged spleen that used to stretch across the pit of the stomach to the liver is thus expressed by her: "I used to say it was as big as a half-quartern loaf." Not only is the lump gone, but she is much stronger; she now wears stays again, and fastens her clothes with comfort. She again gets some cold feeling in the pit of the stomach, but not much.

Her Liver seems considerably enlarged, and there is still too much beating of the blood-vessels (Veins) in the neck. In my opinion the condition of the blood-vessels calls for Ferrum 6, which I now -prescribe, and when that has done its duty-as it surely will - the liver will call for attention. But what I wanted to bring out was the specific affinity of Ceanothus Americanus for the spleen, and its consequent brilliant effects, as the simile only grounded on the homoeopathic specificity of seat, which some say has no existence.

This poor woman thus took Ceanothus during about four months in small appreciable doses: at first the 1x and then the 1 centesimal. The existence of the hypertrophy was ascertained by percussion and palpation; and subsequently I ascertained by the same means that it had ceased to exist. Although patient took the drug for four months I could not find that it affected any other organ-liver, kidney, bowel - save and except the spleen.

The dyspnoea and palpitation were cured certainly, but these arose, I submit, from the engorged condition of the spleen itself.

As far as I could ascertain, the secretions and excretions were not affected in the least degree; the remedial action must, therefore, be considered specific. My conception of the cure is simply this, that the specific Ceanothus stimulus persistently applied restored the spleen tissue to the normal. This homoeopathic specificity of seat suffices only in simple local disturbances; it is only a simile, not a simillimum. The latter would, I apprehend, have affected the liver also and the right heart, and I should then not have needed further detail treatment.

This charwoman continued to attend at my rooms for some months, and Ceanothus Americanus and other indicated remedies cured her of her "incurable heart disease;" and I saw no more of her for some time, when one day she was ushered into my consulting room. She came up to where I was sitting, told me she was perfectly well, could do any work with ease, and-then occurred one of the sweetest things in my whole professional life - the old lady (and what a lady!) put a tiny packet on my desk, tried to say something, burst into tears, and rushed out!

I never saw her again, and have often since wished I had kept that particular sovereign and had it set in diamonds.

In this case, the apparently peculiar symptoms originally attributed to heart disease are fully explainable as merely resulting from mammoth splenomegaly. As such, these symptoms lose their aphorism 153 status as characterizing symptoms, and the only symptoms of genuine note remaining in the case are "massive splenomegaly" and "splenic pain worse pressure (of clothes, etc.)".

The rubric (Abdomen - Enlarged - Spleen) lists 61 remedies in the Quantum view of the Synthesis Repertory (Kent listed 51), with *Ceanothus, China* and *Iodium* in boldtype. (Abdomen - Pain - pressing - Spleen - pressure agg.) lists only *Ceanothus* and *Zincum*. (Abdomen - Pain - Spleen - lying on left side, while) lists *Agar, Cean, Cocc* and *Colch*.

We find in Hering, for Ceanothus, "Enlarged spleen, extending to within an inch of crest of ilium, with severe pain in side." - the only remedy in our materia medica described for such massive enlargement of the spleen, and one of our remedies with a primary "specificity of seat" for the spleen.

Here an 'organopathic' remedy is indicated - not because Burnett made a decision to abandon Hahnemann and resort to organopathy, but because the focal involvement of a particular tissue - a locality - was overwhelmingly the most characterizing feature of the case (Taylor 2001a).

Burnett's Use of Potency

His reputation was for low potencies, but if we take every potency mentioned in, say, Burnett's *'Cure of Consumption'* (1890) we find that he used quite a diverse range of high and low potencies, especially when compared to his contemporaries.

Burnett prefers some higher potencies, occasionally going very high, mainly for nosodes. Only 50.1% of his prescribing is covered by potencies of 3x and lower, and 25% is covered by potencies 6, 12 and 30. The commonest potency he uses is 30 with 18 [20.5%] out of 88 in the whole book; this is followed by 15 at 3x which is 17%; 14 mother tinctures which is 16%, and 13 of 100 potency, which is 13%. The highest potency used is 10M which figures twice in the book (Morrell 2000).

In the case of organ remedies, small material doses act best – indeed brilliantly, such remedies need to be repeated at short intervals. On the contrary, organ hypertrophies from constitutional causes are not curable by the organ remedies at all until the constitutional disease has been cured by infrequently repeated high dilutions of the remedies closely homoeopathic.

I maintain that organopathy is just elementary homoeopathy, the degree of similitude being very small, wherefore small material doses are needed in fairly frequent repetition. As the degree of similitude increases so must the dose of the remedy be lessened. (Burnett 1896)

...the smaller the degree of similitude the lower the dose and the more frequent the repetitions of the dose. My own range of dose is from a few globules of the 200th dilution at eight day intervals down to 10 drops of the mother tincture four times a day (Burnett 1888).

The Organ Remedies

Adapted from Burnett and Ian Watson   Ø = Mother Tincture

Brain and Nervous System	Avena sat Ø	Kali phos 6x	Hyp 6 -cm
Heart	Strophanthus Ø	Cactus Ø	Crat Ø
	Adonis Ø	Convallaria Ø	
Valves	Spongia 6	Naja 6	
Digestion	Alfal Ø	Hydrastis Ø	
Liver	Card mar Ø	Chel Ø – 3x	Taraxicum Ø
	Cholst 6x – 200	Hydrastis Ø – 6x	Mag mur 6
and Gall Bladder			
Spleen	Ceanothus Ø	Quercus Ø	
Urinary	Berb Ø	Urva usi Ø	
Kidneys	Berb Ø	Solidago Ø	
Bladder	Equis Ø	Triticum Ø	
Breast	Phyt Ø - cm		
Uterus	Helon Ø	Caul 6 - cm	Frax Ø
Ovaries	Foll 4 – 9	Ooph 30	
Male	Ag cast Ø	Sel 6	Cal 6
	Chim 6		
Prostate	Sabal 3x	Thuj 6x	Con 6
	Puls 6	Ferrum pic 6	
Blood toxicity	Gunpowder 6	Echin Ø	Pyrog 6
	Bapt 3		
Veins	Vip 30	Hamm Ø	Puls 6
	Calc flour 12		
Arteries	Crat Ø	Bar mur 6	
Skin	Lappa arct Ø	Berb aqu Ø	Skook 3x
Bones	Symph Ø	Calc phos 6x	Hekla I 6
	Phos 6		
Endocrine Pituitary	Pit 6	Bar carb 30	
Thyroid	Fucus ves 3x	Iodum 6 – 30	Thyroid 6
Adrenals	Adr gland 6	Adrenalin 6	
Pancreas	Phos 6	Iris vers 6x	

Random Gems from Burnett, Rademacher and Others

Alcoholism	Spiritus glandium quercus. I thought we might find in our common acorns a notable homoeopathic anti-alcoholic. (Burnett 1895).
Remedies acting upon liver and spleen	Semen cardui mariae (*carduus marianus*) it is excellent in the sympathetic spitting of blood which not seldom accompanies chronic hepatic and splenic troubles.
Nux vomica	Rademacher used this remedy from 1816 to 1819 with much success in diseases of the liver, which appeared either as jaundice or as bilious fevers.
Other spleen remedies	*Galiopsis grandiflora, Rubia tinctorum, Juniper berries, oil of amber*, which is excellent in painful spleen affections, accompanied by hysterical cramps.
Shepherd's purse	Excellent in chronic diarrhoea
Gravel and renal stones	*Magnesia* or *lime water* are excellent remedies for renal calculi.
Thrush of children	*Borax* is the best remedy.
Skin remedies	*Copper* is a good remedy for some cutaneous diseases, as has been seen. *Carbonate of copper* made into a salve with wax removes warts and other vegetations of this kind.

Ash leaves (folia fraxini)	Proved very beneficial in arthritic pains, in podagra and in rheumatism of the external parts of the head; one ounce of the leaves are steeped half an hour in hot water and the infusion is drunk during the day.
Digitalis salve	(Unguent cerae 3i, Extr. *Digitalis* 3ii) rubbed on inflamed joints or limbs in rheumatism, or even in sciatica, wonderfully allays the pains in a very short time.
Rademacher's liver medicines	*Quassia, Chelidonium, Liquor calc. mur., Nux vom., Crocus, and Carduus* (Burnett 1891).
Gallstones:	*Carduus* in the attacks of gallstone colic he recommends from 15 to 30 drops in a teacupful of water or milk five times a day (Burnett 1891).
Iodine	I have used it in tumours of the pancreas with striking effect (Burnett 1888).
Carduus marianus	Haemorrhages, especially connected with hepatic disease. Nose-bleed. Gallstone disease with enlarged liver.
Quercus robur glandium spiritus	Chronic spleen affections; spleen-dropsy.
Zincum metallicum	Effects of night-watching and erysipelas; brain feels sore (Boericke 1927).

Carduus marianus	Pains in left hypochondrium are apt to vomit blood, after which they are relieved.
Solidago virgaurea	"This herb," says Rademacher, "is a very old and good kidney medicine.
Squilla	Rademacher also mentions those so-called "stomach pains" that are made much better by lying on the left side, and probably in reality splenic.
Terebinthinae oleum	Stricture of urethra (Clarke 1900).
Natrium nitricum	A remedy in inflammations. (Hansen 1898).
Zincum aceticum	Rademacher professes to have cured Mania, with diarrhoea.
Cochineal	Kidney remedies (Hempel 1864).
Chelidonium	Par excellence a liver remedy.
Ceanothus	Which chooses the spleen for its action, malign and benign.
Crataegus, Digitalis	These pick out the heart (Tyler 1938).
Pancreatitis	Of the diseases of the pancreas, the only one I can specify is simple inflammation of its substance ... and states that its "organ-remedy" is Iodine (Hughes 1869).

Nosodes

Like most of his contemporaries, he also made extensive use of the newly introduced nosodes, like his own *Bacillinum*, prepared from tuberculous sputum (Allen 1910). These nosodes were used in the 30, 200 and 1M potencies, widely spaced. He swiftly became famous as a doctor who could cure tumours and was reckoned in his obituary in the (Westminster Gazette 1901) to have the largest consulting practice in London. He also introduced to homeopathy many nosodes,

- *Bacillinum testium*
- *Coqueluchinum*
- *Carcinosinum*
- *Epihysterinum*
- *Ergotinum*
- *Morbillinum*
- *Schirrinum*
- *Influenzinum* (Allen 1910).

For and Against

Watson (1991) argued that organ support remedies should be used more widely than they were. He cited the considerable advantages. There are many patients whose entire symptom pictures and pathological processes revolve around the dysfunction of a particular organ. In these cases, the organ weakness may present as an obstacle to the cure, and often it will be found that the indicated constitutional remedy is ineffective until the weakness is rectified. There is some significant clinical evidence to support this theory because so often when an organ remedy is given to patients it will act as if it were a medicine for the whole chronic disease because all of the symptoms of the patient improve significantly.

Furthermore, in some cases, prescribing from this perspective provides an unexpected advantage because patients are used to and often expect a homeopath to discuss with them the site of the problem, the organ that is not functioning properly and so it makes perfect sense to them. Compliance is maintained when you are able to hand them a bottle of medicine which is for a specific problem from their allopathic biomedical perspective. It kills two birds with one stone, and avoids all of the awkwardness of trying to explain the totality of symptoms.

Watson further argued that there were significant advantages because aggravations were reduced. In his experience, all the aggravations following on from constitutional prescriptions could be avoided altogether by the judicious use of organ support remedies. This is a well-made point as we have time after time seen significant aggravations from high potencies used too often in some patients, causing unnecessary suffering, which is far from the advocated rapid, permanent and gentle directives of Hahnemann.

There are other advantages also. One of the attitudes that one has to shift when using this style of prescribing is that there is a possibility of suppressing the vital force of the patient and making the patient worse by focusing on these perceived external aspects of the case. As Watson (1991) argued, and I concur from my own experience of prescribing in Australia, this anxiety about suppression is simply not borne out in practice as most patients feel better in themselves, their energy becomes freed up, they start to sleep better or have more energy, all before receiving any treatment for their chronic condition. Over and over in the treatment of complicated cases where there are issues caused by lifestyle, medical or recreational drug use, I have used organ-orientated prescriptions at the beginning of treatment with the intention of facilitating a more complete symptom picture appearing. Clarity replaces cloudiness with changes noted over a period of days, weeks or months after a prescription taken daily that is orientated to the organ or the seat of the disease. While always aspiring to a prescription based on the broadest and largest totality of symptoms, it is not always possible. Homeopaths around the world know what it is like to take a case, analyse the case, and not be able to decide between one of a number of well-known remedies. This is a daily working reality in practice, and from experience, many homeopaths conclude that best practice is to restrict the working totality and begin with an organ prescription until the case becomes much clearer.

Computers and Burnett

These days with computer software available, it is very simple with a few clicks of a button to be able to understand the organ affinities of any homeopathic remedy. A rubric extraction will quickly and easily tell you at a glance the organ affinities of every remedy.

Burnett's Works

1878:	Natrum Mur As a Test of The Doctrine of Drug Dynamisation
1879:	Gold As a Remedy In Disease
1880:	Curability Of Cataracts With Medicines
1880:	On The Prevention Of Hare-Lip, Cleft Palate, And Other Congenital Defects
1881:	Ecce Medicus, or Hahnemann As a Physician
1881:	The Medicinal Treatment of Diseases Of The Veins
1882:	Supersalinity of The Blood
1885:	Valvular Disease of The Heart From a New Standpoint
1886:	Diseases of The Skin From The Organismic Standpoint (Second edition In 1893 with the title, Diseases of The Skin: Their Constitutional Nature And Cure)
1887:	Diseases of The Spleen
1888:	Fevers And Blood Poisoning, And Their Treatment With Special Reference To The Use of Pyrogenium
1888:	Tumours of The Breast and Their Cure
1888:	Fifty Reasons For Being a Homeopath
1889:	Cataract Its Nature and Cure
1889:	On Fistula and Its Radical Cure By Medicines
1889:	On Neuralgia: Its Causes and Remedies
1890:	Consumption and Its Cure By Its Own Virus (this book was republished in 1894 as "Eight Years Experience In The New Cure of Consumption")
1891:	The Greater Diseases of The Liver
1892:	Ringworm: Its Constitutional Nature and Cure
1893:	Curability of Tumours
1895:	Delicate, Backward, Puny and Stunted Children
1895:	Gout and Its Cure
1896:	Organ Diseases of Women
1897:	Vaccinosis and Its Cure By Thuja
1898:	Change of Life In Women
1901:	Enlarged Tonsils Cured by Medicine

Conclusion

Burnett's extensive contributions to homeopathy include;

- The concept and practice of organopathy
- The extensive use of nosodes
- The treatment of chronic ill-effects of vaccination.

His writings and work offered a bridge between many different schools. With the precedent set by Paracelsus from whom the idea of the doctrine of signatures made its way into herbal medicine, alchemy and some medicine in the Enlightenment, (the idea that the plant shape, colour, habitat and other features indicated its use, such as eyebright, Liver wart, Knit bone, Lung wart, Chaste tree and Blood Root) Burnett married these ideas and the recent writings of Rademacher. Burnett proceeded on the assumption that remedies had specific affinities to certain organs. For some patients, it seems necessary to treat specific organs or systems of the body before treating the whole person or rallying the vitality of the patient to begin to respond to homeopathic remedies.

The technique itself involved prescribing low potencies or even mother tinctures. Watson (1991) advocated prescribing these low potencies and mother tinctures; five drops in a little water to be taken three times daily. He argued that if a patient has taken a mother tincture and experienced any new symptoms this could be a sign that the remedy was well indicated but that the dose was too much. A reduction in the amount prescribed generally produced the required curative response without any discomfort. Watson talked of several patients where they had felt queasy after taking *Crategus* mother tincture but they responded well when the dose was reduced subsequently from 5 to 2 drops. Watson preferred to prescribe an organ remedy before commencing treatment based on any larger totality of symptoms. It is known that some practitioners prefer to give the indicated constitutional medicine in a much higher potency, as well as the organ remedy in a mother tincture or low potency simultaneously. Watson rightly points out that any opportunities for learning about the action of those remedies are lost with two or more substances being active in the body at the same time. Nevertheless, from a practical point of view, it is understandable why a practitioner might need to speed things along.

At the outset however there was no shortage of controversy.

Our late colleague Dr. Sharp proposed (following in the footsteps of Paracelsus and Rademacher) to make seat of action instead of symptoms the basis of our method, which accordingly he would call "organopathy." That remedies so led to may prove effectual is undoubted: we have a good example of them in the ceanothus americanus, which, though never proved on the healthy, and only known to "act upon" the spleen, has been found strikingly effective in pains, enlargements, and other disorders of this organ. But we should never, if possible, rest content with identity of seat between disease and drug: we should aim also at making their kind of action the same, and this can only be done by securing similarity in their symptoms. In this way we elevate the simile to a simillimum, and proportionately enhance its energy in cure (Hughes 1902).

What is clear is that even Hahnemann relied on the information of some herbalists and organopathists. Rademacher is referenced in Hahnemann's work a number of times.

Nux vomica

- Sensation in the face as if innumerable ants were creeping

upon it. [Rademacher, Hufel. Journ.iv, p.573.]
- Objects appear brighter to look at than usual. [Rademacher, l.c.]
- Intolerable itching of the nose. [Rademacher, l.c.]
- It drew the mouth sideways. [Rademacher, l.c.]
- Locking of the jaws with full consciousness. [Rademacher, l.c.]
- Weakness and staggering of the legs, he must sit down. [Rademacher, l.c.] (Hahnemann 1830)

Opium
- Intoxication. [Rademacher, in Hufel. Jour., iv, 3, p.587. - Buchner, Diss. de Opio, Halae, 1748, ° 45.]
- Single twitches in the arms. [Rademacher, l.c.]
- During almost constant slumber, with half-shut eyelids, he has floccilation and feels all about him. [Rademacher, l.c.]
- Anxiety. [Rademacher, -Tralles, l.c.] (Hahnemann 1830).

Burnett juggled the issues with aplomb and at times argued his case with force. In a letter (Burnett 1880), he wrote:

> To the editors of "the organon." Gentlemen, - In your July number you accredit Dr. Sharp, F.R.S., of Rugby, with the discovery of Organopathy. Will you allow me to draw your attention to my paper on Organopathy read at the Malvern Homoeopathic Congress? You will observe that Dr. Sharp's claim is utterly and entirely without foundation, in as much as Loeffler developed the very same doctrine in almost identical words in 1847, he truly regarding it as a mere amplification of the teachings of Paracelsus, and of his disciple Rademacher, whereas Dr. Sharp, twenty years later, poses as a would-be founder of a new system of medicine with the very same material. Of course

Dr. Sharp abuses Paracelsus, and the gentle genial Rademacher, the latchets of whose shoes, etc. - I am, yours faithfully (Burnett 1880).

Further Reading

- Puhlman — *The History of Homoeopathy in Germany*
- Hahnemann — *Materia Medica Pura*
- Hughes — *A Manual of Therapeutics: According to the Method of Hahnemann*
- Hughes — *The Principles and Practice of Homoeopathy*
- Hempel — *A New and Comprehensive System of Materia Medica*
- Boericke — *Pocket Manual of Homeopathic Materia Medica*
- Clarke — *Dictionary of Practical Materia Medica*
- Hansen — *A Text-Book of Materia Medica and Therapeutics of Rare Homeopathic Remedies*
- Hering — *Guiding Symptoms of our Materia Medica*
- Burnett — *Greater Diseases of the Liver*
- Burnett — *Gout and its Cure*
- Burnett — *Tumours of the breast and their treatment and cure by medicines*

Chapter 13

Polypharmacy, Complexes and Combinations

Their beginning was promising, the continuation less favorable, the outcome hopeless. Samuel Hahnemann, Chronic Diseases

If our school ever gives up the strict inductive method of Hahnemann, we are lost, and deserve to be mentioned only as a caricature in the history of medicine. Constantine Hering, in his last address to the profession 1880

Contents

- Definitions
- Literature and Opinion
- Controversy, Mongrelism, Multilation and Perversion
- The Double Remedy Experiments of 1833
- The Technique Itself
- Why NO! Opinions Past and Present
- Contemporary Opposition
- Why Yes! Opinions - Past and Present
- Some Commonly Used Combinations
- When it is Best to Use Polypharmacy

In this chapter you will:

1. Explore the historical and philosophical reasons for the opposition to the method
2. Learn why some strongly advocate the practical, clinical and commercial advantages understand the components of the method
3. Learn about Hahnemann's changing opinion of the method

Chapter 13

Polypharmacy, Complexes and Combinations

Definitions

Yasgur (1994) defines Polypharmacy (Mixology, combination, complex homeopathy) as the administration of more than one remedy at a time either through giving a number of single remedies at the same time or giving a combination homeopathic product.

Literature and Opinion

Very little has aroused such hostility and opposition within homeopathic circles throughout the years as the use of combination remedies or polypharmacy. But there is very little good literature on the subject. In the last decade or so, Medhurst (1994, 2011) and Moskowitz (2011) have written articles that highlight the pragmatic realities and the value of combinations in some situations, and the philosophical opposition to the idea. In addition, David Little at *www.simillimum.com* has written extremely well on the historical controversy and I have quoted him extensively.

Controversy, Mongrelism, Multilation and Perversion

In my own training, the notion of prescribing a combination remedy filled me with horror. I was a good student imbued with the spirit of a single remedy. While I have not changed my view, at least now I understand the arguments, and can respect the judicious use of the occasional combination remedy in certain circumstances. I work in a private college providing degrees in natural medicine in Australia, Endeavour College of Natural Health, and one of the joys and dramas of that work, is to deal daily with non-homeopaths who have no idea, nor care about the nuances of homeopathic prescribing. As our marketing director once said to me with a quizzical look. 'Why don't you just put all the possibilities in a bottle and shake it?' It's a pragmatic approach to problem solving.

However, in the literature we see nothing but reactionary opinion. But actually, as is the case with isopathy and tautopathy, in the early days of homeopathy during the controversies of the 1820s and 1830s, there was broad experimentation. When the policy decisions were being made by Hahnemann and others about what was and what wasn't homeopathy, what was in and what was out, those decisions were mainly being made within the context of ignorant allopathic physicians not grounded in homeopathic method or theory giving frivolous and inappropriate prescriptions. Of course Hahnemann had to draw a line, and he drew it quite clearly - no combinations.

In the *American Homoeopathist* in 1897, Menninger wrote a passionate and a stirring article, *The Eradication of Mongrelism*:

> Nothing has done more to injure the prospects of

homoeopathy than polypharmacy, and nothing will more effectually kill homoeopathy. By polypharmacy we mean any mixture of remedial agents in the treatment of disease, and consequently alternation or rotation, whether of the same or different potencies, as well as that monstrosity, the compound tablet. How is it that in the face of such explicit directions from the founder of homoeopathy, so many have become infected with this blighting innovation? The fault is not all with the pharmacists, yet they have and are exerting a most baneful influence that will work harm to all concerned. They have prepared combinations of homoeopathic remedies in almost countless numbers, and have had the temerity to ask physicians to use them. They have the audacity to send traveling salesmen to all parts of the country, who urge physicians to use them, regardless of all proper indications. There has been an unexpressed feeling that this evil would soon be corrected through the silent protest and lack of patronage of the better class of homoeopathic physicians. It was a false hope and some decided steps should be taken by the profession at large, by the colleges and the teachers. We maintain that the chief cause for this advance of mongrelism is ignorance of how to do better than prescribe the compound tablet (Menninger 1897).

Strong stuff! I was having a conversation once with the historian and collector, Julian Winston, at his dining room table. Looking into the homeopathic library and his significant collection of remedies, books, articles, journals, pictures and other memorabilia was a beautiful print of a stained-glass window, which quite clearly had Samuel Hahnemann on one side. 'Who's the other guy?' I asked Julian. I fully expected it to be an unrecognisable version of Hering or Bönninghausen. 'Oh that's Lutze', says Julian. It was the first time I heard the name. Lutze clearly had a high opinion of himself in order to create such a stained-glass window, side by side with Hahnemann. Later when I wrote to him about it Julian replied:

> The guy in the window is Arthur Lutze who released (what he said was) a 6th edition of the Organon in which Hahnemann OK'd the use of combos. This was stopped by Melanie, and all copies were (as far as I know) withdrawn. The correspondence was with Count Aegidi and Hahnemann. Lutze was not aware that Ageidi stopped the practice after a number of trials. In Lutze book "The Family Advisor" or something like that. I am quite sure the whole thing is discussed in one of the chapters of Haehl's "Life of Hahnemann" set. JW.

The debate about combination remedies that occurred in Hahnemann's own lifetime is best summarized in a great article by Little (2000) *Following in Hahnemann's Footsteps: The Definitive Years 1833-1843* in the *American Homeopath* of 2000. In this article he highlights Hahnemann's own experiments and ultimately the clear policy decision that resulted from them.

The Double Remedy Experiments of 1833

> The method of combining two homoeopathic remedies in mixture originated with Dr. Aegidi, who forwarded Hahnemann 233 cases of his method. Aegidi found a confidant in Baron von Bönninghausen, who used his influence with the Founder to support the new method. The Hofrath was so impressed by the enthusiasm of his disciples that he promised to refer to the double remedies in the 5th Organon, even before trying them! He wrote from Coethen on June 15, 1833:

Do not think that I am capable of rejecting any good thing from mere prejudice, or because it might cause alterations in my doctrine. I only desire the truth, as I believe you do too. Hence I am delighted that such a happy idea has occurred to you, and that you have kept it within necessary limits; 'that two medicinal substances (in smallest doses or by olfaction) should be given together only in a case where both seem homoeopathically suitable to the case, but each from a different side.' Under such circumstances the procedure is so constant with the requirement of our art that nothing can be urged against it; on the contrary, homeopathy must be congratulated on your discovery (Hahnemann in Little 2000).

In other words, administering two remedies at a time was fine where there were two separate and distinguishable diseases.

Hahnemann had not yet tried Aegidi's method but he was very hopeful that it would prove a benefit to his new healing art. For this reason, he promised to take up testing the hypothesis in the clinic as soon as possible. His letter continues:

"I myself will take the first opportunity of putting it into practice, and I have no doubt concerning the good results. I think too, that both remedies should be given together; just as we take Sulphur and Calcarea together when we cause our patients to take or smell Hepar sulph, or Sulphur and Mercury when they take or smell Cinnabar. I am glad that von Boenninghausen is entirely of our opinion and acts accordingly. Permit me then, to give your discovery to the world in the fifth edition of the Organon which will soon be published."

He began his first experiments with the olfaction of a double remedy on June 17, 1833. What was the outcome of the Founder's four months of clinical trials? He wrote the following to Bönninghausen from Coethen, on October 16, 1833:

> "Easily your eloquence would have defeated me, if I were in the same case as you, that is, if I had already been as convinced by several and by so many experiences of the utility, even preference/superiority of the giving of a double remedy as you supposedly had been. But from several trials in this manner only one or two turned out well, which isn't sufficient for the apodictic [irrefutable] proposing of a new theorem." [Emphasis added]

Hahnemann's experiments with the double remedies proved a failure because they did not work as well as the single remedy. He was critical of the double remedies because he could see their limitations in the clinic. The second half of his letter to Bönninghausen offers more information about his conclusions:

> "I was therefore in this practice still too far behind to proceed with full conviction. Therefore it required only a slight moment to induce me to a change of these passages in the new Organon, which results in this, that I concede the possibility that two well-selected, different remedies can be given simultaneously [together] with advantage in some cases, but that this seemed to be a difficult and critical [serious/delicate] procedure." [Translation from the German by Gaby Rottler]

In the beginning, Hahnemann hoped to have "some good results" with the double remedies (his letter of June 1833 to Boenninghausen). In a later letter, dated September 17, he wrote Boenninghausen to say that they were "never, as we know, absolutely necessary." In the end, as he wrote in the letter of October 16, he found "only one or two" of his experiments "turned out well." It was the Founder's experience that one single remedy alone, or in alternation, or as a series of remedies, worked much better than combinations.

The Hofrath had listened pensively to his disciples, Aegidi and Bönninghausen, but with increasing reservation. He was now caught between his own inner convictions, and the enthusiasm of his two students for a simple but less effective method. The meeting of the Central Society on August 10, 1833 offered the Founder a perfect way out of this difficult position. He brought the subject of the double remedies to the floor for a discussion of their ramifications. Bradford reported in his Life and Letters of Hahnemann, page 488:

> "Dr. Aedigi proposed to Hahnemann to administer a mixture of two highly potentized remedies each corresponding to different parts of the disease. In the potentized state the medicines thus mixed would be incapable of chemical reactions, but would each act separately in its own spheres. Dr. Boenninghausen approved of the idea and Hahnemann was induced to present the matter to the meeting of the Central Society in 1833. Hahnemann was persuaded that this would probably lead to the polypharmacy of the old school, and he decided to exclude this doctrine from the new edition of the Organon."

Although Bradford highlighted the political aspects of the situation, Hahnemann's later letter to Bönninghausen in October shows that, in fact, the failure of his double remedy trial was a major factor in the withdrawal of his support at the meeting. All present at that meeting unanimously agreed to remove the passage from the 5th Organon-because the failed method was a political liability that would be abused by the polypharmacists. One month later, Hufeland was given a copy of the passage on the double remedies from the printer calling for quick action by the homoeopaths. At that time, the passage was replaced with a strong caution, in which the Founder called the double remedy trials a "hazardous experiment." Vide aphorism 272 of the 5th Organon:

> "In no case is it requisite to administer more than one simple medicinal substance at one time. 2(a)
>
> Footnote 2(a): Some homoeopathists have made the experiment, in cases where they deemed one remedy homoeopathically suitable for one portion of the symptoms of a case of disease, and a second for another portion, of administering both remedies at the same time; but I earnestly deprecate such a hazardous experiment, which can never be necessary, though it sometimes may be of use."

This footnote expresses the same thoughts Hahnemann wrote in his letter to the Baron in October 1833. He still did not wish to say that Aegidi and Boenninghausen never got any results, but he knew that a homoeopathician could do better with one single remedy at a time. He also realized that there were inherent hazards in giving a double remedy. Since he wanted everyone to be very careful with their patients, he advised against the method. Was this because he had noticed side effects after several months of observation? There was also the concern that those who used double remedies would never learn how to use a single remedy correctly; the method would thus become self-defeating to homoeopathic education. For all of these reasons, all reference to the double remedies were removed and the aphorisms on the single remedy were strengthened even further in aphorism 273 of the 6th Organon:

> "In no case of cure is it necessary to employ more than a single simple medicinal substance at one time with a patient. For this reason alone it is inadmissible to do so. It is inconceivable that there could be the slightest doubt about whether it is more in accordance with nature and more reasonable to prescribe only a single simple, well known medicinal substance at one time in a disease or a mixture of several different ones. In homoeopathy-the only true and simple, the only natural medical art-it is absolutely prohibited to administer to the patient, at one time, two different medicinal substances."

Many have pointed to the radical nature of Hahnemann's Paris period, but in truth, his most controversial experiment took place before the publishing of the 5th Organon, while Hahnemann was living as a widower in Coethen. Indeed, as the Paris casebooks progress to 1843, the Founder uses even less alternations and changes of remedies than he did in 1833. In 1837, he was still mostly using C potencies up to 30C, but by 1843, he had a much bigger pharmacy of around 130 remedies ranging from 30C to 200C, and he had even tested the 1M. He also utilized a full range of the complementary LM potencies, 0/1 to 0/30. This new higher potency pharmacy had an immediate effect on his case management strategies. The Paris casebooks from the period of the 6th Organon [1840-1843] correspond very well to the eyewitness accounts of faithful Dr. Croserio, who practiced with Melanie after Samuel's death. The 6th edition is the Founder's last will and testament and a guidebook to the medicine of the future (Little 2000).

Some further light was shown on the matter in Bradford's *Life and Letters of Hahnemann* (1895).

The intended publication of a new edition of the "Organon," of which Dr. Neidhard speaks, resulted from the following circumstances: When Hahnemann died he left, in his own handwriting, numerous annotations in a copy of the last edition of the "Organon" for a sixth edition, in which it is presumed he had propounded his later medical opinions. Although it was known by the friends of Hahnemann that such a book existed, it was not given to the world. As may be seen, Croserio in his letter mentions this fact and it is mentioned by others. After his death the MSS. remained in the hands of Madame Hahnemann and nothing was done about publishing it. In 1865 Dr. Arthur Lutze published at Coethen a sixth edition of the "Organon," interpolated with certain notes and suggestions of his own. He added the following new paragraph, advising the use of double and triple remedies:

"Section 274 b. There are several compound of cases of disease in which the administration of a double remedy is perfectly Homoeopathic and truly rational; where, for instance, each of two medicines appears suited for the case of disease, but each from a different side; or where the case of disease depends on more than one of the three radical causes of chronic diseases discovered by me, as when in addition to psora we have to do with syphilis or sycosis also. Just as in very rapid acute diseases I give two or three of the most appropriate remedies in alternation; i.e. in cholera, Cuprum and Veratrum; or in croup, Aconite, Hepar sulph. and Spongia; so in chronic diseases I may give together two well-indicated Homoeopathic remedies acting from different sides, in the smallest dose. I must here deprecate most distinctly all thoughtless mixtures or frivolous choice of two medicines, which would be analogous to Allopathic polypharmacy. I must also once again particularly insist that such rightly chosen Homoeopathic double remedies must only be given in the most highly potentized and attenuated doses."

The following foot-note occurs on page 267 of Lutze's "Organon:" "This is the paragraph intended by our Master for the fifth edition of the 'Organon', but suppressed by the senselessness of others, which I had the good fortune to discover, and which I deem it my duty to give to the world in this place, after having already published a chapter on the double remedies in my 'Lehrbuch der Homoopathie.' Dr. Julius Aegidi, at that time physician in ordinary to the Princess Frederica of Prussia, in Dusseldorf, sent Hahnemann the report of two hundred and thirty-three cases of cures effected by double remedies, and the reply of this great thinker, dated Coethen, 15th of June, 1833, of which I possess the original, runs thus:

'Dear Friend and Colleague: Do not think that I am capable of rejecting any good thing from prejudice, or because it might cause alterations in my doctrine. My sole desire is for truth, and I believe yours is also...Permit me, then, to give your discovery to the world in the fifth edition of the 'Organon,' which will soon be published. Until then, however, I beg you to keep all to yourself, and try to get Mr. Jahr, whom I greatly esteem, to do the like. At the same time I there protest and earnestly warn against all abuse of the practice by a frivolous choice of two medicines to be used in combination. Yours sincerely, Samuel Hahnemann.'

Lutze continues:

'After State Councillor Dr. von Boenninghausen, whose

name has been several times honorably mentioned in this book, and our Master himself had tested this practice and found it good, he (Hahnemann) wrote the following letter, the original of which I also possess, to Dr. Aegidi, dated 19th August, 1833: 'I have devoted a special paragraph in the fifth edition of the "Organon" to your discovery of the administration of double remedies. I sent the manuscript yesterday evening to Arnold and enjoined him to print it soon and put the steel engraving of my portrait as a frontispiece. The race for priority is anxiously pursued. Thirty years ago I was weak enough to contend for it.

"But for a long time past my only wish is that the world should gain the best, the most useful truth, let it come from me or from any other."

"The foregoing paragraph is sanctioned by these expressions of the now enlightened spirit. In the Congress of Homoeopathic medical men which took place soon afterwards on the 10th of August, 1833, the Master brought this new discovery before his disciples, but in place of finding willing listeners, he encountered opposition. The narrow mindedness and ignorance of these men went so far as to compare this true Homoeopathic discovery to the polypharmacy of Allopathy, and they drew such a dismal picture to the hoary Master of the harm he would do to his doctrine thereby, that he allowed himself to be persuaded to recall the paragraph he had already sent to the printer, which an eager disciple of not the purest sort undertook to do, and thus the world was for many years deprived of this important discovery."

Lutze continues with examples of this double remedy, and

signs his name at the end. In an editorial in the British Journal of Homoeopathy, of July, 1865, the author says that the letters printed by Lutze are no doubt genuine and thus explains the matter:

Dr. Aegidi proposed to Hahnemann to administer a mixture of two highly-potentized remedies each corresponding to different parts of the disease. In the potentized state the medicines thus mixed would be incapable of chemical reaction, but would each act separately in its own sphere. Dr. Boenninghausen approved of the idea and Hahnemann was induced to present the matter to the meeting of the Central Society for 1833. Hahnemann was persuaded that this would probably lead to the poly-pharmacy of the old school, and he decided to exclude this doctrine from the new edition of the "Organon." Hahnemann in no manner sanctioned alternation after this time.

Jahr afterwards mentioned Aegidi's discovery, and Aegidi answered Jahr in an article published in the Archives for 1834. He disavowed this method in 1857. Hahnemann recommended alternation of remedies in the first edition of the "Organon." Paragraph 145 of this edition reads: "It is only in some cases of ancient chronic diseases which are liable to no remarkable alterations, which have certain fixed and permanent fundamental symptoms, that two almost equally appropriate Homoeopathic remedies may be successfully employed in alternation."

He gives as a reason that the number of remedies at that time proven was not large enough to produce in every case the exact similimum. In the "Chronic Diseases" Hahnemann mentions certain cases in which he alternated remedies in intermittent fever. But it is very certain that Hahnemann's ideas upon alternation were different from those held by certain of his followers. His were rather those of rotation. Hahnemann, instead of recommending alternation in the fifth edition of the "Organon," says in paragraph 272: "In no case is it requisite to administer more than one single, simple medicinal substance at one time." In a note he says: "Some Homoeopathists have made the experiment in cases where they deemed one remedy Homoeopathically suitable for one portion of the symptoms of a case of disease, and a second for another portion, of administering both remedies at the same or at almost the same time; but I earnestly deprecate such a hazardous experiment, which can never be necessary, though it may sometimes seem to be of use." Paragraphs 273, 274 also treat of this matter.

Whatever Hahnemann wrote to Lutze or to Aegidi, or in whatever degree his spirit of experimentation and fairness led him to discuss the plan of alternation, it is very certain that he was not enthusiastic in the matter, and at best considered it a makeshift for careful study.

An interesting article on alternation, by Dr. Aug. Korndoerfer, may be found in the Hahnemannian Monthly for February and April, 1874. This so-called sixth edition of the "Organon," edited and published by Lutze, contains many alternations from the original text, and many important parts are also suppressed. It called forth the opposition of the whole German Homoeopathic Press and the German Homoeopathic Societies protested against such a liberty on the part of Dr. Lutze.

A long article appeared in the Allgemeine hom. Zeitung, Vol. lxx. (April 10, 1865), declaring the book to be spurious and apochryphal and utterly repudiating it. This is signed by Drs. Bolle, Hirschel, Meyer, Cl. Muller. In 1857 Dr. Aegidi had repudiated, in the Allgemeine Zeitung, the practice of alternation, although in his "Lehrbuch," in 1860, Lutze quoted him in its favor. But on the appearance of this "Organon" both Dr. Aegidi and Dr. Boenninghausen denied Lutze's assertions, as follows:

"Explanation. The protest of the honored representatives of the Homoeopathic press, of Germany, against the alleged sixth edition of the "Organon of the Healing Art," published in the Allg. hom. Zeitung of April 10, Hahnemann's birthday, having embraced the mention of my name, yet having omitted to mention that I also participate in the conviction in behalf of which the signers of the protest contend, that, years ago, I loudly and publicly made known my disapproval of the administration of so called double remedies, as an abuse and a mischievous proceeding, I find myself compelled to publish my explanation as it originally appeared in the Allg. hom. Zeitung, 54, 12 (May 18, 1857), and thence copied in the Neue Zeitschrift fur Homoopathische Klinik, 11, 12 (June 15, 1857). It was in the following language:

"The undersigned finds himself compelled to join his voice in the reproaches that have been made, particularly of late, against the Homoeopathic administration of so-called double remedies so much the more in as much as it is he who is charged with having taken the initiative in this mode of acting which is the subject of reprobation. Entirely agreeing with all the arguments adduced against it by competent persons and the refutation of which must be impossible, the undersigned is compelled to make known emphatically and publicly his decided disapproval of such an abuse of our excellent and most serviceable art, as has been lately recommended in an apparently systematic manner and as a rule; to the end, that persons may forbear to take his supposed authority, as a sanction of a mode of treatment which, even as he (Stapf's Archives, 1834, 14) thought he might recommend a modification of it for very rare and exceptional cases, is very far from being the abuse and mischief which it is now made and being made.

"I add to this that I thoroughly agree with the contents of the above-mentioned protest; and that, in my opinion, the practice therein rebuked is not dealt with even as severely as in the interests of our science it should have been.

"Aegidi. "Freienwald, April, 12, 1865."

Dr. Boenninghausen wrote to Dr. Caroll Dunham regarding this affair as follows:

"Munster, March 25, 1865.

"To Dr. Carroll Dunham, New York.

"My Very Dear Friend and Colleague: I have just to-day received your letter of the 2nd instant. The passage which you quote concerning the 'combined doses containing two different remedies' imposes on me the duty of replying without a moment's delay.

"It is true that during the years 1832 and 1833, at the instance of Dr. Aegidi, I made some experiments with combined doses, that the results were sometimes surprising, and that I spoke of the circumstance to Hahnemann, who after some experiments made by himself had entertained for awhile the idea of alluding to the matter in the fifth edition of the 'Organon,' which he was preparing in 1833. But this novelty appeared too dangerous for the new method of cure, and it was I who induced Hahnemann to express his disapproval of it in the fifth edition of the "Organon," 1833, in the note to paragraph 272. Since this period neither Hahnemann nor myself have made further use of these combined doses. Dr. Aegidi was not long in abandoning this method, which resembles too closely the procedures of Allopathy, opening the way to a relapse from the precious law of simplicity, a method, too, which is becoming every day more entirely superfluous from the augmentation of our Materia Medica.

"If, consequently, in our day, a Homoeopathician takes it into his head to act according to experiments made thirty years ago, in the infancy of our science, and subsequently rebuked by unanimous vote, he clearly walks backwards, like a crab, and shows that he has not kept up with nor followed the progress of science.

"Supposing that it may interest you to know the origin of the above-mentioned method, I add the following: There was about this time (1832 and 1833), at Cologne, an old physician named Dr. Stoll, himself a constant invalid and hypochondriac, who, distrusting the old medical doctrine, but having only a superficial smattering of Homoeopathy, had conceived the idea of dividing the remedies into two classes, the one of which should act upon the body and the other on the soul. He thought that these two kinds of medicine should be combined in a prescription in order to supplement each other.

"His method making some noise in Cologne, and Dr. Aegidi, then at Dusseldorf, having in vain endeavored to discover the essential secret of this novelty, the latter induced me to endeavor to find it out. I succeeded in doing so. Although the idea of Dr. Stoll was utterly devoid of foundation, it nevertheless induced us to make experiments in another way; namely, that above recited, but which, as I said before, was utterly rejected long, long ago.

"Yours very sincerely,

C. von Boenninghausen."

The Homoeopathic Medical College of Pennsylvania held a meeting on May 20, 1865, and entered a solemn protest against Lutze's book, which was declared "to be mutilated and perverted." The Homoeopathic profession in Europe and America refused to have anything to do with Lutze's edition of Hahnemann's "Organon" (Bradford 1895).

Searching through the literature provides a wealth of story myth and further controversy. The following passage is written in *The Homeopathic Physician* 1890 (Cahis 1890):

> Dr. Gailliard related the discovery of the use of complex medicines: Aegidi, friend of Hahnemann, wanted to administer two or three medicaments together having a similar action, and made vain attempts to form a school. Later, Lutze actually practiced this method. But only after thirty years do we find that the polypharmacists have completely systematized their methods. About the year 1850, a poor abbé of Turin, named Soleri, practiced Homoeopathy, availing himself of the small manual of Jahr. One day he gave a miserable peasant several different powders to take successively for a period of forty days. His patient, desiring more speed than certainty, swallowed it all at once, and was cured before the forty days had expired. To the abbé this seemed a miracle, and forthwith he advocated the complex system, and proclaimed the superiority of it over Hahnemannism.

He formed a partnership in 1861 with his nephew, Dr. Belotti. They classified remedies in twenty-six series, the cerebral, medullary, great sympathetic, vascular, lymphatic, etc. In 1866, Dr. Finella simplified Belotti's method and created new formulas, specifics against worms, etc. Signor Mattei, who was then an unbeliever, conceived his idea of Electro-Homoeopathy. This method was revealed to him by Providence, the secret of which he guarded with great care, no doubt by Divine command. We know today, thanks to Sauter and other brotherly enemies, the composition of his pills for scrofulosis, aneurisms, etc., and his electric solutions, red, green, etc. The latest incarnation of complete polypharmacy has been revealed to us in the year of grace 1888, in that "Homo-homoeopathist," Dr. Conan. This "Homo-Homoeopathy" comprehends twenty-six series of medicines, all specifics; anti-febriles, specifics for inflammatory diseases, acute or chronic diseases of the cerebrum, meningitis, etc., etc. Each series of medicines contains invariably six groups and each group embraces from twelve to thirty remedies. The groups should be alternated on various occasions each day-that is to say, the series should be alternated and be employed successively in divers dilutions; and, finally, from time to time as an intercurrent, the urinary simillimum dynamized in a very high dilution the thirtieth, one hundredth, two hundredth, three hundredth (Cahis 1890).

The Technique Itself

Watson (1991) defines polypharmacy as any prescribing technique in which two or more remedies are prescribed either in alternation with each other or as a combined formula. I am not sure that I agree with his definition because in homeopathy, especially where there are two separate diseases present in the same patient, there are plenty of precedents of using alternating remedies depending on the dominant symptom picture. Nonetheless, the point is well made. Polypharmacy is giving two things at the same time. Watson (1991) argues that polypharmacy may be individualised whereby single remedies are given concurrently according to indications in each individual case, or it could be diseased based whereby multiple remedies prescribed solely on the basis that they all have some degree of similarity to the particular disease process without due regard for the individualities. Generally, but not always, low potency is a given. Conversations with manufacturers of combinations revealed that they tend to look for some kind of evidence either in a trial, even a small one, or clearly indicated symptoms that emerge from well-conducted provings as the basis for constructing their combinations. Some have even argued to me that their choice of potency is based on the proving or trial from which the evidence came.

Watson (1991) identifies two charismatic individuals who, in more modern times prescribed successfully using polypharmacy. Ellis Barker in the 1930s and 40s achieved some notoriety with brilliant cures in some hopeless and complex cases. The system seemed to involve astonishing remedy prescriptions in quick succession without much obvious justification. An example from Watson, if a patient presented with chronic constipation, indigestion and flatulence, a history of adverse reactions to vaccinations and a tubercular family history, the first prescription would typically involve, *Cabo veg* 6x twice-daily in alternation with *Nux vomica* 6x twice daily,

Thuja 30 each Saturday and *Bacillinum* each Wednesday.

The other homeopath is Jouanny from France who has written and taught that giving a fundamental constitutional remedy together with an intercurrent miasmatic nosode, plus one or more low potency remedies as well, is a legitimate strategy.

Why NO! Opinions Past and Present

So it is clear there was to be no compromise regarding combination possibilities or multiple drugs in a bottle. Ultimately, there are two fundamental arguments against polypharmacy. The first is that our remedies were proven singly, and therefore they should be given singly. The rationale for this argument is that no one can predict how several remedies will act on an individual when given simultaneously. This argument is grounded in the scientific realities of homeopathy. Nevertheless, the implication here is that misery and suffering will result from such deviations from these traditional methods. Many a homeopath has examples of patients having bad reactions to a combination remedy, either prescribed by another homeopath, or taken over the counter, and which has upset our treatment plans. Watson (1991) argues that this argument is theoretically sound but in practice the fears turn out to be unfounded. In reality the worst that usually happens after combination prescription is that nothing happens, and that the patient didn't get any better. Ironically, the same thing that often happens after the administration of a single remedy!

The second argument is that the practitioner will be uncertain as to which remedy worked, assuming a curative response takes place at all. This is a significant problem with the use of polypharmacy. There is such an ease and simplicity of case management by being able to chart the action of the single remedy once it has been administered to the patient. This capacity to know what has happened and what to do next is completely diminished by combination remedy, and the long term treatment of patients is rendered impossibly complex. Of course this doesn't matter at all to patients, but it sure matters to the astute homeopath trying to do good work.

Those arguments and many others have been put forward for 200 years. Because of their vehemence, I have quoted in full the best of them.

> Hahnemann says, "The question now arises: Is it good to mix various kinds of medicine in a prescription? The human mind never understands more than one thing at a time and can hardly determine accurately the causes resulting from two simultaneous forces acting on one object. How can medicine attain a higher degree of certainty, when the doctor seems to be intent only on allowing a number of miscellaneous forces to be exerted at the same time on a pathological state? ... I take it upon myself to avow that of two and two medicines put together, no single one will exert its own particular effect on the human body, but almost always an effect quite different from that of the two separately. This is a middle effect, a neutral effect, if I may borrow the expression of chemical compounds."—Aesculapius in the Balance, 1805 (as quoted in Resonance, Ju/Aug. 1996, p. 4).

> "Homoeopaths do not follow the objectionable practice of mixing several drugs together, trusting to the discriminating powers of the stomach to discard the unsuitable and appropriate the suitable one. They endeavour to prescribe with precision, by administering one medicine only at a time." Ruddock, The

Lady's Manual (Yasgur 1994).

In Fundamental Laws of Therapeutics, Bernoville wrote, 'for the selection of the simillimum remedy the psychic symptoms should dominate over physiological symptoms, the general characteristics should dominate over the particulars, the universal modalities over the particulars or the local modalities. For this reason, it will be often difficult for us to find the indications exclusively of one remedy excluding others. This fact authorises us to use a complex...there is almost nothing common between the mode of action of a dynamised medicament acting on the subtle spheres of the organism and the mode of action of a non-dynamised substance acting in gross doses because of its immediate properties' (Mukerji 1975).

No greater crime can be committed against the human economy than to aid and abet these suppressions, for these may be the direct cause of many constitutional diseases, and the symptoms are, in their natural state, always the expression of constitutional conditions. Suppression is the source of many functional disturbances (Roberts 1934).

Purveyors of polypharmacy often attempt to justify the use of these remedies by claiming they offer "temporary" relief, thus begging the question: What is the effect on the chronic disturbance while the vital force is being relieved "temporarily"? This is one of the most common features of all suppressive use of dynamized substances under the misnomer "Homeopathy". Pain, inflammation and fever are not the real disease nor the real object of treatment. To view them as such tends logically and inevitably to mere palliation or suppression of symptoms, than which there are no greater medical evils. It is based upon a false and illogical interpretation of the phenomena of disease which mistakes results for causes...Homoeopathy is opposed to polypharmacy. It depends for all its results upon the dynamical action of single, pure, potentiated medicines, prepared by a special mathematico-mechanical process and administered in minimum doses (Close 1924).

When asked upon what authority they base their combinations, polypharmacists become tongue-tied. They become as unable to speak as the symptoms they have themselves suppressed: As surely as the voice of the symptoms is hushed, so surely does the physician put out of his way the opportunity for selecting a homeopathic remedy. When the index to the remedy is spoiled, the ability of the physician to benefit his patient is destroyed....The man who does these things is a homeopathic failure (Kent 1900).

In short, nothing has caused more positive evil after apparent good (Caroll Dunham in Bedayn 1995).

Prejudice the chief obstacle to the scientific investigation of posology in clinical medicine (HC Allen 1881). The single remedy is the remaining corollary of vital importance to a successful application of the law of cure in scientific medicine. Polypharmacy lays it down as a rule that we must select our remedies according to the effect which each produces singly, and then combine them with reference to the effect which we wish to produce in a given case, which is usually a modification of the action of one or the other. Hydrargyrum cum creta, Calomel and Opium, and Dover's powder, are familiar examples of the prevailing practice. But this does not always work well. The scientific objection is that there is a theory at both ends; the practical objection-the bedside objection-is that it is a failure in practice. It lacks all the elements of scientific prevision of which a system based on a law of cure can boast. Our Materia Medica is the record of the symptoms obtained in the proving of each drug individually, not in alternation or in rotation, or of two or more drugs mixed together, (not a chemical union). We have no pathogenesy of Arsenic and Nux vomica, of Aconite and Belladonna, of Rhus tox. and Bryonia in alternation, nor do the demands of science require it. Dr. Sorge says, "The practice of alternation as it exists among homoeopathicians is only another form of mixing remedies with the intention of getting an effect compounded of the action of the two or more drugs that are alternated." Given, the "totality of the symptoms" of a properly recorded case, two or more drugs cannot be the similimum. We have no such record in our Materia Medica. Suppose the case to be one of intermittent fever, where pathology can afford us no aid, some remedy is more similar to the aggregate of symptoms than any other, for the best of all reasons, that no two drugs are alike in their action. It may be Arsenic or Nat. muriaticum, but it cannot be both. If one be like the array of symptoms presented the other cannot be, as no two remedies are identical in their action. Our law of the similars is a universal guide for the selection of the remedy, and it is the universal application which constitutes homoeopathy the "science of therapeutics." On the other hand it is absolutely impossible to formulate a rule or rules for the selection of remedies to be given in alternation. The practice leads directly to polypharmacy, routinism and theorizing; but an imperfect knowledge of our Materia Medica and the underlying principles of our science, combine to keep it alive (Allen 1881).

At all times there have been homoeopaths who, in imitation of Aegidi and Lutze, and in order to simplify the therapeutic diagnosis, had taken to exhibit two or three remedies mixed in the same draught; but for the last thirty years complexism has been held as a principle, and, a fact worthy of remark, it was initiated by unprepared laymen without any medical learning, and who acted as by inspiration: the Abbé Soleri, Doctors Bellotti and Finella, Count Mattei, and afterwards a long list of manufacturers, dowagers, some apothecaries, and very few medical men, all of them eager for novelties and enamoured of mysteries, since, it must be said, the formulae of these complex remedies has been kept secret by their inventors. The last incarnation of complexist polypharmacy was revealed in the year of grace 1888. This is the homo-homoeopathy of Dr. Conan. Let us hope it will remain the final one. All these methods are kindred to homoeopathy only by the use of Hahnemannian triturations and dilutions. The alternatist polypharmacists make use of the very name of Hahnemann, who, indeed, said, in the first edition of the Organon: "It is only in some cases of inveterate organic diseases that one may sometimes alternate with success two homoeopathic remedies." But this passage is found in no other edition of the Organon. It is related that Hahnemann himself had twice or thrice made some alteration in the decline of his career, when more than eighty years of age, and soon after his second marriage. This is possible, and of but little consequence, but what is certain is, that not one of Hahnemann's writings bears any trace of approbation of alternation. Richard Hughes writes: "I have had sometimes such results as these: "The medicine A has improved the case in a manner, then the medicine B had to supplement it; after the exhaustion of its effects there seemed to be no better similia than A, which again improves the case for a while, and then medicine B comes back, until a complete cure is effected." It is evident that, so understood, alternation departs only apparently from the principles of monopharmacy. In such conditions it has been applied at every epoch by the truest and strictest Hahnemannian physicians; and actually it is applied by the most unquestioned authorities, like Drysdale and Dudgeon in England, P. Jousset and Léon Simon in France, De Moor and Torez in Belgium. Such alternation is absolutely actuated by Hahnemann's teaching, and I cannot make it better understood than by quoting Léon Simon's following declaration, which obtained so great applause at the Congress of Paris: "By applying these rules to the alternation-of-medicines question our brother, Dr. Gailliard, has just been treating so magisterially, I shall say that it cannot be condemned in the lump. Indeed, we alternate in acute diseases characterized by a rapid course and transformations often so startling. It is what Dr. Boyer has proposed to do in diphtheria, against which he makes use of cyanide of mercury alternated with bromized water. In such circumstances, with Dr. Gailliard, I will say: I also alternate! I alternate, because in such cases the action of medicines is rapidly exhausted, and so there is no inconvenience in multiplying the doses and in giving two substances, one after the other at short intervals. In chronic diseases the case is quite different; here the transformations are going on slowly, the effect of therapeutic agents is protracted during many days, and there is no interest to intermingle actions in such a manner that it becomes impossible to make them out. Consequently, I repel as illogical and contrary to the principles I have called to mind the practice of administering one kind of medicine at morning, a second at eleven o'clock, a third at four o'clock in the afternoon, a fourth at bedtime, and of recommencing thus during a certain number of days. To act so is putting ourselves in the impossibility of following the action of medicines, and also of deriving advantage from those we have been making use of; such a proceeding must decidedly be given up" (Gailliard 1891).

H. C. Allen said, 'I object to giving a student an Allopathic drill before he studies Homoeopathy. Why should the Homoeopathic colleges let their students first be loaded with Allopathic theories and methods before they know Homoeopathy thoroughly?' It is wrong. It is not what the student pays for; it is dishonest, it is a criminal assault on our school; it is a practical abjuration of our principles; why not give him what he comes for, a Homoeopathic education de nova? The colleges are primarily responsible for polypharmacy, alternation, combination tablets and the hypodermic syringe. The shame belongs to the teacher, not to the student. There is no interest to intermingle actions in such a manner that it becomes impossible to make them out. Consequently, I repel as illogical and contrary to the principles I have called to mind the practice of administering one kind of medicine at morning, a second at eleven o'clock, a third at four o'clock in the afternoon, a fourth at bedtime, and of recommencing thus during a certain number of days. To act so is putting ourselves in the impossibility of following the action of medicines, and also of deriving advantage from those we have been making use of; such a proceeding must decidedly be given up (Wesselhoeft 1901).

We assuredly do entertain the belief that "two or more medicinal forces (or, we prefer to say "morbific forces") cannot together act upon the economy without so modifying each other that neither shall produce the effect it would if only one were acting." This belief has prevailed among medical men from the earliest ages. It is the foundation of the practice of polypharmacy in all its varieties, from the complex prescriptions of the seventeenth century to the alternations of our own colleagues. For we hold, with Dr. Sorge (by no means a Hahnemannian, let us add), that "the practice of alternation, as it exists among homoeopathicians, is only another form of mixing remedies with the intention of getting an effect compounded of the action of the two or more drugs that are alternated." We say, this belief is the foundation of polypharmacy. The rationale of a compound prescription we take to be the following: the drug which is regarded as the one chiefly indicated possesses, let us suppose, certain properties which would be hurtful to the patient. Another drug is conjoined with it for the purpose of antidoting those hurtful properties. Again, it lacks the power to produce certain effects which are deemed desirable. Another drug is added to supplement this deficiency, and so on, ad infinitum. This entire procedure rests on the belief that these medicinal forces will so modify each other in the economy that neither shall produce the effect it would if only one were acting (Dunham 1877a).

Do you alternate the high potencies, or do you rely upon the single remedy? Here again our friend confounds a principle and quantity. If it be right and advantageous to alternate the low, it is right and advantageous to alternate the high potencies. But, in fact, we do not alternate at all. We always rely on the single remedy at one time. Dr. Drysdale says that everybody alternates, and, therefore, there must be some necessity for the practice. But his illustrations are so far fetched, and his definition of alternation is so contrary to the conceptions which all other homoeopathicians, from Hahnemann down, have had on the subject, that, notwithstanding our respect for Dr. Drysdale, we must repeat, in the very face of his learned paper, that we do not alternate. Our understanding of the practice of alternation, and our objections to it were stated, as well as we are able to state them, in the American Homoeopathic Review, June, 1863, vol.

iii., No. 12. 1. We are opposed to it in theory, and we abjure it in practice. It is an abominable heresy. As a shot-gun maims where the rifle would kill, so alternation may change and modify and maim the disease, but it never does nor can effect the clean, direct and perfect cure that a single remedy, exactly homoeopathic, will accomplish. As a relic of the polypharmacy which has been the stumbling-block of the Old School, we loathe it. As a refuge of the careless prescriber and slothful student, we despise it. As an anomaly in homoeopathic practice, a fatal obstacle to progress in the clinical portion of our Materia Medica, we deplore it (Dunham 1877b).

Grimmer concluded, In the name of sick humanity, let us turn from a sloven, soulless routinism originated by the old school and weakly followed by too many of our own. Be homeopaths in heart and soul, as in name: cast aside clumsy, lazy methods of alternation and polypharmacy that end only in disappointment and suffering; pursue the path enlightened by the great law of Hahnemann: administer the single indicated remedy under the accurate life-sustaining methods of truly scientific medicines. So shall we maintain the steady march toward our goal: complete and universal recognition and acceptance of God's best gift of healing to sick mankind - the Law of Similars (Grimmer 1997).

In chronic diseases we generally confine ourselves to one remedy at a time. The method of alternating two medicines at regular intervals is generally resorted to in acute cases only. We may alternate Aconite and Belladonna, or Aconite and Bryonia, or Aconite and Phosphorus, Belladonna and Nux, Phosphorus and Arsenic, etc. It should be remarked, however, that, in many cases, this method of alternation is an expedient shift rather than a usage necessitated or justified by principle (Hempel 1864).

Hughes was vehement as usual. Hahnemann very early came to entertain a strong aversion to the polypharmacy so prevalent in his day. This was the proposal of two of Hahnemann's immediate disciples Lutze and Ægidi, and almost (it is said) secured the master's own expressed approval. I am far from saying that such mixtures would be ineffective; but their use would be fatal to the simplicity of the homoeopathic method, and would embark us once more on the confused and unscientific polypharmacy from which we have so happily escaped. Still more strongly does this apply to the complex blendings of our remedies lately advocated by Drs. Pinella and Conan. All good purpose to be served by such combinations can be better obtained by the successive, or if need be the alternate, administration of their component drugs (Hughes 1902).

Similarly Clarke in the *Prescriber* noted,

The revision of this little handbook means much to the Homeopath. We had occasion to criticise the first edition for teaching polypharmacy. In the preface to this edition the author says: "Where formerly two remedies were advised to be given in alternation, the particular indications when to give the one and when the other are now supplied. The indications will be found to be more symptomatic and less pathological than formerly." In other words, it is more homeopathic. The author still considers it his duty to advise a low potency and frequent repetitions of the remedy, an error which he should have dropped when he dropped alternation (Clarke 1885).

Roberts summarises the issues.

Here we are faced with another problem in physics which has to do with the single remedy or polypharmacy. There is a reason for the single remedy even more profound than that practical one first advanced by Hahnemann and his followers: that since we know from careful provings what the single remedy will do, we can depend upon its uniformity (within certain limitations), but no one can predict the action of more than one remedy in combination or in alternation or in close proximity to each other. This is an observation, not an explanation. Modern physics may give us the solution in the "wandering neutron"; and neutrons are evidently loosed when certain elements of low atomic weight are combined even with an infinitesimal weight of radiations of an element of high atomic weight, and these neutrons in turn readily combine with other elements with which they come in contact; and while these elements of the third state do not necessarily become changed, they become unstable and again subject to further changes. Millikan quotes the case of "a bit of beryllium mixed with an infinitesimal amount of radium emanation..." where one of the neutrons released enters the nucleus of an atom of silver and thus raises the atomic weight of the silver one unit, the silver becoming extra heavy, still retaining its chemical properties, but becoming unstable and proceeding to throw out a negative electron and transforming itself into cadmium. To be sure, these changes were the result of experimental procedures, but we cannot be assured that any combination of elements might not produce just as profound changes, either constructive or destructive. This would be particularly true when we consider the methods we employ to release the inherent energy in seemingly inert substance. If our methods are sufficient to release energy we cannot be assured that they might not be transmuted (Roberts 1936).

Polypharmacy was abandoned first by Paracelsus, then by Rademacher, and lastly Hahnemann went further and gave us the law by which the selection of the single curative drug could be found. Prescribing the autogenous toxin complex is not exactly a homeopathic preceding as given us by Hahnemann, the remedy being proved in the patient's own body. The toxin complex of the disease gives us the symptom complex of the patient. There is not a single process which the stock vaccine undergoes in the laboratory that adds to its therapeutic value. On the other hand every single step in its progress through the laboratory alters its therapeutic character (Duncan 1913).

Contemporary Opposition

The 1960s saw no alteration in pitch or opposition.

The simultaneous incursion into the body of multiple medicaments could only result in metabolic confusion. Moreover it would be impossible to attribute any effects produced to the action of any particular ingredient, thus making accuracy in prescribing an impossibility. If more than one drug is given in one prescription the possibility of synergistic action cannot be ruled out, but it cannot be argued that the effect will be the sum total of the effects of the separate drugs. Rather will the combination function as a single drug. The ingredient drugs may supplement one another or may antagonize one another, they may even result in inter-reactions that have adverse effects in the body. It is a matter of experience that certain groups of drugs, grouped chemically, botanically or biologically, may possess the power to evoke somewhat similar effects on the tissues. While each member of the group has its own individual character and genius yet the similarity of action shared in some respects may make the members complementary to one another. Such complementary remedies given in sequence, and possibly in differing potencies, appear at times to enhance the curative effect, but they are always to be given singly and not in the same dose. A mixture of more than one remedy in a single dose would constitute a new remedy which would require to be proved as such for a proper estimate of its probable effects. A warning: The temptation to repeat remedies one after the other in quick succession and in high potency must be sedulously resisted. This form of polypharmacy may easily produce a most confusing picture of drug-induced symptoms plus original disease symptoms, all mixed up, and render accurate prescribing well-nigh impossible (Miller 1966).

In 1988 Chatterjee argued:

A definite trend is now discernible amongst homoeopaths to favour polypharmacy in the treatment of a disease or mixing of remedies to cover parts of the disease and not the whole. In fact, combination of homoeo-drugs is being thought of more frequently and is being ingeniously devised to meet a particular disease situation. Examples in point are: (a) mixture of China and Cynodon dyctylon in 3x, 6x, 30 or 200 potencies for diarrhoea, dysentery and colitis; (b) mixture of Hydrastis, Chelidonium, Cheonanthus, in low potency, for treatment of jaundice and as mother tincture for diseases of liver and spleen; (c) mixture of Thuja and Pulsatilla or of Thuja and Calcarea carb in 30, 200 or 1M potencies for diseases of menstrual periods; (d) mixture of Sulphur, Silicea and Carbo-veg in 6 or 200 potency for treatment of acne; (e) mixture of Phosphorus 6, Calcarea carb 6 and Thuja 30 for high Cholesterol count in blood; (f) mixture of Ruta, Rhus-tox and Arnica in 30 potency for Tennis-elbow. Patently, the concept behind polypharmacy or mixing of remedies in the treatment of a disease whether as a whole or in part runs counter to the Hahnemannian approach of Single Remedy, based on the logic of Totality of Symptoms and the Law of Similars. At the same time, it is difficult to resist their application to individual cases merely because they are non- Hahnemannian in concept, particularly when they have proved a success. But this apparent success is due to the fact that potentised medicines are not subject to the laws of neutralisation and will, therefore, act unless they are mutually anti-doting. However, it needs to be emphasised that the so-called cure is not "cure" in Hahnemannian sense and that such an attempt is frought with the dangers of palliation and drug-miasm which may ultimately lead to the incurability of the disease sought to be cured. Either of the methods-Polypharmacy or Combination of remedies - tends to cripple the vital dynamis permanently, making the body prone to disease dynamis (Chatterjee 1988).

The late David Warkentin wrote:

Fringe therapies like polypharmacy would benefit us all by attempting to define themselves clearly, and then developing appropriate doctrines. Having done so they could rename themselves with titles which more accurately reflect the principles (if any) upon which they are founded. Personally, I would be fine with combinations if they just weren't called "homeopathy". I think that they are homeopathic remedies being used allopathically (Warkentin 1994).

Interviews with contemporary homeopaths in the *Amercian Homeopath* find no shortage of opinion either. Sheilagh Creasy when asked:

AH: Have you ever seen a seriously disrupted case from combination remedies, or damage done? Creasy: Oh, yes, combination remedies are terrible! I have in mind straight away a case where the person had been given polypharmacy for years. She had a very disrupted case and it took me six years to straighten her out. AH: What message would you give homeopaths about using combination remedies. Creasy: The message is: absolutely DO NOT use combination remedies! Learn the principles through the literature. Once you have absorbed the philosophy, and you have a right mind in your head, you cannot possibly see otherwise. This is where the training and philosophy comes in. Hahnemann says in the Organon, very clearly, do not use more than one remedy, ...which some people seem to be very happily twisting into some self-serving idea or another that does their patients no good. However it has been awfully good for the people who manufacture and sell them... This is almost like preaching the whole time, I really don't like it, I would prefer if there was a general understanding of homeopathy, an alignment in thought and practice (Creasy 1997).

Misha Norland in 2000 argued:

AH: When you are using the term classical homeopathy, are you holding the same chain as other disciplines of practice, such as polypharmacy, for instance? What is your stance there? MN: I use the term classical homeopathy to honor George. He was the first person to coin this phrase, as far as I know. What he meant by it was "homeopathy as described by ..." He has a list of people whom he considers to be classical, in order to define what he means, such as Boenninghausen, Kent, Boericke, Farrington, Hering. He is not okay with other viewpoints, not happy with the Miasm theory expounded by Ortega, or the insights of Sankaran or Scholten or the provings of Sherr. He has his classical group of homeopathic writers that he feels comfortable with. They have stood the test of time and their information is reliable. Polypharmacists (by which I take it you refer to those who use mixtures of many remedies) are coming from somewhere else.

Generally speaking a polypharmacist is viewing homeopathy in a more traditional medical light, through therapeutic application: a pile of remedies for treating a pile of bits. It's not a synergistic view (Norland 2000).

Morrison's view was:

> But such clarification rarely occurs. Why is it that most people who champion the consumption of combination remedies are those who stand to gain monetarily by their sales? It is a well-kept secret that impulse-packaged (ah, pretty!) polypharmacy outsells homeopathic pharmacy by a factor of one-hundred. This excess of commercialism appears to have replaced good sense and proof of efficacy. There are many cases of patients who have taken a course of combination remedies and either suppressed their disease or taken on proving symptoms, thus corrupting their health. We have seen some disrupted cases from patients proving symptoms of each of the remedies in the combination they have been taking, making accurate prescribing next to impossible.
>
> The use of combination remedies can actually be quite dangerous. A case in point is the nationally marketed "Colds and Flu" combination that contain Allium cepa. It is common knowledge that All-c. can be a severe suppressant of coryza, potentially resulting in a pharyngitis, a bronchitis, or asthmatic attacks. It should be mentioned that injudicious use of this remedy (Allium cepa) in common colds may in some instances suppress this minor annoyance only to precipitate acute asthmatic attacks or severe throat infections. Severe bronchitis or asthmatic attacks which result from the suppression of coryza with Allium cepa often respond to Phosphorus. Severe pain with constant disposition to swallow after suppression of coryza with Allium

cepa is antidoted by Mercurius corrosivus (Morrison 1993).

Hahnemann maintained that such palliation actually masks the vital force to the point where the chronic complaint is suppressed and the patient's health declines. True homeopathy can be likened to organic gardening, where a weak soil is carefully tended and strengthened so that its fruits will proliferate with vitality and in such a way that weeds, bugs, and blights, etc. are discouraged. Whereas suppressive or would-be homeopathy is like mowing the weeds, but leaving the soil untended so that the weeds grow back, often more obstinate -such is palliation. Finally, allopathic medicine is like gardening with herbicides, chemical fertilizers, and a bulldozer; forever corrupting the terrain through the ensuing toxicity and erosion -this is frank suppression. Consider, from among this escalation that threatens to overrun our homeopathic estate, the use of combination remedies (polypharmacy) for disease indications. Polypharmacy, as a practice, violates nearly every principle of homeopathy i.e, selecting the simillimum, the use of a single substance, individuality, totality, case management, posology, the assessment of chronic as over acute -to mention just a few. In one way, this is not surprising: it is not homeopathy. If a child takes a carpenter's level from the toolbox of a craftsperson and proceeds to hammer screws with it, this will not convince anyone the child is actually practicing the trade of carpentry nor dissuade anyone from continuing to benefit from that trade. Unfortunately, in the absence of greater knowledge in the lay public, the use of "homeopathic remedies" by many of these garbled versions can be sufficient to dissuade people from homeopathy itself. Despite the great number of homeopaths in the US, Kent was dissatisfied with the quality of homeopathic practice. Most of these physicians utilized the homeopathic remedies in a mechanistic and reductionistic manner similar to the way in which orthodox physicians prescribed drugs. Frequently, these "homeopaths" violated many basic tenets of classical homeopathy by prescribing more than one remedy at a time, by recommending frequent repetition of doses, and by prescribing a remedy based upon a person's disease rather than his or her individualized symptoms (Ullman 1979).

The complexes started round about the 1830's. It came and went and it came again in the late 1870's and it disappeared and in France now, or even in Germany it is very, very wide spread. It is a branch that exists strongly today. But you will notice, all the people that practise complexes are basically practising an allopathic type of practice, it is not a homeopathic type of practice. It is a change of symptoms they are trying to do. They are not basing the prescription on the most similar remedy, it is just a change of symptoms, there is no direction of cure, no basic principle. They are really, really far away from the basic principle (Saine 1999).

Wright-Hubbard wrote of polypharmacy:

Furthermore, the simillimum is a personality having a rhythm, one might almost say a permeating aura of its own, and in the fleeting instant of its administration it takes complete possession of the patient, thereby buoying up the vital force so that it can carry on the restorative process. To have two or more remedies would be to introduce two separate rhythms, partial and disharmonious factors. Moreover, if more than one remedy be used the doctor cannot know which element was curative and one source of future guidance is thereby obscured. Lastly, since only one remedy can possibly be proved at a time, so only one can cure at a given moment. Some mongrel homoeopaths when in doubt give mixed prescriptions. This means that they are merely prescribing symptomatically, one remedy for one symptom or organ, and another for another. Each of these if homoeopathically chosen may wipe out the fragmentary illness at which it was aimed but that which is profound, total, and primal, of which all these symptoms are but manifestations and will remain untouched and simply crop out through other channels as subsequent symptoms. Other half-hearted homoeopaths, and even some with a wide knowledge of the materia medica but a relatively feeble grasp of the philosophy alternate remedies. This practice can not be too strongly condemned as it seesaws the patient into temporary ups without real progress (Wright-Hubbard 1977).

The single remedy is the third member of the essential homoeopathic trilogy. The reason for this is obvious: only one remedy can be the most similar at any given time with the condition of any given patient. If the physician can not decide between two remedies he has not gotten the totality of the symptoms, or the remedies which he has chosen are merely superficially akin to fragments or aspects of the case. Many modern French homoeopaths give a main deep acting remedy and one or more so-called drainage remedies with it, the chronic remedy in high potency and the drainage remedies in low potency, the idea being that the drainage remedy opens up an outlet for the exodus of the disease. These drainage remedies aim at the production of a discharge or the stimulation of the secretory organs, etc. This is a recent variant and does not appear in Hahnemann, the old masters, or Kent, and the self-styled purists of today do not approve of it (Wright-Hubbard 1977).

In *Homoeopathic Links* (2000), Vithoulkas wrote:

When, 35 years ago, I was fighting against polypharmacy - the form of homeopathy practiced at the time by the majority of homeopaths all over the world - there were similar outcries, and even threats, demanding that they should expel me from LIGA, arguing that polypharmacy is very effective, is actually a modern way of practicing homeopathy. Actually Christian Boiron in a letter to me wrote: 'we promote.... Modern Homeopathy'! The outcries then were worse than today's outcries but homeopaths eventually understood the importance of what I was saying and turned to classical homeopathy in masses (Vithoulkas 2000).

Why Yes! Opinions - Past and Present

Can there be any justifiable grounds therefore? It is easily available over-the-counter in combination form: Sinus-plex this, hayfever-plex that, menstrual-plex this, backpain-plex that. Students often ask the very legitimate question, 'what's the big deal?' Some even more astute practitioners and students argue the case that any advertising is good advertising. If homeopathy is seen anywhere in the marketplace, it is an advertisement for their own private practices.

As long as homeopathy has existed, the temptation has also existed to combine several remedies together and prescribe them for a specific disease. There is no need when an individual patient has crystal clear symptoms, strong characteristics, and a couple of strange, rare and peculiar symptoms to boot. The remedy just screams to be given. But for those of us working in the 21st century where things seem much more complex, and symptom pictures are less clear, the temptation whispers in our ears. The theoretical advantage (Watson 1991) is that by combining say five of the most commonly prescribed remedies for an earache, the practitioner is able to bypass the necessity to individualise each case, and give every earache patient the same prescription. The assumption is that the combination will cover a remedy most similar to the earache and it will act, and the other non-indicated remedies will do nothing. Robert Medhurst of Brauer's Pharmacy in Australia cites numerous examples where this has been the case. As Watson argues (1991),

> 'I have tried many of the disease orientated combination formulas for problems such as hay fever, pain, varicose veins and so on and generally the results have been disappointing with a few notable successes. As far as I can ascertain, when prescribed routinely these combination seemed to work palliatively or not at all in a fairly high percentage of cases and curative leap in a small number. But for this reason I would prefer to prescribe a single remedy over a multiple prescription on the basis of an individualised basis wherever possible as the results seem to justify the extra effort required.'

Some Commonly Used Combinations

The following table highlights and describes some of the commonly used combinations of homeopathic remedies:

Remedies and Potencies Combined	Description
Sulphur 6x, Silica 6x, Carbo veg 6x	Reputation as being useful in acne and as a cleanser of the blood.
Arnica 6x one part, Crategus mother tincture two parts, Kali mur 3x one part	Used for post-apoplectic patients to promote reabsorption of clots and reduce the tendency to further strokes and deal with the resulting weakness of the heart and arteries.

Ambra grisea 6x, Anacardium 6x, Argentum ntitricum 6x	Useful for peace of mind and those suffering in anticipation of some ordeal or who are troubled and worried about many things. They are all over the High Street, Boots in England, in Australia in Martin and Pleasance and Brauers, and in the US at Pharmica (Watson 1991).

Medhurst (1994) asks the question:

Can complexes be considered homeopathic? The short answer to this is no, and the long answer has a lot to do with what defines Homoeopathy. Homoeopathy can be defined as the art and practice of the application of similars, ie determining what substance in nature can cause the signs, symptoms and experiences of the patient in front of us, and the application of smaller amounts of that same substance in accordance with the principles laid down by the designer of the system, Dr Samuel Hahnemann. Inherent in these principles is the use of one dose of a single remedy matched to the individual. The ingredients used in complexes may also be selected on the basis that some single remedies have been found to have a high degree of specificity for a particular disease. The remedy Syzygium has been found to be very useful in the treatment of diabetes and so may be used for this in a complex. Thiosinimum, a remedy made from the oil of the Mustard seed has been found to be very useful for the resorption of old scar tissue, and the remedy, Anas barbariae has been shown to be extremely effective in the treatment of influenza. Clearly then, the use of multiple ingredients, selected for use with a disease rather than with the individual, and repetition of dose would tend to rule complexes out as strictly "homoeopathic".

Once he establishes that combinations are not homeopathic,

he then presents defences the five usual arguments against their use and employment.

1. A patient's use of complexes will mask the symptoms upon which a constitutional diagnosis can be made. Certainly - but so will any other form of intervention. Some forms of intervention are more problematic than others, and given the choice, and at the end of the day, one needs to make a decision about risk versus benefit and the patient's quality of life in the short and long term.
2. Complexes have not been proved, and they therefore offer little more than symptomatic relief which will disappear once the patient stops using the medicine. Although most remedies traditionally used in Homoeopathy have been proved, there are some that have not, such as Adonis, Aethiops and Corudalis amongst others, and yet these continue to be used. There is a great deal of experimental anecdotal evidence to support the case that complexes can cure, and some therapists in Australia spend in excess of twice the average annual national wage per year on complexes, one of whom has been using these products for over 40 years.
3. The complexes often contain remedies that are inimical or antidotal, and so will have limited or no therapeutic activity. It has been found in clinical practices all over the world that remedies which are indicated as inimical to each other in the texts, do not appear to be so when combined at low potency. I have yet to see this theory refuted.
4. We don't know what's working in a complex- it could be that mixing creates a whole new entity. Many people who've looked into this issue (including me) are of the opinion

that if Homoeopathic medicines are energistic replicas of the mother tincture from which the remedy was made, complexes are mixtures containing separate and distinct vibratory spectra that relate to the original tincture. I had some interesting confirmation of this recently at a conference where a very well known user of bioenergetic medicine devices was demonstrating a new diagnostic device that has the capacity to determine the specific homoeopathic medicine required by the patient. The device indicated that the person on whom the demonstration being carried out needed a certain single remedy. This was unavailable on its own so she was supplied with a complex that contained this remedy- on re-testing the device indicated that her requirement for the single remedy had been fulfilled by the complex which contained it.

5. Classical/constitutional Homoeopathy is the only Homoeopathy. Sure, but what is "Classical Homoeopathy"? The Hahnemannian approach? The Kentian approach? Or the approach taken by many others such as Seghal? There are some Homoeopaths who prescribe almost entirely on the basis on mental symptoms, others who prescribe solely on generals, some who prescribe on keynotes and so on. They all call themselves Classical Homoeopaths but there seems to be little agreement on what this actually means.

Ultimately, I don't think that anyone who has ever had anything to do with Homoeopathy would deny that nothing could replace the Similimum for depth and breadth of cure. However, in a world where the Natural therapist or even the Homoeopath is increasingly being seen as just one amongst many other healthcare providers, anyone failing to take a less than pragmatic approach to prescribing- ie hoping that the patient will be happy to wait for 2 weeks while the single remedy (if it is actually the correct one) takes effect, may well lose the patient to someone else who's happy to provide a pharmaceutical product, herb, supplement or complex to get the situation under control in the short term (Medhurst 1994).

When Is it Best to Use Polypharmacy?

Some have argued that there is a strong place for them in professional and medical homeopathy. While homeopathic prescribing with HIV and AIDS is no different from any other condition, (take the case and give the indicated remedy), some such as Baker, Fox, Groot & Honan (1994) have argued the place for the combination remedy holds some significant pragmatic value. However, there are some aspects characteristic of HIV and AIDS that do represent a particular challenge to the homeopath.

1. There is often a complex miasmatic background, both inherited and acquired.
2. Allopathic treatment for past and present illnesses can be substantial and there are often the side effects of current treatment to be taken into account.
3. There is frequently a history of emotional, physical or sexual abuse, with deep, unresolved grief and anger.
4. The fear and anxiety produced as a result of the HIV/AIDS diagnosis usually creates additional symptoms, both emotional and physical.
5. A variety of treatments, both orthodox and alternative may be in use simultaneously and can result in confusion over the

effectiveness of chosen remedies.

6. Sometimes multiple opportunistic infections run into one another and present problems in terms of case management, the assessment of remedy reactions and the need for rapid and continuous prescribing. Of course, homoeopathy is not without the tools with which to respond. Careful and long-term constitutional prescribing, together with suggestions about life-style changes may be all that is required, but we have also found the need to incorporate other methods, using for example the smaller specific remedies, organ remedies, polypharmacy and tautopathy, as appropriate, with good results. For those who have been recently diagnosed there is often an acute state of fear and grief. In these cases, remedies such as Aconite, Arsenicum, Ignatia and Gelsemium in high potencies may offer great benefit. In situations where there is a history of drug use (both prescribed and recreational) the combination of Nux vomica and Sulphur has helped as has Nux vomica alone in high potency. Many homoeopaths have successfully used particular drugs in potency to alleviate side effects and this seems not to interfere with concurrent constitutional treatment. AZT and Septrin are very commonly prescribed and both can undermine the action of remedies, whilst AZT, in particular can have serious side effects. AZT 30 can be given once or twice weekly both alongside current drug treatment or if the effect lingers once treatment is stopped. Pentamidine as an alternative to Septrin for allopathic prophylaxis of PCP is generally felt to be preferable and seems to interfere less with remedies. Acyclovir for herpes and Fluconazole for thrush are also commonly used, but their effects seem not to be so problematic. The most common chemotherapy regime

for Kaposi's Sarcoma is Vincristine and Bleomycin. Again these drugs can be used in potency (a 6 or 12 seems most helpful) during chemotherapy and this often alleviates the side effects without negating any beneficial effects. A side-effect of AZT can sometimes be anaemia and in these cases Lecithin 6 in repeated doses can help to avoid the trauma of a blood transfusion. When transfusions are given, either as a result of drug use or because of opportunistic infections like MAI (Mycobacterium avium intracellulare), it can sometimes be necessary to give the major nosodes in quick succession to clear the resulting problems. In cases of Kaposi's Sarcoma both Lachesis and Phosphorus are frequently indicated, though results of homoeopathic treatment of this condition are not particularly encouraging. Results with the treatment of PCP vary, but early cases, in particular, often respond to remedies like Bryonia, Silica and Phosphorus. (Baker, Fox, Groot & Honan 1994).

Watson (1991) argues that polypharmacy is best suited to serious cases, particularly where the disease is manifesting in several different ways, and in cases where palliation is more desirable because cure is unlikely to happen. This point, plus the reality that in 21st century prescribing, compliance is a massive issue give some credence to this point. But it is also a rare circumstance that it could be justified to a homeopath prescribing on Hahnemann's principles.

Further Reading

- Yasgur   *Homeopathic Dictionary*
- Menninger   *The Eradication of Mongrelism*

- Little — *Following in Hahnemann's Footsteps: The Definitive Years 1833-1843*
- Chatterjee — *Fundamentals of Homoeopathy and Valuable Hints for Practice*
- Roberts — *The Principles and Art of Cure by Homoeopathy*
- Close — *The Genius of Homeopathy*
- Dunham — *The Science of Therapeutics. A Collection of Papers*
- Hempel — *A New and Comprehensive System of Materia Medica*
- Hughes — *The Principles and Practice of Homoeopathy The administration of the similar remedy*
- Clarke — *The Prescriber*
- Roberts — *The Principles and Art of Cure by Homoeopathy*
- Ullman — *Forward to Kent's Lectures on Homeopathic Philosophy*
- Morrison — *Desktop Guide to Keynotes and Confirmatory Symptoms*
- Saine — *Psychiatric patients*
- Bradford — *Life and Letters of Hahnemann*

Chapter 14

Conclusion

Method and Totality

In this book I have introduced a range of prescribing methods used in homeopathic medicine. It is not an exhaustive list. I have described the background, the method, situations for use, and some advantages and disadvantages of each of those methods chosen. There is no agreed or specific classification of all of the possible ways of prescribing. They are many and varied. They often overlap. After all, just what is the difference between constitutional and essence prescribing or centralist or central disturbance prescribing, specific or organ prescribing, characteristic totality or keynote characteristic prescribing? These are all methods and variations of method that have been described in the homeopathic literature over the years.

What is important to remember is that the classification used in this book has been based upon an understanding of totality. And it is this concept expressed in many and varied ways which has given rise to the range of methods used in homeopathy. Every homeopath, everyday, asks in any given clinical situation, 'what is the meaningful totality in this case'?

'What is the best totality to use that as can lead to cure in the shortest possible time and in the gentlest way?' Will it be the quantum approach, all of the symptoms of a patient cured with one prescription, the big bang, the golden bullet? Or will it be a constitutional, a situational, an aetiological, a therapeutic or an organ remedy approach? Should I use the legs of the stool? What about using the symptom similarity of the whole person, the essence, the central disturbance? Should I be treating the constitutional state? Will it be treating the whole person on all levels, mental or emotional and physical? A meaningful attempt has been made to untangle all of these terminologies, and render more clearly the fundamental issues faced by prescribers at the coalface of homeopathic medicine.

The message of this book is that method is determined by totality. The perception of the homeopath determines the size of the 'totality of symptoms'. This issue of totality is fundamental to understanding why different homeopaths prescribe in different ways why they have different methods as such. In the daily practice of homeopathy, practitioners expand and constrict their totalities depending on who is talking to them. In other words, this idea of totality is relative and relative to the specific facts in front of them. In any case, be it acute, chronic, simple or dramatic the necessary rule is to keep that totality meaningful. As articulated by Jeremy Sherr, this means that totality is relative in time and in space in any given situation.

To state it plainly, the issue confronting every homeopath in all clinical situations is which symptoms of all that are presented do we choose and use. If the patient gives you some presenting symptoms, and that's all that you can see, and those presenting symptoms are clear and sharp, then by all means prescribe upon them. This is what Hahnemann and Bönninghausen did, and it constitutes effective prescribing in homeopathic medicine. If however you can see those symptoms in the context of something much larger, and it is equally as meaningful, then you must prescribe on that larger totality. If further still, you see a greater totality, where all the symptoms in the case or the life of patient seem to hold together in one coherent, whole thread, mind, body, emotions and it is meaningful, then you must prescribe on it. This is what aphorisms 9 and 12 in the *Organon of Medicine* tell us.

Remember though that just because we choose a large totality, choosing thousands of symptoms is not going to find you the accurate remedy. The size of the totality will determine the questions that you ask. Homeopathy at its best is really about the size of the totality upon which we prescribe base on how we perceive the patient. Sometimes it is entirely appropriate to prescribe on the smallest and most minute totality. But often the totality based on mental and emotional symptoms is larger still and gets more lasting and deeper change. Miasms constitute a greater totality still. Constitutional prescribing also represents a greater totality. Treating the epidemic is an example of an even larger totality of symptoms generalised across a population, and in this situation we treat the epidemic 'as if one person' (Sherr 1993).

It is the homeopath's job to prescribe towards the largest and most meaningful totality perceived. The more similar the remedy, the less force is required. That prescription for the sore throat will need to be repeated again and again and again. The prescription for the broad chronic picture may only need to be prescribed just the once. To my mind, this point has been articulated beautifully in the chapters in this book by Gadd and Bhouraskar. But many homeopathic authors have taken this point one stage further and argued, that in as much as the prescription is for a smaller totality, it will suppress. Furthermore they assert the more a prescription is based on a part of the totality, the more it will suppress. This is the fundamental difference between the different schools of homeopathy; it is the different perception of the size of the totality.

Hahnemannian prescribing is characterised by an attempt to find the complete symptom. A subjective symptom with clear modifications, the location and concomitant are the underpinnings of this method. So simplistic in its conception it still does represent the cornerstone of thriving homeopathic practice. But, it is less useful when there are uncharacteristic emotional symptoms in the case. Still, its advantages are its replicability and its simplicity.

Kentian prescribing involves the totality of all the characteristic symptoms of a person, taking into account mental and emotional symptoms, the generals and the physicals. A strong feature of this method is to use a repertory that was designed specifically for this purpose, to then differentiate and prescribe the best possible remedy match. The prescribing style is rounded out with the use of the single remedy, a single dose, mostly with a high potency using the centesimal scale and infrequent repetitions of that remedy, with perhaps a follow-up at four or six weeks. It is argued that this style of homeopathy is best in chronic functional disorders where there are well-marked mental and emotional symptoms and physical generals. It seems that the style is less useful in more advanced and degenerative conditions where there is severe

Conclusion

pathology and where there are a lot of medications. One of the clear advantages is that when it works it produces change at all levels and there is an ease of use with the single remedy and infrequent follow-ups. Yet a heavy emphasis on mental and emotional symptoms often leads to a reliance on very few remedies with well-developed profiles. It is also found that single doses quite often don't hold as well because of the stresses of the 21st century. In addition, it is time-consuming with long case taking and evaluations. Furthermore, anecdotal evidence suggests that when poorly used, practitioners go too deep too soon and the case taking process can be perceived as unduly invasive.

Etiological prescribing can be so useful and yield dramatic results. The prescription is simply based on the cause and the choice of remedy determined on those few remedies where we have clear causation in the profile. It is best to use when there is a direct or clear link to the cause. Of course this may well be hidden or deep in the past but nevertheless if it emerges in the consultation process then that information should undoubtedly be used. It becomes harder to use when there are multiple causations. An advantage is that it can be used in a whole range of cases from simple acute, simple chronic or complex chronic diseases. Of course a disadvantage is that many cases have very unclear causations and another limitation is that those causations are sometimes not well represented in our repertories.

Keynote prescribing can be exemplified with the idea that the remedy in a given case is based on the constellation, or clear characteristic symptoms of the case. The final choice of a remedy may be from a single but preferably from a number of keynotes. This is so useful where those key indications are strong. Acute cases that lack symptom clarity but have one or more strong keynotes lend itself to the style. One-sided cases may also respond well. It is quick and effective especially in acute prescribing and palliative care but a strong disadvantage is its tendency to create laziness and sloppy habits in prescribers.

Isopathy is that style of prescribing where the remedy given is made from the causative agent. It may be the diseased tissue from which the remedy is manufactured. Very often low potencies are prescribed and it is often used as a last resort when other methods have been attempted. But nevertheless it is incredibly effective in situations where there may be hypersensitivities or allergic conditions, miasmatic influences or a lack of response when well indicated remedies have tried and been unsuccessful. A significant advantage is that it is so simple to use and it is based on a clear diagnosis. Long case taking is often not required. But in this advantage is its single greatest disadvantage in that it leads to laziness.

It is the same with tautopathy, where the drug or toxin is potentised and given to the person who has been suffering from the effects of a drug. Often used in low potencies, it has been used for many years now in homeopathy, after vaccination for example, or the effects of drugs or toxins and definitely in drug withdrawal. It is clearly valuable in those cases that are not responding well to totality prescriptions and can be used to support deeper acting polycrest prescriptions. But there's no doubt that it does not treat the whole person and can lead to some superficial prescribing.

Organ orientated prescribing is based upon the idea that remedies have specific affinities for organs in the body. A reality of practice, this understanding that some remedies have affinities for the heart, liver, valves, nerves etc mean that we have a legitimate option in those cases where clear symptoms or a broader totality is not to be found. Characterised by the use of low potencies and often mother tinctures, the method identifies the seat of the disease, the main complaints and orientates itself to supporting the organs of the body in the initial stages of treatment while the vital force rallies. It is a quick method and an effective one. It is very helpful in supporting deeper treatment and especially useful where deeper acting remedies have failed to act. Of course it can be superficial, lazy and one of the practical difficulties is determining the optimal repetition and management and administration of the remedy chosen.

These different methods highlighted, explored, unpacked and deconstructed, the last word goes to Richard Pitt.

To American homeopaths Richard needs no introduction. He was a driving force behind the development of the certification process in the USA. He's been a pivotal figure with the C.H.C. and driving their profession forward in difficult times. Running a college in the Bay area, practicing and being involved at a political level in the profession for more than a decade, he's made a considerable mark. What struck me when I first met Richard was not just his scholarship but his openness. Often those two things don't go together. Scholars and academics often hear a new idea and say 'No' as an immediate reaction or a default position. What is striking about Richard is that he maintains his critical thinking capacity while remaining open to the new.

His work with individual substances such as tobacco,

and his perspective on broad issues impacting heavily on homeopathy at a professional level and at an educational level are incredibly valuable at this time. I'm deeply grateful for Richard's permission to re-publish his article on method and the way forward in homeopathic education, which to me go hand in hand.

If You Meet Hahnemann on the Road, Kill Him

Richard Pitt - CCH, RSHom (NA)

Don't be afraid; you won't do either—not literally, anyway. The zen-inspired title of this essay is adapted from the book *If You Meet The Buddha On The Road, Kill Him,* by psychologist Sheldon Kopp. The premise of Kopp's book is the necessity of finding one's own inner truth rather than relying on any external authority, of moving beyond a spiritual or therapeutic relationship based on an abdication of personal autonomy. The relevance of Kopp's premise to homeopathy lies in the fact that the aura of Hahnemann hangs over homeopathy as strongly today as it did 100 years ago. Indeed, the very identity of homeopathy is so inextricably linked with the influence of Hahnemann that it is difficult to imagine an alternative approach.

I do not mean to suggest that there is anything essentially wrong with acknowledging the unique contribution of Hahnemann to the establishment of the homeopathic method and the elucidation of its main philosophical positions; his writings are a vital part of homeopathic thinking and a pioneering contribution to medical thought. At the same time, however, it is apparent that Hahnemann's personality dominates the profession to the extent that it has incorporated, along with his ideas, vestiges of his personal issues and of cultural dynamics peculiar to the time in which he lived. It can be argued, in light of this, that the collective identity of our profession resembles that of a cult of personality as much as it does that of a medical art, giving rise to distinctly religious overtones in the expression of homeopathic thought and philosophy as expounded by Hahnemann, Kent and others, and rendering the system of homeopathic practice an extension of Hahnemann's profound influence.

In Constantine Hering's preface to T.L. Bradford's biography, *The Life and Letters of Hahnemann*, he suggests that Hahnemann should be judged on the basis of his own words and actions, and that a biographer should be careful not to make assertions regarding his character that could be abused or taken out of historical context. The purpose of this essay is neither to pathologise Hahnemann nor to minimise in any way his impact on homeopathy and medical thought, but to attempt to understand his impact on homeopathy *today*, and to explore the issues we face as an evolving professional community—particularly those related to our professional heritage, which inevitably includes Hahnemann as a man and an historical figure.

The Influence of Hahnemann

The practical consequences of Hahnemann's impact are manifold. As indicated above, the most important of these is a perception of the very identity of homeopathy as an extension of one man's influence, which tends to confine it, in the minds of many, to a realm of quasi-religious doctrine as opposed to that of a full-fledged scientific methodology. While this may be a result of conflicting dynamics within Hahnemann's personal development, and of the contextual influences of the religious and scientific cultures of the 18th and 19th centuries, it perpetuates a contemporary tendency to seek confidence in what we do in the authority of living teachers, and to choose teachers and schools of thought that satisfy our emotional needs. While there is nothing wrong with learning homeopathy from more experienced teachers, there is a tendency in the profession to confer authority on such teachers—and to establish hierarchical relationships with them in which they are put on pedestals and treated like gurus—that is similar to the intensity of devotion that Hahnemann demanded of his own students. Interestingly, some of these students had received theological as well as medical training, another indication of the strong religious dynamics characteristic of homeopathic thought during his lifetime.

The influence of Hahnemann on homeopathy, even today in the 21st century, is intrinsic to its very identity, and may be one reason why homeopathy has struggled to "find itself" and to achieve a greater level of recognition within the spectrum of medical modalities. Homeopathy is not alone in having its roots in the founding contributions of a single powerful figure; Chiropractic, Osteopathy, Rolfing, Feldenkrais, and Alexander Technique have each followed a similar pattern and may struggle to some degree with some of the same issues that homeopathy does. In homeopathy, however, the ongoing influence of Hahnemann is perhaps stronger than that of the founding figures of these other healing professions, and to that extent, ours has inherited both the wisdom and the shadow of the man himself.

Conclusion

One of the characteristics of many influential historical figures is their willingness, founded in the uniqueness of their vision, to take great risks and to challenge the *status quo*. While this strength allows them to resist the stream of convention, it is often accompanied by an intolerance of dissent and a demand for obedience from followers. This is a dynamic seen in many cults and religions, as well as in political movements in which the dynamics of power, control and conformity may be more obvious. Such individuals often have great charisma and an unusual intensity of purpose—which can be seductive to those searching for profound answers to life's fundamental questions—and homeopathy has historically attracted practitioners interested in the formulation of a comprehensive narrative of the world and its workings, encompassing as it does both the overtly religious/spiritual concerns and the anti-conventional elements inherent in such a quest.

Hahnemann's own story is characterised by intellectual tenacity and a determination to pursue his purpose at great personal expense, both to himself and to his family. He accepted discomfort and refused to be impeded by social and political constraints. He exhibited highly unusual capacities, qualities often found in those who have a far-reaching impact on the world. However, the shadow side of such personalities often leaves a trail of damage that raises many questions as to the motives and psychological dynamics that fuel their behaviour. In his seminal book on charismatic spiritual leaders, *Prophetic Charisma: The Psychology of Revolutionary Religious Personalities*, psychologist Len Oakes explores the dynamics of such personalities in search of a deeper psychological understanding of their underlying motivations. In his introduction, he cites the following passage from William James's *Varieties of Religious Experience:*

> When a superior intellect and a psychopathic temperament coalesce—as in the endless permutations and combinations of human faculty they are bound to coalesce often enough—in the same individual, we have the best possible condition for the kind of effective genius that gets into the biographical dictionaries. Such men do not remain mere critics and understanders with their intellect. Their ideas possess them; they inflict them, for better or for worse, upon their companions or their age.

While we would not want to use the term "psychopathic" to describe Hahnemann, it is nevertheless apparent that he does conform to many of the descriptions proffered by James. Oakes suggests that what all such "prophets" have in common is their opposition to convention and their ability to inspire others with their visions. While Hahnemann may not conform to Oakes definition of a prophet as someone who attracts followers that look to him or her for guidance in their daily lives, it is clear that he did demand a high degree of adherence and conformity to his way of thinking, and expended great energy in the condemnation of those who refused to see the wisdom of homeopathy, and of the so-called "mongrels" (his word) who practiced various hybrid forms of medicine. He also exhibited many of the qualities that Oakes lists as key attributes of a prophetic personality:

- Enormous energy for life
- Grandiose self-confidence
- Optimism and positivity, leading to delusions of optimism and refusal to compromise or hear criticisms—a blindness

to others and fixation on revolutionary vision
- The use of moral absolutes, to amplify a sense of crisis in which the sinfulness of the world is described in absolute terms

While Hahnemann does not seem to have attempted to use the power of his personality to influence his followers in a direct way, he did insist on adherence to a philosophical purity rooted, in his estimation, in a divine source, and his intolerance of even his closest followers engagements with practices that deviated from his formulation of "pure" homeopathy is well known. This tendency can perhaps be rationalised as a manifestation of the inevitable growing pains of a system in the process of self-definition in an historical context of adverse social and political forces, but it has also been an essential expression of many charismatic political and religious leaders throughout history—"You are either with me or against me."

While we need to be careful not to unduly pathologise Hahnemann, who sacrificed so much to develop and promulgate homeopathy in the wider world, it is not inappropriate, in my estimation, to examine the dynamic influence of his legacy as it finds expression in homeopathy over 200 years later. Within homeopathy, Hahnemann is revered both as a profound thinker and as the founder of its system: we still study the Organon as the bible of homeopathy; we still adhere to his philosophical guidelines, accepting them as the foundation of classical homeopathy; and while we may not practice as Hahnemann practiced in his time, in general we still measure what we do against his example, and engage in considerable debate when practitioners methods deviate from his. Among a large number of the more conservative "classical" homeopaths, Hahnemann's dictates are regarded as impervious to challenge, and the whole of the system of homeopathy is seen through his experience and writings.

In our profession, then, the influence of Hahnemann is alive and well, and while it offers us the coherence of tradition and principle, it is also reasonable to ask whether—and if so to what degree—this coherence also constitutes an impediment. Are we like children who can't escape the dominion of our parents? Is the widespread influence of one man, with all his issues, inhibiting the growth of the profession itself? And does this influence perpetuate a cult of personality, and replicate patterns associated with it, within the field of homeopathy?

The Implications of Individualism in Homeopathy

As we all know, homeopathy is focused on that which individualises each particular case. We explore the unique qualities, sensations and personality of each client. This individualisation of our cases, embracing both objective and subjective phenomena, in turn focuses more attention on the individual ability of the practitioner. The relationship between homeopath and patient can be vital to the creation of an atmosphere that allows the case to unfold. This focus on the individual homeopath as a reflection of the system of homeopathic practice is part of the creative tension and exploration within homeopathy, as it is in many other arts and sciences. There will always be Einstein-like figures that challenge the accepted principles of conventional wisdom; but in homeopathy, it may be necessary to ask whether too much weight is given to the influence of certain individual practitioners as opposed to the collective wisdom of homeopathic science, and whether this perhaps reflects the lack of an objective system within homeopathic practice, giving greater significance to its "artistic" expression through individual practitioners than to scientific principles and guidelines of practice.

Much contemporary debate in homeopathy addresses this concern—with emphasis on the question of whether individual practitioners are delving into interpretive, speculative or subjective realms in unwarranted opposition to the so-called scientific tradition of homeopathy represented by Hahnemann and other "masters." One of the more interesting aspects of this debate, however, is its largely unquestioned focus on the famous individual practitioners and "masters" that seem to dominate the consciousness of the profession, in light of which the system of Homeopathy can come to seem less significant than the individuals who formulate it. Is this a problem in the development of homeopathy? Is our apparent need for "masters"—dead or alive—to show us the way a reflection of a collective immaturity on the part of our community and of certain narcissistic tendencies in its central figures?

I use the term *narcissism* here to refer both to a self-centered focus in general and also to those psychological characteristics, said to be attributes of the narcissistic personality, outlined by Oakes. Drawing on the formulations of traditional psychology, Oakes classifies six key characteristics of the second developmental phase of so-called narcissistic personalities: 1) not belonging to any group, 2) construction of a personal "myth of calling," 3) splitting of the personality, 4) radical autonomy, 5) conflicts with authorities, and 6) the acquisition of practical skills appropriate to a later prophetic career. Without engaging in an excessive analysis of Hahnemann's psychology or restricting our understanding of him to that of a classically defined narcissistic personality, it is nevertheless apparent that some of these attributes are consistent with Hahnemann's personality to a degree sufficient, perhaps, to have influenced the developing identity of the homeopathic profession down to the present day.

The scholar and teacher Alfonso Montuori describes a model of learning that suggests a related but alternative understanding of the concept of narcissism. Montuori suggests that the apparent polarisation of so-called "Reproductive/Rationalistic" and "Narcissistic" models of learning can be balanced by a third learning modality that he refers to as "Creative Inquiry":

> By "Reproductive" I mean an approach to education that sees the source of knowledge as almost exclusively outside the knower, and focuses almost exclusively on the accurate reproduction of that knowledge by the knower. It is about reproducing the content one has received; reproducing the disciplinary organization, instructional pedagogy, and power structures that generates this knowledge; reproducing the standard, accepted ways of conducting inquiry; reproducing the societal/industrial expectations for what a good member of the workforce is; reproducing the existing social and academic order.
>
> Narcissistic Education emerges as an important corrective to the dry, limited view of traditional Reproductive Education. But if in the process it rejects high academic standards, if it does not involve dialogue with the larger scholarly community, if it is not grounded in the literature, if it is not open to challenge and critique, if it defies the laws of science and common sense, we

end up with a narcissistic world of navel-gazing that adds little if anything of value to the field, "process" replaces "content," and an entirely new set of oppositions is created.

Creative Inquiry is designed to integrate the best of traditional scholarly inquiry and also expand what we mean by education and inquiry by including an ongoing process of self-inquiry that recognizes the role of the knower in inquiry. Creative Inquiry in the educational process is not merely an accumulation of facts and figures, the development of an academic specialization and expertise in a given topic, but can also be an opportunity to transform oneself, one's world, and the process of inquiry itself.

We can see characteristics of both Montuori's Reproductive/Rationalistic model and his Narcissistic model in contemporary homeopathic learning and practice; in fact his formulation is, in my estimation, an accurate representation of some of the fundamental issues that we face as practitioners in defining the science and art of homeopathy. On one level we have a "scientific" emphasis on homeopathic philosophy and practice—examination based on objective criteria for remedy knowledge and methods of analysis—and on the other, the "unknown" qualities of the client/practitioner relationship and the "intuitive" abilities of the practitioner, who seeks an understanding of the individual subjective realities of the client. Both methods have validity and it is precisely the integration of the two that allows for success in practice. However, undue emphasis on either one can lead to a dry, sterile, reductionistic form of practice, or a highly subjective, self-reflective form of practice that seeks no rational comparison or justification.

My use of the term narcissistic here also encompasses homeopathy's emphasis on central figures and its tendency to foster institutional factionalism and the perpetuation of a cultic orientation both within homeopathy and in relation to the world at large. As mentioned earlier, contemporary devotion to living teachers partakes of qualities similar to the kind of relationships Hahnemann cultivated with his students. While it is clear that Hahnemann was a medical genius and a great thinker, he also exhibited qualities of rigidity and authoritarianism that evoked strong devotion and aversion in equal measure. Perhaps these qualities were necessary prerequisites of the construction of the phenomenal system we know as homeopathy; a less rigid person might not have had the tenacity, determination and mental discipline to achieve what Hahnemann did. Does this mean, however, that we are bound to replicate the same inflexibility and doctrinal rigidity? Some of the profession's more "conservative" contemporary commentators seem at times to embody the role of the Catholic priests of old, imparting the wisdom of the "masters," always looking to the past for their authority and questioning any ideas or methods that do not adhere to pre-established doctrine. In contrast, some of the more "progressive" homeopaths act more like born-again Christians, identifying themselves as bringers of a new paradigm with all the passion and zeal of those who believe they have found the light.

In terms of relations with the world at large, it is apparent that many systems that exist on the margins of social acceptability tend to maintain rigid ideas of identity in response to real or perceived threats from the established powers. Homeopathy has had this type of adversarial relationship to conventional medicine since Hahnemann's time, and one can as easily assert that its fortifying adherence to the foundational principles laid down by Hahnemann is also a weakness to the extent that it isolates us unnecessarily from more mainstream thinking.

Teachers in Contemporary Homeopathy

External pressure during Hahnemann's time may also have contributed to the underlying "cultic" dynamic within homeopathy, especially with respect to Hahnemann's insistence that his students adhere to his dictates. Today, there are a number of teachers who evoke, consciously or not, a similar level of devotion. Perhaps the most significant of these are Rajan Sankaran and others of the Bombay Group. For quite a number of years, Sankaran in particular has attracted a passionately devoted group of followers who treat him like a guru and who tend to accept less than critically the positions he articulates in his writings and seminars. Many of these students now identify themselves as practitioners of the "Sensation Method," making a distinction between themselves and other homeopaths. While this may not necessarily represent a conscious attempt to separate their practices from others in the homeopathic community, the effect is to establish a clear distinction that tends to suggest feelings of uniqueness and superiority.

While Sankaran's ideas obviously merit serious study and experimentation, the identity dynamics thus created are potentially problematic. After all, homeopathy is homeopathy. There are many ways to find the simillimum within the homeopathic method, but to identify oneself as an adherent of one method within the broader homeopathic system raises certain questions. Many practitioners now say, for example, that they conduct all their cases according to this method—as if one methodology, however wonderful, is complete in and of itself. Is it valid to assert that an attempt to systematise a particular style of case taking and analysis represents a new and more complete homeopathic "method"? While Sankaran's systematisation exemplifies an interesting dynamic with respect to the challenge of addressing the subjective nature of homeopathic practice, to the extent that every case demands a unique approach it remains open to question. As neophyte practitioners uncritically adopt Sankaran's method of seeking the "Vital Sensation," they may unwittingly reduce the art of homeopathy to a specific system of case taking and analysis whose results will be difficult to replicate in other situations. Further, such systematisation may be unnecessary and superfluous to the extent that what Sankaran is advocating is at its root simply good homeopathy, i.e., knowing when to ask the question that elicits the most revealing response, which is after all the goal of all homeopathic practice.

The fact that a large number of teachers have become involved with Sankaran's ideas and identify themselves accordingly creates interesting challenges in the teaching of homeopathy to students. Some now recommend the teaching of Sankaran's method fairly exclusively from the beginning of training, theorising that it is no longer necessary to attend to the fundamentals of homeopathic case taking and practice as they have been developed over the last 200 years. For these people, Sankaran's method is *it*, and one need only learn it well to practice homeopathy with greater success than anyone else.

Such total conviction is perhaps the inevitable result of commitment to inspiring ideas that seem to offer secure answers to the challenges of practicing an art as subjective as homeopathy. At the same time, however, the tendency to identify oneself not just as a homeopath but as, for example, a practitioner of the "Vital Sensation System," creates an illusion of separation and hierarchy within homeopathy as a whole. As philosopher Ken Wilber explains in *A Brief History of Everything*, new ideas and systems often arise from a desire not to build on an earlier method but to supersede or subsume an extant paradigm so as to be able identify oneself as the creator of something distinct from it. My intent here is not to dismiss Sanakran's ideas so much as to question social and political constructs that have evolved around them and that have caused considerable consternation within our profession.

Method or No Method

As homeopathy is an art as well as a science, in the end we all have to find our own way. It is important to realise that even if we learn a great deal from various teachers, we ultimately have to leave the teacher as we forge our own identity, gaining the necessary confidence from our own practice and experience. To the extent that we insist on imposing any "system" on the organic process of the homeopathic art, we court the risk of a rigidity in our style of thought and practice that disempowers us as unique individual practitioners. Our "method" then replaces the experience of being a simple witness for the patient's story, and the agenda of getting to the "vital sensation" may be inappropriately imposed on our relationship with the patient. Similarly, the "seven-level" model espoused by Sankaran (similar to many other esoteric models of levels of consciousness), can foster a desire to "get to" each of the seven levels, even if the remedy picture has become very clear at level one or two. While this approach may work in the hands of a skilled practitioner, when attempted by inexperienced homeopaths it can create more confusion than clarity. The simple beauty of just listening without a particular agenda, which can effortlessly lead one to a deeper understanding of a person and therefore the correct remedy, can be undermined by a relentless style of inquisition in which the client is required to express feelings and thoughts until "the truth" is revealed.

Sankaran's philosophy can be seen as a continuation of a Kentian stream of thought with distinct connections to the esoteric aspect of spiritual thought adapted by Kent from Swedenborg. From this perspective, the central "spiritual" core is seen as the holy grail of understanding, in contrast to the more "mundane" objective methodologies of "scientific" homeopathy, especially the more non-classical styles practiced in France and other countries. This is just one more example of the subjective/objective dichotomy in homeopathic practice. While the concept of individualisation lies at the centre of Hahnemann's revelations and is also central to our concept of the simillimum and holistic principles, the vulnerability of Sankaran's method lies in its potential for subjective interpretation of individual dynamics by different homeopaths in a manner that could be construed as "Narcissistic" according to Montuori's classification. The quest for a "systemic" approach in which objective methodology and subjective process can come together is the continuing challenge of homeopathy that Sankaran, along with the rest of the profession, is striving for. The goal of finding the correct remedy through our knowledge of *materia medica* is a formulation of an objective process in the context of an uncompromising embrace of the uniqueness of every individual and of the many ways by means of which it is possible to discover the simillimum. The fascinating conundrum surrounding Sankaran's method of establishing the Vital Sensation, as well as his system for examining families and miasms, is his search for an objective "method" of homeopathic analysis through the utilisation of highly *subjective* processes. The issue is not that it doesn't work, as enough people have used it successfully it to confirm its validity; the problem rather lies in the adoption of any method as *the* method.

From a philosophical point of view, Sankaran's thought and methodology represents the esoteric perspective within homeopathy—the other, more objective side being represented by the "medical" wing of homeopathic practice and history. Ironically, Hahnemann's own practice was strongly medically based, whereas one could say that Kent and the other Swedenborgian homeopaths were more influenced by underlying esoteric theories, even if their practices included extensive medical analysis. The implication in Sankaran's philosophy seems to be that there is only one correct remedy for each person, and that the goal of the interview process is to figure out the unique pattern within one remedy image. While it can be said, however, that at any given time there is only one correct remedy that will work the best, this does preclude the possibility of identifying additional remedies that may be necessary at various times in a given case. Even if Sankaran and his colleagues in India don't believe that only one remedy is necessary for a cure, this remains a common assumption among those who subscribe to his philosophy as a whole.

One of the difficulties of devoting ourselves to the teachings of a single theorist is that doing so can cause us to deviate from own independent development as practitioners; it can give rise to a conscious or unconscious abdication of autonomy, as well an isolation from other theorists and practitioners. Identification with a particular method inevitably creates some degree of separation. Given the historical tendency for homeopaths to squabble among themselves, and given the schisms that exist even within the broader "classical" family, it is interesting to observe the impact that Sankaran's thinking is having on contemporary dialogue within homeopathy. It does not constitute a wholesale denial of the validity of his ideas to question the wholesomeness of the impact—similar to that of some authority figures in other walks of life—of his personal psychological dynamics on the broader homeopathic *gestalt*.

One of the contentions of this article is that we ought perhaps to question our need to have a "guru" to tell us what to do or think, and our need to seek such direction from certain charismatic teachers. There will always be a need for teachers, but their role must be questioned more closely in terms of the impact they have on others and the motivations underlying their desire to occupy it. While Sankaran and his colleagues have enjoyed great success in the promulgation of their ideas, it remains to be seen whether their philosophy will encourage or stifle further innovation and originality, and to what extent it will become part of the mainstream of homeopathic practice. While there are many other innovators in homeopathy today, for some reason the energy around Sankaran and the Bombay Group partakes of the "cultic" dynamic described above to a greater degree than seems to be the case with most other teachers. It may be that this reflects variations within the professional community with respect to the need for guidance and authority.

Implications for Practice

The ultimate goal of this discussion is an examination of the process of developing self-knowledge and evolution in the homeopathic practitioner. While like most human beings we can be quite neurotic and still function somewhat effectively in our profession, it is also true that homeopathy is a journey for all of us, and that our ability to function competently as homeopaths is connected to some degree to how well we know ourselves. But there is an even more compelling question that pertains to the structural influences of homeopathy itself: When we immerse ourselves in the system, philosophy, history and practice of homeopathy, we become part of the hologram of homeopathy; we inherit the "miasm" and energy of the whole system and its entire history. Part of the spirit of Hahnemann is in us, and the question is, what do we do with it all?

Obviously, we want to do the best work we can, and it seems to me that our work should force us to look into ourselves, to question our own processes and to use homeopathy to help us in our own evolution. We cannot separate this personal evolution from that of our patients. We are implicated by our actions and our relationship with our patients and fellow practitioners. We have to strive to "Know Thyself" and, in that endeavor, to respect others. We have to cultivate caution against pride and vanity, which will rebound on us individually and on our profession as a whole. We have to recognise that our actions have consequences and that the future of homeopathy as a viable profession is dependent on how we conduct ourselves as practitioners. Our own willingness to evolve personally will affect our capacities as healers. The fact is, most people come to see us because of who we are as human beings, not because of which system or method we practice. Regardless of the system, "guru" or method to which we subscribe, it is by our humanity that we will ultimately be measured, rather than our brilliance with respect to case taking, materia medica, or analysis. As Van Morrison so famously put it—"No Guru, No Method, No Teacher."

References

Agrawal, Y.R. (1995) *A Comparative Study of Chronic Miasms*, Vijay, New Delhi, India.

Allen, H.C. (1881) 'Prejudice the Chief Obstacle to the Scientific Investigation of Posology in Clinical Medicine', *American Institute of Homoeopathy*, accessed in Radar Opus 2011.

Allen, H.C. (1910) *Allen's Keynotes and Characteristics with Comparisons with Bowel Nosodes*, B. Jain Publishers (P) Ltd., New Delhi, India.

Allen, H.C. (1910) *The Materia Medica of Some Important Nosodes*, Boericke & Tafel, Philadelphia.

Allen, H.C. (1931) *Keynotes and characteristics with comparisons of some of the leading remedies of material medica with bowel nosodes*, 6th edn., Boericke & Tafel, Philadelphia.

Allen, H.C. (1910) *Allen's Keynotes and Characteristics with Comparisons with Bowel Nosodes*, B. Jain Publishers (P) Ltd., New Delhi, India.

Allen, J.H. (1994) *The Chronic Miasms: Psora and Pseudo-Psora*, B. Jain Publishers (P) Ltd., New Delhi, India.

Allen, J.H. (1994) *The Chronic Miasms: Sycosis*, B. Jain Publishers (P) Ltd., New Delhi, India.

Allendy, R. (1912) *Alchemy and the medicine: Thesis*, Chacornac, Paris.

Anshutz, E.P. (1900) *New Old and Forgotten Remedies*, Boericke & Tafel, Philadelphia.

Antoniou, A. (2006) 'The Five Therapeutic Relationships', *Clinical Case Studies*, October 2006, 5: 437-451.

Bailey, P.M. (1995) *Homeopathic Psychology: Personality Profiles of the Major Constitutional Remedies*, North Atlantic Books, Berkeley.

Bailey, P. (1998) *Carcinosinium: A Clinical Materia Medica*, Palmyra, Western Australia.

Baker, A., Fox, K., Groot, C. & Honan, N. (1994) 'Working and living with AIDS and HIV', *Homoeopathic Links*, accessed in Radar Opus 2011.

Baldwin, W.W. (1898) 'Homoeopathy and Drug Miasms', *Hahnemannian Advocate*, Vol. XXXVII: Chicago, accessed in Radar Opus 2011.

Banerjea, S. (1991) *Miasmatic Diagnosis: Practical Tips with Clinical Comparisons*, B. Jain Publishers (P) Ltd., New Delhi, India.

Barker, E. (2003) *Miracles of healing and how they are done how to cure the incurable*, Reprint edn., B. Jain Publishers (P) Ltd., New Delhi, India.

Barker, E.J. (1940) 'Gallstones', *Heal thyself*, February Vol. LXXV (890) accessed in Radar Opus 2011.

Baum, M. & Ernst, E. (2009) 'Should we maintain an open mind about homeopathy?', *Am J Med*, 122 (11): 973-4.

Bedayn, G. (1995) 'Hew to the line', *American Homeopaths*, accessed in Radar Opus 2011.

Bedayn, G. (1997) 'Something Happen', *American Homoeopaths*, accessed in Radar Opus 2011.

Bellavite, P. & Signorini, A. (1995) *Homeopathy: A frontier in medical science*, Berkeley, California, North Atlantic Books.

Bennett, J. & Pope, A. (2008) *The Pill: are you sure it's for you?*, Allen and Unwin, Australia.

Bentley, G. (2003) *Appearance and Circumstance*, Pennon Publishing, Melbourne, Australia.

Bentley, G. (2006) *Homeopathic Facial Analysis*, Pennon Publishing, Australia.

Bentley, G. (2008) *Soul and Survival: The common human experience*, Pennon Publishing, Australia.

Bernoville, F. (1933) 'Fundamental laws of therapeutics', *l'Homoeopathie Moderne*, (17 & 19) accessed in Radar Opus 2011.

Bernoville, F. (1934) 'Drainage and Canalisation in Homoeopathic therapeutics', *l' Homoeopathie Moderne*, (19) accessed in Radar Opus 2011.

Bernoville, F. (1940) *Syphilis and Sycosis*, accessed in Radar Opus 2011.

Bernoville, F. (1960) 'What We Must Not Do In Homeopathy', *Journal of Homeopathic medicine*, accessed in Radar Opus 2011.

Bertani, S. & Lussignoli, S. (1999) 'Dual Effects of a Homoepathic Mineral Complex on Carageenan-induced Oedema in Rats', *British Homoepathic Journal*, Vol. 88: 101-105.

Bettelheim-March (1998) *General, Organic & Biochemistry*, Saunders College Publishing, United States of America.

Bhanja, K.C. (1993) *Constitution: Drug Pictures & Treatment*, 3rd edn., National Homoeo Laboratory, Calcutta, India.

Bhouraskar, S. (2010) *The Quest For Simillimum*, HomeoQuest, available at http://www.homeoquest.com/books/tqfs/

Blackie, M. (1986) *Classical homoeopathy*, Beaconsfield Publishers Ltd., Berkshire, UK.

Boericke, W. (1927) *Pocket Manual of Homeopathic Materia Medica*, 9th edn., Boericke & Runyon, Philadelphia.

Boger, C. (1964) *Studies in the Philosophy of Healing*, accessed in Radar Opus 2011.

Boger, C.M. (1915) *Synoptic Key of the Materia Medica*, accessed in Radar Opus 2011.

Boger, C.M. (1941) *The Study of Materia Medica and Taking the Case*, Roy & co, Mumbai, India.

Boger, C.M. (1998) *Boger-Boenninghausen Characteristics and Repertory*, B. Jain Publishers (P) Ltd., New Delhi, India.

Bonnerot and Bernoville (1934) *Ulcer of the Stomach and Duodenum*, accessed in Radar Opus 2011.

References

Bradford, T.L. (1895) *The Life and Letters of Dr. Samuel Hahnemann*, Roy Publishing House, Calcutta, accessed in Radar Opus 2011.

Brotteaux (1947) *Homoeopathy and Isopathy*, Peyronnet, Paris.

Burnett, J.C. (1887) *Diseases of the Spleen and their Remedies Clinically Illustrated*, Epps: London, accessed in Radar Opus 2011.

Burnett, J.C. (1888) *Tumours of the Breast and their Treatment and Cure by Medicines*, Epps: London, accessed in Radar Opus 2011.

Burnett, J.C. (1890) *Five Years Experience In The Cure Of Consumption By Its Own Virtue (Bacillinum)*, Homeopathic Publishing Co., London, accessed in Radar Opus 2011.

Burnett, J.C. (1891) *Greater Diseases Of The Liver*, Hahnemann Publishing House, Philadelphia, accessed in Radar Opus 2011.

Burnett, J.C. (1895) *Gout and its Cure*, Boericke & Tafel, Philadelphia, accessed in Radar Opus 2011.

Burnett, J.C. (1896) *Organ Diseases of Women, Notably Enlargements and Displacements of the Uterus and Sterility: Considered Curable by Medicines*, Homeopathic publishing Co., London, accessed in Radar Opus 2011.

Burnett, J. (1888) *Fifty Reasons for Being a Homeopath*, accessed in Radar Opus 2011.

Burnett, J. (1893) *Curability of Tumours*, accessed in Radar Opus 2011.

Burnett, J. (1896) *Organ Diseases of Women*, accessed in Radar Opus 2011.

Burnett, J.C. (1880) 'Letter from J. C. Burnett', *The Organon*, Anglo-American Journal of Hom. Medicine and Progressive Collateral Science, accessed in Radar Opus 2011.

Burnett, J.C. (1898) *Curability of Tumours*, Boericke & Tafel, Philadelphia, accessed in Radar Opus 2011.

Cahis, M. (1890) 'Electro-homoeopathy', *The Homeopathic Physician*, Vol. X, accessed in Radar Opus 2011.

Cahis, M. (1890) 'Polypharmacy and the single remedy', *The Homeopathic Physician*, Vol. X (*The International Homoeopathic Congress of Paris*, Aug 1889, Summary of its proceedings), accessed in Radar Opus 2011.

Campbell, A. (1981) 'The Concept of Constitution in Homeopathy', *British Homeopathic Journal*, 183-188.

Carleton, E. (1896) 'Hahnemann vs. Isopathy', *Hahnemannian Advocate*, Vol. XXXV (11), Chicago, accessed in Radar Opus 2011.

Case, E.E. (1916) *Some Clinical Experiences of E. E. Case*, accessed in Radar Opus 2011.

Castonuay, L. (2006) 'The Working Alliance Where are We', *Psycotherapy Theory Research Practice Training*, Vol. 43 (3): 271-279.

Chalmers, A.F. (1994) *What is this thing called science? An assessment of the nature and status of science and its method*, 2nd edn., 13-14, University of Queensland Press, St. Lucia Qld, Australia.

Chatterjee, T.P. (1988) *Fundamentals Of Homoeopathy And Valuable Hints For Practice*, B. Jain Publishers (P) Ltd., New Delhi, India.

Choudhuri, N.M. (1929) *A study on Materia Medica*, 2nd edn., Das, Calcutta, India.

Choudhury, H. (2005) *Indications of Miasm*, B. Jain Publishers (P) Ltd., New Delhi, India.

Clarke, J.H. (1900) *Dictionary of Practical Materia Medica*, Homeopathic Publishing Co., London, accessed in Radar Opus 2011.

Clarke, J.H. (2001) *Grand Characteristics of the Materia Medica*, B. Jain Publishers (P) Ltd., accessed in Radar Opus 2011.

Clarke, J.H. (1885) *The Prescriber: A Dictionary Of The New Therapeutics*, Keene & Ashwell, London, accessed in Radar Opus 2011.

Clarke, J.H. (1902) *The Life and Times of Dr. Burnett*, accessed in Radar Opus 2011.

Clarke, J.H. (1904) *A Clinical Repertory of the Dictionary of Materia Medica*, Homeopathic publishing Co., London, accessed in Radar Opus 2011.

Clarke, J.H. (1925) *Constitutional Medicine With Especial Reference to the Three Constitutions of Von Grauvogl*, Homeopathic publishing Co., London, accessed in Radar Opus 2011.

Clarke, J.H. (1985) *Homoeopathy Explained*, B. Jain Publishers (P) Ltd., New Delhi, India.

Close, S. (1898) 'Homoeopathy and Drug Miasms', *Hahnemannian Advocate*, Vol. XXXVII (3), Chicago, accessed in Radar Opus 2011.

Close, S. (1924) *The Genius of Homeopathy – Lectures and Essays on Homeopathic Philosophy*, Reprint edn., B. Jain, New Delhi, India.

Collet, D. (1898) *Isopathic-Methode of Pasteur for Internal Use*, Baillere, Paris.

Coulter, C.R. (1998) *Portraits of Homoeopathic Medicines: Psychophysical Analyses of Selected Constitutional Types*, Quality Medical Publishing Inc., St Louis, Missouri.

Creasy, S. (1997) 'Interview with Sheilagh Creasy', *American Homeopath*, accessed in Radar Opus 2011.

D'Aran (2008) Lecture, Sydney, Australia.

D'Aran, K. (1997) 'Totality of the Whole Person or Totality of the Whole Diseased Person', *Journal HANSW*, 1 (1) April, Australia.

Danciger, E. (1993) 'The Wounded Healer', *The Homeopath*, Journal of the Society of Homeopaths, (51) UK.

Davidson, J., Fisher, P., Van Haselen, R., Woodbury, M. & Connor, K. (2001) 'Do constitutional types really exist? A further study using grade of membership analysis', *British Homeopathic Journal*, Vol. 90 (3): 138-147.

De Rosa, C. (2011) *Mappa Mundi method and its application to homeopathy*, available at http://www.similima.com/gen254.html, http://hpathy.com/, and http://www.claudiaderosa.com/ last accessed September 2011.

De Schepper, L. (2003) *Homeopathy and the Periodic Table*, Full of Life Publications, Sante Fe.

De Schepper, L. (1999) *Hahnemann Revisited: Hahnemannian Textbook of Classical Homeopathy for the Professional*, Full of Life publishing, Santa Fe.

Desai, B.D. (2005) *How to find the Similimum with Boger-Boenninghausen's Repertory*, B. Jain Publishers (P) Ltd., New Delhi, India.

References

Dewey, W.A. (1934) *Practical Homeopathic Therapeutics* (3rd ed.) accessed in Radar Opus 2011.

Dimitriadis, G. (2007) 'Bogus Bönninghausen', *American Journal of Homœopathic Medicine*, Vol. 100 (1): 50-58, available at http://www.hahnemanninstitute.com/bogus_bonninghausen.pdf last accessed Sept 2011.

Dimitriadis, G. (2000) *The Böenninghausen Repertory: Therapeutic Pocket Book Method*, Hahnemann Institute, Sydney, Australia.

Dimitriadis, G. (2004) *Homoeopathic Diagnosis*, Hahnemann Institute, Sydney, Australia.

Dimitriadis, G. (2005) *The Theory of Chronic Diseases According to Hahnemann: a critical examination and objective analysis of Hahnemann's model*, Hahnemann Institute, Sydney.

Dudgeon, R.E. (1853) *Lectures on the Theory and Practice of Homoeopathy*, Leath & Ross, London, accessed in Radar Opus 2011.

Duncan, C.H. (1913) 'Auto-therapeutic technique', *Transactions of The Homeopathic Medical Society of the State of New York*, accessed in Radar Opus 2011.

Dunham, C. (1877a) *The Science of Therapeutics*, A Collection of Papers, editorial remarks on alteration (suggested by a contribution by Dr. H. to the American homoeopathic review, Vol. V), excessed in Radar Opus 2011.

Dunham, C. (1877b) *The Science of Therapeutics*, A Collection of Papers, reply to a letter on high potencies, accessed in Radar Opus 2011.

Eizayaga, F.X. (1991) *Treatise on Homeopathic Medicine*, Ediciones Marecel, Buenos Aires.

Eizayaga, F.X. (1996) 'Homeopathic treatment of bronchial asthma: retrospective study of 62 cases', *British Homeopathic Journal*, Vol. 85: 28-33.

Eizayaga, J. (2002) 'Obituary: Dr Francisco X Eizayaga', *Homeopathy*, 91: 269.

Ernst, E. (2002) 'A systematic review of systematic reviews of homeopathy', *Br J Clin Pharmacol*, 54: 577-582.

Eyre, P. (1999) *Proving of Mobile Phone Radiation*, accessed in Radar Opus 2011.

Farrington, E.A. (1908) *Clinical Materia Medica*, Archibel, S.A. Belgium.

Foubister, D.M. (1967) 'The Carcinosin Drug Picture', *British Homoeopathic Journal*, accessed in Radar Opus 2011.

Foubister, D.M. (2001) *The Significance of Past History in Homoeopathic Prescribing*, B. Jain Publishers (P) Ltd., New Delhi, India.

Fraser, P. (2002) *The AIDS Miasm Contemporary Disease and the New Remedies*, Winter Press, United Kingdom.

Fraser, P. (2004) *Using Mappa Mundi in Homoeopathy*, Narayana, Kandern, Germany.

Fraser, P. (2008) *Using Miasms in Homoeopathy*, Winter Press, West Wickham.

Frei, H. (2009) 'Polarity analysis, a new approach to increase the precision of homeopathic prescriptions', *Homeopathy*, 98: 49-55.

Furlenmeier, M. (1992) 'The 'Constitution' in Homeopathy', *Zschr Klass Homöop*, 36: 180-86.

Gailliard, B. (1891) 'A critical inquiry concerning the exhibition of complex and alternate medicines in the homoeopathic treatment of disease', *American Institute of Homoeopathy*, accessed in Radar Opus 2011.

Galatzer, N. (1949) 'Eight Years in China', *The Homeopathic Herald*, Jan Vol. IX (10), accessed in Radar Opus 2011.

Gamble, J. (2005) *Mastering Homeopathy*, Karuna, Australia.

Gauley, N. (1998) *Counseling Difficult Clients*, Norton Sage Publications.

Ghegas, V. (1994) 'About the practical use of miasm and layers', *Homoeopathic Links*, accessed in Radar Opus 2011.

Ghegas, V. (1996) 'The classical homeopathic lectures of Dr Vassilis Ghegas', Vol. D, *Homeo-Study*, Gent, Belgium.

Gibson, D. (1987) *Studies of Homoeopathic Remedies*, Beaconsfield, Berkshire, UK.

Gnaiger-Rathmanner, J., Schneider, A., Loader, B., Böhler, M., Frass, M., Singer, S.R. & Oberbaum, M. (2008) 'Petroleum: a series of 25 cases', *Homeopathy*, 97 (2): 83-88.

Goldberg, B. (1942) 'Homoeopathy and the nosodes', *Homeopathic Herald*, Oct Vol. V (8), accessed in Radar Opus 2011.

Gray, A. (2010) *Case Taking*, B. Jain Archibel, Assesse, Belgium.

Grimmer, A.H. (1997) 'The Collected Works of Arthur Hill Grimmer', *Hahnemann International Institute for Homoeopathic Documentation*, Norwalk Conn & Greifenberg, Germany, accessed in Radar Opus 2011.

Grimmer, A.H. & Bernoville, F. (1965) *Homoeopathic Treatment of Cancer*, accessed in Radar Opus 2011.

Guernsey, H. (1868) 'The Keynote System', *The Hahnemannian Monthly*, Vol. III (12): 561-569, available at http://www.homeoint.org/articles/reis/guerkeyn.htm last accessed August 2011.

Guernsey, H.N. (1867) *The application of the principles and practice of homeopathy to Obstetrics and the disorders peculiar to women and young children*, Boericke & Tafel, Philadelphia.

Gunavante, S.M. (1994) *The "Genius" of Homoeopathic Remedies*, B. Jain Publishers (P) Ltd., New Delhi, India.

Gupta, A.C. (1989) *Organon of Medicine: At a glance*, B. Jain Publishers (P) Ltd., New Delhi, India.

Haehl, R. (2006) *Samuel Hahnemann His Life and Work*, Reprint edn., B. Jain Publishers (P) Ltd., New Delhi, India.

Hahnemann, S. (1830) *Materia Medica Pura*, 3rd edn., Vol. I, Kothen, English translation, Messrs Homoeopathic Publishing Co., London, accessed in Radar Opus 2011.

Hahnemann, S. (1843) 'Cases Communicated by Letter', dated 24th April, 1843, to Dr. von Boenninghausen, *Neues Archiv*, Vol. I. 1844, accessed in Radar Opus 2011.

Hahnemann, S. (1922) *Organon of Medicine*, Boericke & Tafel, Philadelphia.

Hahnemann, S. (2005) *Organon of Medicine*, 5th & 6th edn. combined, B. Jain Publishers (P) Ltd., New Delhi, India.

References

Hahnemann, S. (2005) *The Chronic Diseases: Their Peculiar Nature & Their Homoeopathic Cure*, Vol. 1 & 2, B. Jain Publishers (P) Ltd., New Delhi, India.

Handley, R. (1990) *Homeopathic Love Story*, Beaconsfield Publishers.

Handley, R. (1997) *In Search of the Later Hahnemann*, Beaconsfield Publishers.

Hansen, O. (1898) *A Text-Book of Materia Medica and Therapeutics of Rare Homeopathic Remedies*, Copenhagen, accessed in Radar Opus 2011.

Hempel, C.J. (1848) *The True Organisation of the New Church as indicated in the writings of Emanuel Swedenborg and demonstrated by Charles Fourier*, New York.

Hempel, C.J. (1864) *A New and Comprehensive System of Materia Medica*, 2nd American edn., Grand Rapids, Kent Co., Michigan, accessed in Radar Opus 2011.

Hering, C. (1875) 'Hahnemann's Three Rules Concerning the Rank of symptoms,' *Analytical Therapeutics*, Vol. 1: 21, Boericke and Tafel, Philadelphia.

Hering, C. (1997) *The Guiding Symptoms of Our Materia Medica*, B. Jain Publishers (P) Ltd., New Delhi, India.

Herscu, P. (2005) *Homoeopathic Treatment of Children – Pediatric Constitutional Types*, Reprint edn., B. Jain Publishers (P) Ltd., New Delhi, India.

Heudens-Mast, H. (2005) *The Foundation of the Chronic Miasms in the Practice of Homeopathy*, Lutea Press, Florida.

Howard, W. (2003) 'Bringing Back the Baron', Originally published in UK Society of Homeopaths' journal, *The Homeopath*, Apr, (89): 16-22, available at http://www.morphologica.com/english/reference/baron.htm last accessed 2011.

Hughes, R. (1869) *A Manual of Therapeutics: According to the Method of Hahnemann*, William Radde, New York, accessed in Radar Opus 2011.

Hughes, R. (1991) *The Principles and Practice of Homoeopathy*, 4th Reprint edn., B. Jain Publishers (P) Ltd., New Delhi, India.

Jackson, R. (1998) *American Homeopath*, Archibel S.A., Belgium.

Jahr, G. (1867) 'Forty Years of Practice', in *Taylor*, available at www.wholehealthnow.com | http://www.wholehealthnow.com/homeopathy_pro/wt7.html last accessed September 2011.

Joardar, R.R. (2002) *The Dictionary of Organon*, 3rd edn., Chhaya Joardar, Calcutta, India.

Jouanny, J. (1994) *The Essentials of Homoeopathic Therapeutics*, Boiron, Lyon, France.

Julian, O.A. (1962) *Biotherapics and Nosodes*, Maloine, Paris.

Julian, O.A. (1997) *Materia Medica of Nosodes*, B. Jain Publishers (P) Ltd., New Delhi, India.

Kanjilal, J.N. (1977) *Writings on Homoeopathy*, Das, Calcutta, India.

Kent, J.T. (1900) *Lectures on Homeopathic Philosophy*, B. Jain Publishers (P) Ltd., New Delhi, India.

Kent, J.T. (1904) *Lectures on Homeopathic Materia Medica*, Boericke & Tafel, Philadelphia.

Kent, J.T. (1921) *Lesser Writings*, accessed in Radar Opus 2011

Kent, J.T. (1926) *New Remedies: Clinical Cases, Lesser Writings, aphorisms and percepts*,

Erhart & Karl, Chicago.

Kent, J.T. (2005) *New Remedies, Clinical Cases, Lesser Writings*, B. Jain Publishers (P) Ltd., New Delhi, India.

Klein, L. (2009) *Miasms and Nosodes*, Narayana Publishers, Germany.

Kurz, C. (2005) *Imagine Homeopathy: A book of Experiments, Images & Metaphors*, Thieme, New York.

Launsø, L. & Rieper, J. (2005) 'General practitioners and classical homeopaths treatment models for asthma and allergy', *Homeopathy*, 94(1): 17-25.

Lesigang, H. (1990) 'Some Aspects Of Magnesia Fluorica', *Liga Medicorum Homoeopathica Internationalis*, accessed in Radar Opus 2011.

Lesser, O. (1934) 'Constitution and constitutional treatment', *British Homeopathic Journal*, 24: 230–244.

Lesser, O. (2001) *Textbook of Homeopathic Materia Medica*, Reprint edn., B. Jain Publishers (P) Ltd., New Delhi, India.

Little, D. (1998) *What are miasms?*, available at http://www.wholehealthnow.com/homeopathy_pro/dl-miasms-03.html last accessed July 2011.

Little, D. (2011) *Hahnemann a Comparison of the Centesimal and LM Potency*, available at http://www.simillimum.com/education/little-library last accessed July 2011

Little, D. (1996-2007) 'Hahnemann on Constitution and Temperament' Part 3, *Constitution and Predisposition*, available at http://www.simillimum.com/education/little-library/constitution-temperaments-and-miasms/hct/article01.php last accessed July 2011.

Little, D. (1996-2007) 'Hahnemann on Constitution and Temperament' Part 4, *Mappa Mundi*, available at http://www.simillimum.com/education/little-library/constitution-temperaments-and-miasms/hct/article01.php last accessed July 2011.

Little, D. (1996-2007) 'Hahnemann on Constitution and Temperament', Part 1, *Constitution, Temperament and Diathesis*, available at http://www.simillimum.com/education/little-library/constitution-temperaments-and-miasms/hct/article01.php last accessed July 2011.

Little, D. (1996-2007) 'Hahnemann on Constitution and Temperament', Part 2, *The Phlegmatic Temperament*, available at http://www.simillimum.com/education/little-library/constitution-temperaments-and-miasms/hct/article01.php last accessed July 2011.

Little, D. (1996-2007) available at http://www.wholehealthnow.com/homeopathy_pro/dl0.html or http://www.simillimum.com/education/little-library/index.php last accessed July 2011.

Little, D. (1998) 'Dose and Potency According to The Organon', *The American Homoeopath*, Journal of the North American Society of Homoeopaths,128.

Little, D. (2000) 'Following in Hahnemann's Footsteps: The Definitive Years 1833-1843', *American Homeopath*, accessed in Radar Opus 2011.

Little, D. *The 6th Organon and the Paris Casebooks*, available at http://www.simillimum.com/education/little-library last accessed July 2011.

References

Little, D. The Prevention of Epidemic Diseases by Homoeopathy, available at http://www.simillimum.com/education/little-library last accessed July 2011.

Lonely Planet (2011a) available at http://www.lonelyplanet.com/germany/saxony last accessed August 2011.

Lonely Planet (2011b) available at http://www.lonelyplanet.com/germany/saxony/dresden last accessed August 2011.

Maiwald, V.L. & Weinfurtner, L. (1988) *Therapy of the Common Cold with a Homoeopathic Combination Preparation in Comparison with Acetylsalicylic Acid*, Arzneimittelforschung, Apr 38 (4): 578-582.

Mas, R.D. (1912) 'Foreign exchange notes', *The Homoeopathician*, Vol. 2, accessed in Radar Opus 2011.

Master, F.J. (2006) *Homoeopathy in Cancer*, B. Jain Publishers (P) Ltd., New Delhi, India.

Master, F.J. (2005) *Tumours and Homeopathy*, B. Jain Publishers (P) Ltd., New Delhi, India.

Mastin, J.W. (1905) *The Critique Volume XII*, The Denver Journal Publishing Company, United States of America.

Mathur, K.N. (1975) *Principles of Prescribing*, B. Jain Publishers (P) Ltd., New Delhi, India.

Medhurst, R. (2011) *Research in Homeopathy – There's Lots of It!*, available at http://homeopathyplus.com.au/robert-medhurst-research/ last accessed September 2011.

Medhurst, R. (1994) *Brauer Professional News*, Brauers Tanunda, Australia.

Menninger, C.F. (1897) 'The eradication of Mongrelism', *Hahnemannian Advocate*, Vol. XXXVI, Chicago, accessed in Radar Opus 2011.

Merry, T. (1995) *Invitation to Person Centered Psychology*, Whurr Publishers, London.

Milgrom, L. (2010) *Beware scientism's onward march!*, available at http://www.anh-europe.org/news/anh-feature-beware-scientism's-onward-march

Milgrom, L. (2009) *Under Pressure: Homeopathy UK and Its Detractors*, Homeopathy Research Institute, London, UK.

Milgrom, L.R. (2008) 'Homeopathy and the New Fundamentalism: A critique of the critics', *J Altern Complement Med*, 14: 589.

Miller, G.B. (1966) 'Elements of homoeopathy', *British Homoeopathic Association*, London.

Miller, G.B.,(1911) 'On the comparative value of symptoms in the selection of the remedy', *British Homoeopathic Journal*, Vol. I (2) accessed in Radar Opus 2011.

Mohanty, N. (1983) *Text Book of Homeopathic Materia Medica*, Bhubaneswar, India

Moore, J.H. (1903) *Our materia medica*, accessed in Radar Opus 2011.

Moroweiec-Bajda, A., Lukomski, M. & Latkowski, B. (1993) *The Clinical Efficacy of Vertigoheel in the Treatment of Vertigo of Various Pathology Panminerva Medica*, Jun 35 (2): 101-104.

Morrell, P. (2000) *British Homeopathy During Two Centuries*, available at http://www.homeoint.org/morrell/british/clarke last accessed September 2011.

Morrell, P. (1996) *Hahnemann's Miasm Theory and Miasm Remedies*, available at http://

www.homeoint.org/morrell/articles/index.htm

Morrison, R. (1987) *Seminar Burgh Haamstede,* accessed in Radar Opus 2011.

Morrison, R. (1993) *Desktop Guide to Keynote & Confirmatory Symptoms,* Hahnemann Clinic Publishing, California.

Morrison, R. (2006) *Carbon: Organic & Hydrocarbon Remedies in Homeopathy,* Hahnemann Clinic Publishing, USA.

Moskowitz, R. (2011) *Single Remedies, Combination Remedies Options for Homeopathic Self-Care,* available at http://www.healthy.net last accessed September 2011.

Mukerji, R.K. (1975) 'History Of Drainage', *The Hahnemannian Gleanings,* Vol. 42 (11), accessed in "Fundamental laws of therapeutics" by Dr Forties Bernoville, Published by Indian Books & Periodical Publishers, Reprint edn. 2001, Delhi.

Murphy, R. (2007) *Case Analysis & Prescribing Techniques,* B.Jain Publishers (P) Ltd., New Delhi, India.

Nash, E.B. (1988) *Leaders in Homeopathic Therapeutics,* B. Jain Publishers (P) Ltd., New Delhi, India.

Nebel, A. (1901) 'Contribution to the history of Isopathy', *Journal Belge d'Homoeopathy,* Archives fur die Homoeopathische Heilkunst of Stapf, Vol. 10 (3 & 4), 1831, accessed in Radar Opus 2011.

Norland, M. (2000) 'An interview with Misha Norland', *American Homeopath,* accessed in Radar Opus 2011.

Norland, M. (2003) *Signatures Miasms Aids – Spiritual Aspects of Homeopathy,* Yondercott Press, UK.

Oberbaum, M. (2008) 'Petroleum: A series of 25 cases', *Homeopathy,* 97(2): 83-88.

Ortega, P.S. (1980) *Notes on the Miasms,* National Homoeopathic Pharmacy of Homeopatia de Mexico A.C., accessed in Radar Opus 2011.

Owen, D. (2007) *Principles & Practice of Homeopathy: The Therapeutic & Healing Process,* Churchill Livingstone Elsevier.

Parrot, R. (1967) *Individual Isotherapy,* Doin, Paris.

Patel, R.P. (1988) *What is Tautopathy Hahnemann,* Homoeopathic Pharmacy, India.

Phatak, S.R. (1993) *Materia Medica of Homoeopathic Medicines,* B. Jain Publishers (P) Ltd., New Delhi, India.

Priestman, K. (1988) *Introduction to Borland's Homœopathy in Practice,* Borland.

Puhlman, G. (1880) 'The History of Homoeopathy in Germany', *American Institute of Homoeopathy,* Vol. II (I) accessed in Radar Opus 2011.

Pulford, D. (1936) 'Why Do We Take The Case ?', *Homoeopathic Recorder,* Mar Vol. LI, accessed in Radar Opus 2011.

Rademacher, J.G. (1841) *Universal and Organ Remedies,* Originally published in German, abridged and translated by Ramseyer A.A., 1975, 2nd Indian edn., Haren & Brother, Calcutta, accessed in Radar Opus 2011.

Rapou, A. (1847) *History of the Doctrine of Homoeopathy,* Vol. 2, Baillere, Paris.

References

Rehman, A. (1997) *Encyclopedia of Remedy Relationships*, Thieme, Heidelberg.

Reves, J. (1993) '24 Chapters in Homeopathy', *The Homeopath*, (51): 120.

Roberts, H.A. (1936) *The Principles and Art of Cure by Homoeopathy*, Homœopathic Publishing Co., London, accessed in Radar Opus 2011.

Saine, A. (1999) *Psychiatric Patients I*, 2nd edn., Eindhoven, Netherlands.

Sankaran, R. (1999) 'Glimpses of a System', *American Homoeopaths*, accessed in Radar Opus 2011.

Sankaran, R. (2000) *The System of Homeopathy*, Homeopathic Medical Publishers, Mumbai, India.

Sankaran, P. (1978) *Some Notes on the Nosodes*, Homeopathic Medical Publishers, Mumbai, India.

Sankaran, P. (1996) *The Elements of Homoeopathy*, Homoeopathic Medical Publishers, Mumbai, India.

Sankaran, R. (1991) *The Spirit of Homoeopathy*, Homeopathic Medical Publishers, Mumbai, India.

Sankaran, R. (1994) *The Substance of Homoeopathy*, Homoeopathic Medical Publishers, Mumbai, India.

Sankaran, R. (1997) *The Soul of Remedies*, Homeopathic Medical Publishers, Mumbai, India.

Sankaran, R. (1998) *Provings*, Homoeopathic Medical Publishers, Mumbai, India.

Sankaran, R. (2002) *An Insight into Plants,* Vol. I & II, Homoeopathic Medical Publishers, Mumbai, India.

Sankaran, R. (2004) *The Sensation in Homeopathy*, Homoeopathic Medical Publishers, Mumbai, India.

Sankaran, R. (2005) *Sankaran's Schema*, Homoeopathic Medical Publishers, Mumbai, India.

Sankaran, R. (2007) *Sensation Refined,* Homoeopathic Medical Publishers, Mumbai, India.

Sankaran, R. (2008) *The Other Song*, Homeopathic Medical Publishers, Mumbai, India.

Sankaran, R. (2011) *Survival Reptile,* Vol. I & II, Homoeopathic Medical Publishers, Mumbai, India.

Saxton, J. (2006) *Miasms as Practical Tools*, Beaconsfield Publishers, Beaconsfield.

Schmolz, M. & Metelmann, H. (1999) *Modulation of Cytokine Synthesis in Human Leucocytes by Individual Components of a Combination Homeopathic Nasal Spray Biomedical Therapy*, 17 (2): 161-75

Scholten, J. (2005) *Secret Lanthanides,* Stichting Alonnissos, The Netherlands.

Scholten, J. (1993) *Homeopathy and Minerals* Stichting Alonnissos, Utrecht, The Netherlands.

Scholten, J. (2000) *Homeopathy and the Elements,* Stichting Alonnissos, The Netherlands.

Scholten, J. (2010) *Schema of the Periodic Table,* Archibel S.A., Belgium.

Shang, A., Huwiler-Müntener, K., Nartey, L., Juni, P., Dorig, S., Sterne, J.A., et al. (2005)

'Are the clinical effects of homoeopathy placebo effects? Comparative study of placebo-controlled trials of homoeopathy and allopathy', *Lancet,* 366: 726–32.

Shore, J. (1990) *Homoeopathic Remedies from the Avian Realm,* Seminar 1989, Seminar 1990, Seminar 1991, Seminar, accessed in Radar Opus 2011.

Souk, A.P. (1993) *The Contemporary French Provings,* accessed in Radar Opus 2011.

Souter, K. (2006) 'Heuristics and bias in homeopathy', *Homeopathy,* 95 (4): 237-244.

Speight, P. (1961) *A Comparison of the Chronic Miasms,* Health Science Press, Rustington.

Suijis, M. (2008) *Actinides the 7th Series of the Periodic Table,* Archibel S.A., Belgium.

Swan, S. (1872) 'Isopathy and Homoeopathy', *The Hahnemannian Monthly,* (1): 1871-1872, accessed in Radar Opus 2011.

Swayne, J. (2002) 'The starting point: pathography', *Homeopathy,* 91(1): 22-25.

Taylor, W., (2001) *Specificity of Seat - James Compton Burnett and the Generalization of Locality,* available at http://www.wholehealthnow.com/homeopathy_pro/wt6.html last accessed Sept 2011.

Taylor, W. (2001) *Taking the Case,* available at http://www.wholehealthnow.com/homeopathy_pro/wt7.html last accessed September 2011.

Teixeira, M. (2008) 'Homeopathic Practice in Intensive Care Units: objective semiology, symptom selection and a series of sepsis cases', *Homeopathy,* 97: 206-213.

Tomlinson, M. (1996) 'The Complex Approach', *Similia,* (9) Australian Homeopathic Association.

Treuherz, F. (1984) 'The Origins of Kent's Homoeopathy', *Journal of the American Institute of Homoeopathy,* Vol. 77 (4).

Truzzi, M. (1979) 'On the Reception of Unconventional Scientific Claims', *The Reception of Unconventional Science,* I25-137, Westview Press, Boulder, Colorado.

Twentyman, R. (1975, 1978) 'The Evolutionary Significance of Samuel Hahnemann', *British Homeopathic Journal,* (64): 144-5 and Editorial 'The History of Homeopathy', *British Homeopathic Journal* 67(2).

Tyler, M.L. (1927) *Different ways of Finding the Remedy,* Quinquennial Homoeopathic International Congress, Transactions of the ninth congress, accessed in Radar Opus 2011.

Tyler, M.L. (2005) *Homoeopathic Drug Pictures,* B. Jain Publishers (P) Ltd., New Delhi, India.

Tyler, M.L. (1928) *Different Ways Of Finding The Remedy,* John Bale Sons and Danielsson Ltd., London, accessed in Radar Opus 2011.

Tyler, M.L. (1938) 'Editorial', *Homeopathy,* Feb Vol. VII (2), accessed in Radar Opus 2011.

Tyler, M.L., in Clarke, A.G. (1925) *Decachords,* available at www.homeoint.org/seror last accessed Sep 2011.

Ullman, D. (1979) *Kent's Lectures on Homeopathic Philosophy,* Reprint edn., North Atlantic Books, California.

van Haselen, R.A., Cinar, S., Fisher, P. & Davidson, J. (2001) 'The Constitutional Type

References

Questionnaire: validation in the patient population of the Royal London Homoeopathic Hospital', *British Homeopathic Journal*, 90 (3): 131–137.

Vannier, L. (1931) *Doctrine de l'Homoeopathie francaise*, Doin, Paris.

Vannier, L. (1960) *The origins and future of Homoeopythy*, Doin, Paris.

Vannier, L. (1992) *Typology in Homoeopathy*, Beaconsfield, England.

Vannier, L. (1998) *Homoeopathy: Human Medicine*, Reprint edn., B. Jain Publishers (P) Ltd., New Delhi, India.

Varma, P.N. & Indu, V. (1997) *Encyclopaedia of Homoeopathic Pharmacopoeia*, 2nd edn, accessed in Radar Opus 2011.

Vickers, A. & Zollmann, C. (1999) 'ABC of complementary medicine', *BMJ*, 319: 1115-1118.

Vithoulkas, G. (1980) *The Science of Homeopathy*, Grove Press, Weidenfeld.

Vithoulkas, G. (2000) 'Guidelines for authors', *Homoeopathic Links*, accessed in Radar Opus 2011.

von Lippe A. (1882) *Keynotes of the Homoeopathic Materia Medica*, B. Jain Publishers (P) Ltd., New Delhi, India.

von Lippe, A. (1881) *Key Notes and Red Line Symptoms of the Materia Medica*, B. Jain Publishers (P) Ltd., New Delhi, India.

von Lippe, A. (1881) *Isopathy: A Fatal Error, The Homoeopathic Physician*, No. 11, accessed in Radar Opus 2011.

Wadia, S.R. (1977) *Homeopathy Cures Asthma*, 3rd edn., The Homoeopathic Medical Publisher, Mumbai, India, accessed in Radar Opus 2011.

Warkentin D.K. (1994) *HomeoNet Alerts*, Kent Associates, accessed in Radar Opus 2011.

Watson, I. (1991) *A Guide to the Methodologies of Homeopathy*, Cutting Edge Publications, Kendal, UK.

Websters Dictionary (1999) *Random House Webster's Concise College Dictionary*, Random House, New York.

Weisenauer, M. & Gaus, W. (1989) *Efficacy of Homoeopathic Preparation Combinations in Sinusitis Arzneimittelforschung*, May 39 (5): 620-625.

Weisser, M., Strosser, W. & Klein, P. (1998) *Homeopathic vs Conventional Treatment of Vertigo Arch Otolaryngol Head Neck Surg*, Aug 124 (8): 879-885.

Wesselhoeft, C. (1888) 'Proceedings of the Boston Organon Society', (7) *The Homoeopathic Physician*, accessed in Radar Opus 2011.

Wesselhoeft, C. (1901) 'On the faith in the efficacy of remedies', *American institute of homoeopathy*, accessed in Radar Opus 2011.

Winston, J. (1999) *The Faces of Homeopathy*, Tawa, Wellington, New Zealand.

Winston, J. (2004) 'Uh oh, Toto. I don't think we're in Kansas any more', *Homeopathy in Practice*, Jan: 32-39.

Wright-Hubbard, E. (1977) *A Brief Study Course In Homoeopathy*, Formur, St. Louis, MO.

Wright-Hubbard, E. (1940) 'Strange, rare and peculiar symptoms', *Homoeopathy Herald*,

Nov Vol. III (9) accessed in Radar Opus 2011.

Wurmser, L. (1957) *What is an Isotherapic? La documentation homoeopathique*, L.H. F. de France, No. 38.

Yasgur, J. (1994) *A Dictionary of Homeopathic Medical Terminology*, 3rd edn., Van Hoy Publishers, Greenville, accessed in Radar Opus 2011.

Zee, H. (2000) *Miasms in Labour*, Stichting Alonnissos, The Netherlands.

Zell, J., Connert, W., Mau, J. & Feuerstake, G. (1989) Treatment of Acute Sprains of the Ankle, *Biological Therapy*, 7 (1).

Zenner S., Metelmann, H. (1994) 'Therapy Experience with a Homeopathic Ointment', *Biological Therapy*, 12 (3).

Index

A
Aegidi 472, 473, 475, 476, 479, 480, 481, 482, 483, 484, 485, 486, 493, 499
Allopathic Drugs 123, 397, 405, 425
Allopathy; a warning to all sick persons 40
Aphorisms 32, 58, 59, 60, 61, 62, 65, 87, 89, 92, 93, 121, 128, 158, 160, 225, 234, 280, 281, 283, 287, 288, 290, 296, 297, 315, 316, 350, 368, 399, 400, 439, 441, 453, 476, 477, 521
Archibel 244
Arsenicum album 64, 126, 145, 152, 165, 263, 422
Australia 6, 18, 31, 32, 40, 80, 107, 108, 223, 244, 349, 422, 460, 470, 510, 511, 512

B
Belladonna 35, 41, 49, 50, 53, 54, 55, 146, 177, 178, 324, 341, 440, 445, 493, 498
Berberis 69, 178, 327, 455
Bhouraskar 181, 182, 185, 522
Blackie 106, 113, 116
Boger 70, 71, 277, 310, 322, 328, 334, 342, 343, 378, 408
Bon 22
Bönninghausen 19, 20, 24, 29, 30, 31, 33, 62, 63, 64, 65, 66, 70, 71, 72, 75, 83, 84, 124, 190, 277, 280, 287, 291, 302, 310, 324, 360, 408, 436, 471, 472, 473, 474, 475, 476, 479, 481, 483, 484, 486, 504, 521
Bradford 475, 478, 486, 527
Bryonia 40, 48, 49, 50, 60, 178, 326, 328, 329, 341, 493, 498, 516
Buddhism 3, 22
Burnett 14, 15, 131, 134, 364, 378, 429, 430, 431, 432, 433, 434, 435, 436, 437, 440, 441, 442, 443, 444, 445, 446, 447, 448, 449, 454, 455, 456, 457, 461, 462, 463, 465, 466

C
Calc carb 114, 126, 135, 153, 165, 166, 174, 252, 253, 266, 293, 325, 377, 419
CAM 6
Camphor 40, 146, 375, 416
Canada 7, 66
Carbonic 151, 153, 154, 155
Carbo-nitrogenoid 97, 111, 133, 134, 145, 146
Case Management 44, 97, 161, 192, 232, 237, 239, 423, 477, 490, 506, 515
Cases 9, 17, 18, 19, 20, 21, 26, 29, 30, 44, 45, 46, 48, 51, 53, 55, 57, 66, 69, 70, 73, 74, 77, 80, 82, 100, 105, 107, 108, 116, 117, 118, 120, 124, 135, 140, 141, 142, 146, 147, 160, 177, 183, 194, 198, 212, 216, 221, 222, 226, 231, 233, 239, 248, 251, 252, 254, 255, 260, 261, 262, 263, 271, 272, 273, 278, 279, 280, 284, 285, 291, 295, 297, 298, 303, 304, 307, 321, 325, 326, 327, 328, 329, 330, 332, 334, 335, 339, 340, 342, 343, 345, 353, 362, 364, 371, 372, 374, 375, 381, 383, 385, 397, 402, 406, 407, 413, 416, 419, 420, 424, 429, 449, 459, 460, 461, 472, 474, 476, 478, 479, 481, 482, 484, 488, 494, 495, 498, 503, 505, 510, 515, 516, 523, 524, 525, 532, 537
Castro 113
Causation 29, 59, 72, 75, 160, 162, 235, 288, 317, 445, 523
China 49, 52, 144, 145, 177, 178, 191, 192, 193, 356, 366, 453, 502
Cholera 40, 324, 375, 391, 446, 478
Choleric 157, 161, 163, 164, 166, 167, 168, 176, 178, 291

Chronic Diseases 24, 32, 39, 42, 43, 47,
   58, 60, 88, 90, 94, 114, 116, 123, 128,
   129, 131, 135, 156, 157, 163, 178,
   222, 223, 225, 226, 227, 229, 234,
   236, 237, 238, 239, 240, 263, 281,
   286, 290, 294, 304, 331, 347, 366,
   399, 401, 411, 460, 467, 478, 481,
   487, 495, 498, 523
Clarke 9, 111, 113, 118, 132, 133, 134, 144,
   148, 228, 229, 248, 310, 325, 339,
   340, 364, 432, 446, 458, 499
Classification of Diseases 272, 285
Classification of Symptoms 272, 278, 284
Close 14, 127, 408, 411, 492
Collett 345, 365
Combination 134, 189, 254, 405, 469, 470,
   472, 479, 489, 490, 496, 500, 501,
   502, 503, 504, 505, 506, 509, 510,
   514, 515
Complaint 52, 57, 63, 64, 65, 68, 70, 72,
   75, 99, 101, 114, 144, 158, 171, 194,
   199, 207, 278, 282, 283, 302, 304,
   316, 317, 336, 338, 385, 421, 422,
   506, 525
Complete Symptom 29, 57, 63, 64, 65, 461,
   522
Complexes 467, 469, 507, 511, 512, 513
Constitution 17, 21, 37, 111, 112, 113, 114,
   115, 116, 119, 125, 126, 127, 128,
   129, 130, 131, 133, 134, 135, 141,
   144, 145, 149, 150, 152, 153, 155,
   156, 157, 158, 160, 162, 163, 164,
   170, 171, 172, 173, 174, 175, 176,
   177, 179, 190, 191, 193, 237, 238,
   262, 279, 290, 291, 292, 304, 330,
   332
Constitutional Layer 194, 272, 290, 294
Constitutional Prescribing 11, 14, 20, 111,
   112, 113, 116, 118, 119, 120, 121,
   129, 155, 176, 177, 178, 515, 521
Cope 243, 244, 247, 414
Cöthen 34, 39, 40, 41, 43
Cuprum 40, 145, 146, 324, 375, 448, 478
Cure 29, 36, 61, 62, 76, 236, 241, 242, 454,
   462, 466, 517

D
d'Hervilly 41, 43

Dimitriadis 71, 75, 222
Disease 5, 20, 24, 25, 29, 30, 31, 32, 39,
   42, 43, 45, 46, 47, 48, 50, 52, 57, 58,
   59, 60, 61, 62, 63, 64, 65, 70, 73, 74,
   75, 77, 79, 80, 81, 88, 90, 91, 93, 94,
   97, 98, 99, 103, 114, 115, 116, 121,
   122, 123, 126, 128, 129, 131, 132,
   133, 134, 135, 136, 139, 141, 142,
   143, 145, 148, 149, 150, 151, 152,
   155, 156, 157, 158, 159, 160, 161,
   162, 163, 171, 175, 176, 178, 183,
   189, 190, 191, 192, 193, 194, 208,
   213, 214, 218, 222, 223, 225, 226,
   227, 228, 229, 230, 233, 234, 235,
   236, 237, 238, 239, 240, 248, 251,
   254, 258, 259, 261, 263, 271, 272,
   276, 278, 279, 280, 281, 283, 285,
   286, 287, 288, 289, 290, 291, 292,
   293, 294, 297, 303, 304, 315, 316,
   317, 318, 319, 322, 327, 328, 330,
   331, 332, 333, 340, 347, 348, 353,
   355, 356, 357, 360, 361, 362, 363,
   365, 366, 368, 369, 372, 373, 374,
   375, 376, 377, 378, 380, 387, 388,
   399, 400, 401, 402, 403, 406, 407,
   408, 409, 410, 411, 412, 413, 414,
   415, 416, 417, 421, 431, 434, 436,
   437, 439, 440, 441, 442, 443, 444,
   445, 446, 447, 448, 449, 450, 453,
   454, 456, 457, 458, 460, 461, 462,
   464, 467, 471, 473, 475, 476, 477,
   478, 481, 482, 487, 488, 491, 494,
   495, 498, 501, 502, 503, 505, 506,
   507, 508, 509, 510, 511, 516, 523,
   525
Double Remedy Experiments 468, 472
Dreams 18, 60, 186, 195, 197, 198, 199,
   201, 208, 209, 211, 266, 329
Dresden 34, 357, 358
Dunham 84, 329, 484, 492, 497, 498

E
Eizayaga 194, 271, 272, 275, 277, 278,
   279, 280, 281, 284, 285, 286, 287,
   288, 292, 293, 294, 295, 296, 297,
   303, 304
Elements 150, 168, 174, 176, 237, 243,
   245, 250, 252, 253, 255, 256, 257,

Index

258, 259, 260, 261, 267, 277, 291, 492, 500, 507, 529
Emerson 27
Endeavour College of Natural Health 6, 223, 244, 422, 470
Epidemic Diseases 30, 73, 74, 375

F
Flexner Report 80
Fluoric 151, 153, 154, 155
Fraser 163, 174
Fundamental layer 194, 272, 287, 289, 290, 292, 294, 302

G
Gadd 27, 271, 275, 522
Genus epidemicus 11, 73, 74, 375
Germany 7, 15, 22, 33, 35, 40, 42, 82, 84, 124, 125, 359, 447, 483, 507
Golden 32, 40, 79, 383, 520
Gray 32, 57, 248, 285
Gross 39, 360, 361, 368, 373
Gunavante 307, 316, 317, 318, 322, 324, 325, 327, 328, 329, 332, 334, 335, 336
Gypser 85

H
Haehl 35, 42, 43, 360, 373, 472
Hahnemann 9, 13, 14, 15, 16, 17, 23, 24, 29, 31, 32, 33, 34, 35, 36, 37, 38, 39, 40, 41, 42, 43, 44, 45, 56, 57, 58, 59, 60, 61, 62, 63, 65, 66, 72, 73, 74, 79, 81, 84, 85, 86, 87, 89, 90, 94, 97, 114, 119, 121, 123, 125, 127, 128, 129, 130, 131, 133, 134, 135, 144, 145, 146, 149, 156, 157, 158, 160, 161, 167, 175, 176, 181, 188, 189, 190, 221, 222, 223, 225, 226, 227, 228, 229, 230, 233, 234, 237, 238, 239, 240, 247, 248, 249, 250, 251, 262, 280, 281, 283, 287, 290, 291, 293, 294, 297, 309, 314, 315, 316, 317, 318, 329, 331, 347, 350, 357, 358, 359, 360, 361, 362, 364, 365, 366, 368, 369, 370, 373, 374, 375, 378, 399, 400, 403, 411, 425, 426, 427, 428, 432, 435, 436, 439, 441, 443, 447, 448, 454, 460, 462, 464, 465, 467, 468, 470, 471, 472, 473, 474, 475, 476, 477, 478, 479, 480, 481, 482, 483, 484, 485, 486, 490, 494, 495, 497, 498, 499, 500, 501, 504, 506, 508, 511, 516, 521, 526, 527, 528, 529, 530, 531, 532, 533, 534, 536, 537, 540, 541, 543
Handley 45, 176, 221, 222
Health 5, 6, 19, 25, 29, 36, 43, 49, 57, 58, 59, 60, 91, 115, 121, 124, 138, 148, 160, 162, 175, 187, 201, 214, 222, 223, 238, 244, 247, 289, 292, 304, 353, 368, 399, 401, 403, 404, 422, 470, 505, 506
Hering 43, 75, 83, 84, 160, 161, 162, 230, 235, 238, 325, 342, 345, 347, 357, 358, 360, 361, 364, 378, 408, 416, 453, 467, 471, 504, 527
Homeopaths 5, 6, 7, 8, 9, 11, 13, 15, 17, 20, 22, 23, 24, 25, 26, 27, 32, 37, 40, 44, 57, 58, 59, 60, 61, 71, 72, 75, 79, 80, 81, 82, 84, 86, 91, 97, 106, 115, 118, 120, 122, 123, 124, 149, 151, 156, 160, 163, 177, 181, 182, 185, 186, 187, 188, 190, 191, 192, 194, 212, 214, 215, 216, 217, 220, 222, 223, 225, 226, 229, 230, 233, 235, 237, 238, 239, 244, 247, 248, 249, 253, 255, 262, 271, 275, 279, 280, 283, 287, 290, 291, 296, 303, 311, 312, 314, 316, 317, 326, 350, 351, 361, 366, 380, 385, 401, 402, 403, 419, 432, 443, 447, 460, 461, 462, 470, 472, 489, 490, 498, 499, 503, 504, 506, 507, 509, 514, 516, 519, 520, 525, 532, 536, 537, 539, 540, 541, 542, 543
HomeoQuest 182
Hughes 85, 131, 435, 446, 447, 458, 464, 466, 494, 499
Hydrogenoid 111, 133, 134, 135, 141, 142, 144, 149, 172, 174

I
Intercurrent prescribing 231, 233, 235, 397, 419
Isopathy 11, 20, 26, 230, 233, 235, 245,

347, 348, 350, 351, 352, 354, 356, 360, 361, 362, 363, 364, 365, 366, 367, 368, 369, 370, 371, 372, 373, 374, 376, 377, 378, 379, 382, 385, 401, 411, 422, 470, 524

K
Kanjilal 130, 131, 405
Kent 9, 14, 23, 24, 66, 70, 77, 78, 79, 82, 83, 84, 85, 86, 87, 88, 89, 90, 91, 92, 93, 94, 95, 96, 97, 98, 99, 106, 113, 114, 119, 120, 181, 190, 194, 228, 249, 250, 251, 252, 279, 280, 296, 297, 321, 322, 325, 333, 372, 373, 395, 453, 492, 504, 506, 508, 517, 527, 540, 541
Kentian 13, 15, 19, 25, 31, 66, 78, 79, 81, 114, 119, 120, 122, 176, 178, 190, 192, 206, 207, 208, 243, 279, 287, 292, 513, 522, 540
Keynote 14, 185, 186, 187, 307, 308, 309, 310, 311, 312, 313, 314, 315, 316, 317, 318, 319, 320, 321, 322, 326, 328, 332, 335, 336, 338, 339, 340, 341, 342, 343, 513, 519, 523, 524
Keynote Prescribing 307, 308, 309, 311, 312, 314, 316, 318, 321, 336, 339, 342, 343, 523
Kopp 526

L
Layers 11, 163, 194, 216, 271, 272, 277, 278, 287, 288, 289, 290, 292, 293, 294, 295, 302, 304, 445
Leipzig 34, 35, 38, 39, 127, 357, 358, 359, 360
Lesser 92, 96, 100, 111, 113, 114, 131, 132, 149, 150, 151, 216, 251, 326
Levy 14, 15
Little 63, 111, 113, 114, 125, 127, 129, 156, 159, 160, 163, 164, 167, 174, 175, 177, 228, 469, 472, 473, 477
Locality 376, 429, 439, 441, 454
Location 57, 63, 64, 68, 71, 72, 75, 287, 316, 444, 522
Lutze 472, 478, 479, 480, 481, 482, 483, 486, 493, 499
Lux 345, 352, 358, 359, 360, 361, 364, 366, 373, 378, 379

M
Mappa Mundi 111, 163, 166
Materia Medica 21, 35, 38, 39, 72, 75, 81, 83, 96, 163, 179, 207, 216, 230, 232, 236, 237, 239, 249, 250, 251, 252, 254, 259, 260, 297, 303, 309, 310, 312, 313, 314, 317, 325, 336, 338, 341, 342, 352, 353, 357, 358, 364, 365, 371, 374, 378, 405, 416, 453, 485, 493, 498, 508, 540, 544
Materia Medica Pura 38, 39, 312
Mathur 3, 9, 14, 119, 120, 318
Medorrhinum 70, 219, 221, 232, 365, 380, 388, 391, 392, 396
Meissen 33, 34
Methodologies 3, 10, 15, 32, 182, 251, 262, 527, 538, 540, 541, 558
Miasmatic layer 271, 272, 278, 293
Miasmatic prescribing 11, 219, 223, 224, 225, 226, 230
Modality 33, 63, 64, 65, 68, 75, 80, 284, 287, 326, 341, 534
Modification 63, 64, 378, 484, 492, 522
Montmartre 44
Morell 228
Mumbai 19, 117, 185, 187
Murphy 226

N
Naprosyn 397, 418, 419
Natrum muriaticum 18, 103, 104, 109, 151, 152, 174, 177, 205, 206, 208, 210, 211, 252, 334, 462, 493
Nebel 149, 151, 352, 357, 365, 383
New Zealand 7, 23, 80, 351
Norland 21, 163, 174, 504, 505
Nosode 9, 219, 220, 221, 224, 230, 231, 232, 233, 234, 235, 236, 294, 295, 345, 347, 348, 351, 352, 358, 361, 365, 366, 370, 372, 373, 376, 378, 379, 380, 387, 389, 390, 393, 394, 395, 396, 429, 435, 454, 459, 463, 489, 516
Nux vomica 49, 50, 51, 52, 135, 138, 139, 142, 143, 144, 146, 164, 178, 278, 381, 402, 416, 456, 457, 464, 488,

Index

O
493, 498, 515
Objective 5, 63, 64, 68, 71, 129, 153, 160, 187, 284, 296, 441, 444, 532, 533, 535, 540, 541
Organon of Medicine 24, 38, 45, 47, 50, 59, 62, 403, 521
Organopathy 15, 440, 441, 442, 448, 454, 463, 464
Organ Prescribing 429, 431, 434, 519
Organ Remedies 11, 401, 429, 435, 440, 447, 454, 455, 460, 463, 464, 515
Osborne 219, 223, 225
Oxygenoid 111, 134, 144, 145, 149

P
Paris 29, 41, 42, 43, 44, 118, 157, 176, 222, 354, 447, 477, 495
Peculiarity 25, 29, 57
Phlegmatic 157, 159, 161, 163, 166, 167, 168, 169, 170, 171, 172, 173, 174, 175, 176, 177, 291
Phosphoric 21, 151, 152, 153, 154, 155, 341
Phosphorus 21, 101, 115, 118, 135, 145, 146, 151, 152, 177, 178, 256, 259, 293, 337, 408, 444, 445, 498, 502, 505, 516
Physical General 11, 32, 33, 72, 99, 196, 215, 253, 304, 316, 325, 329
Pitt 14, 27, 525, 526
Plant Kingdom 245, 260
Polypharmacy 11, 343, 467, 468, 469, 471, 473, 475, 479, 480, 487, 488, 489, 490, 491, 492, 493, 494, 496, 497, 498, 499, 502, 503, 504, 505, 506, 507, 509, 514, 515, 516
Posology 261, 272, 295, 492, 506
Post-Kentian 19, 79
Potencies 10, 90, 96, 295, 296, 351, 369, 382, 383, 405, 422, 434, 447, 454, 459, 460, 463, 471, 477, 497, 501, 502, 515, 524, 525
Potency 54, 69, 81, 89, 96, 97, 98, 123, 151, 192, 199, 222, 232, 235, 261, 262, 266, 282, 295, 296, 369, 371, 383, 385, 402, 408, 409, 410, 411, 417, 418, 419, 422, 429, 447, 454, 464, 477, 488, 489, 499, 502, 508, 512, 515, 516, 522
Prescribing 8, 9, 11, 12, 14, 16, 17, 18, 19, 20, 21, 22, 24, 25, 27, 31, 33, 39, 68, 69, 70, 71, 75, 81, 82, 97, 99, 106, 111, 112, 113, 116, 118, 119, 120, 121, 123, 124, 129, 155, 176, 177, 178, 186, 191, 192, 194, 219, 220, 221, 222, 223, 224, 225, 226, 230, 231, 233, 235, 243, 245, 249, 254, 261, 262, 271, 272, 279, 294, 296, 307, 308, 309, 311, 312, 314, 315, 316, 318, 319, 321, 326, 336, 339, 342, 343, 348, 351, 385, 419, 422, 423, 424, 429, 431, 434, 435, 454, 460, 463, 470, 487, 501, 502, 505, 507, 508, 513, 514, 515, 516, 519, 521, 522, 523, 524
P Sankaran 14, 404, 406, 416, 419
Pulford 335, 336, 340, 341
Pulsatilla 49, 50, 51, 52, 63, 96, 104, 118, 135, 166, 174, 175, 176, 177, 178, 195, 206, 207, 233, 324, 334, 377, 402, 455, 502

R
Rademacher 133, 144, 149, 429, 433, 434, 435, 436, 440, 442, 447, 448, 456, 457, 458, 463, 464, 465, 466, 500
Red-line Symptoms 310, 317
Repertory 65, 66, 70, 81, 83, 95, 96, 160, 161, 174, 219, 220, 250, 272, 277, 279, 296, 312, 319, 321, 325, 330, 332, 334, 335, 338, 340, 341, 416, 437, 438, 453, 522
Rhus tox 40, 49, 146, 177, 233, 303, 341, 372, 493, 502
Roberts 27, 106, 236, 322, 376, 377, 491, 499, 500

S
Sankaran: 14,6,24,124,181,186,191,192,194,198,204,205,214,220,238,248,251,254,260,268,378,379,404,406,407,408,416,417,419,443,504,537,538,539,540,541,542.
Saxony 33, 38, 357, 358
Scholten 14, 191, 243, 245, 247, 254, 256, 260, 262, 267, 268, 443, 504
Schroyens 7, 27

Schüssler. 149, 150, 151
Sensation 26, 51, 53, 55, 57, 60, 63, 64, 68, 71, 72, 75, 99, 102, 138, 140, 173, 191, 192, 193, 194, 198, 204, 205, 207, 213, 214, 215, 216, 217, 280, 286, 287, 316, 333, 337, 338, 340, 421, 464, 532, 539
Sherr 21, 60, 163, 504, 520, 521
Similitude 272, 278, 280, 281, 282, 320, 321, 338, 436, 454, 455
Society of Homoeopaths 121
Specificity of Seat 429, 436, 437, 438, 440, 446, 452, 453
Sri Lanka 22
Stapf 39, 312, 358, 361, 484
Subjective 5, 58, 63, 64, 68, 160, 284, 285, 441, 445, 522, 532, 533, 535, 538, 540, 541
Sulphur 54, 56, 96, 103, 104, 113, 118, 132, 133, 145, 146, 151, 164, 177, 178, 220, 221, 222, 230, 233, 263, 291, 293, 316, 332, 337, 399, 408, 473, 502, 510, 515
Swedenborg 77, 78, 83, 84, 85, 86, 88, 89, 90, 93, 243, 250, 540
Syphillinum 178, 220, 232, 372, 373, 380, 387, 392, 396

T
Taffler 14, 27
Taylor 310, 311, 312, 314, 316, 318, 320, 321, 336, 338, 339, 432, 436, 437, 438, 439, 441, 442, 443, 445, 446, 449, 454
The Pill 108, 397, 418
Therapeutic Pocketbook 29, 65, 66, 68, 72, 75, 83, 302
Tibetan Buddhism 22
Totality 13, 15, 17, 20, 26, 29, 31, 58, 61, 70, 71, 73, 74, 79, 82, 108, 111, 116, 121, 126, 149, 175, 177, 185, 192, 206, 237, 238, 251, 272, 277, 282, 283, 287, 288, 296, 301, 310, 311, 316, 317, 318, 320, 322, 324, 327, 335, 338, 342, 349, 401, 417, 423, 435, 443, 461, 506, 519, 520, 521, 522, 524, 525

Totality of Symptoms 16, 20, 30, 57, 58, 63, 82, 91, 120, 121, 149, 236, 249, 272, 277, 278, 282, 283, 316, 320, 323, 338, 339, 429, 435, 443, 460, 461, 463, 502, 508, 520,
Totality of the Characteristics of the Person 77, 79, 80
Treuherz 86, 90, 92, 93, 94, 95
Tuberculinum 219, 351, 364, 372, 373, 380, 389, 394, 395, 396
Twitter 39
Tyler 9, 10, 14, 77, 82, 92, 96, 106, 118, 249, 328, 333, 334, 449, 458

U
UK 7, 17, 18, 19, 80, 107, 120, 121, 405, 432
US 7, 80, 83, 120, 199, 405, 416, 506, 511

V
Vaccinations 355, 369, 397, 401, 402, 413, 416, 463, 524
Veratrum album 38, 324, 375, 478
Vital force 59, 61, 81, 89, 93, 125, 177, 191, 228, 233, 234, 235, 297, 330, 400, 460, 491, 506, 507, 525
Vital Sensation 181, 185, 191, 193, 538, 539, 541
von Bönninghausen 29, 30, 62, 63, 472, 473, 479, 486
von Grauvogl 133, 134, 149, 172, 339
von Lippe 310, 375, 376

W
Watson 9, 10, 11, 12, 13, 14, 33, 58, 69, 72, 75, 106, 113, 119, 120, 121, 124, 219, 220, 221, 222, 401, 402, 419, 420, 422, 423, 455, 459, 460, 463, 464, 487, 488, 489, 509, 510, 511, 516
Whitmont 23, 124
Winston 35, 40, 44, 279, 471

Y
Yasgur 309, 310, 348, 352, 400, 449, 469, 491